Population, Health and Environment

International Institute for Population Sciences, Mumbai

Vision

To position IIPS as a premier teaching and research institute in population sciences responsive to emerging national and global needs based on values of inclusion, sensitivity and rights protection.

Mission

The Institute will strive to be a centre of excellence on population, health and development issues through high quality education, teaching and research. This will be achieved by (a) creating competent professions, (b) generating and disseminating scientific knowledge and evidence, (c) collaboration and exchange of knowledge, and (d) advocacy and awareness.

Population, Health and Environment

Edited by
Sayeed Unisa, T.V. Sekher, Chander Shekhar, Abhishek Singh, L.K. Dwivedi and M.R. Pradhan

International Institute for Population Sciences, Mumbai

RAWAT PUBLICATIONS
Jaipur • New Delhi • Bangalore • Guwahati • Kolkata

ISBN 978-81-316-0811-1

Published by
Prem Rawat for **Rawat Publications**
Satyam Apts, Sector 3, Jawahar Nagar, Jaipur 302 004 (India)
Phone: 0141 265 1748 / 7006 Fax: 0141 265 1748
E-mail: info@rawatbooks.com
Website: www.rawatbooks.com

New Delhi Office
4858/24, Ansari Road, Daryaganj, New Delhi 110 002
Phone: 011 2326 3290

Also at *Bangalore, Guwahati* and *Kolkata*

Typeset by Rawat Computers, Jaipur
Printed at Chaman Enterprises, New Delhi

Contents

Section II
Health and Health Care Services

Section III
Maternal Health Care

Section IV
Population Dynamics and Environment

Acknowledgements

It gives us great pleasure to acknowledge the help, support, encouragement and guidance we have received from the people and organizations involved in the preparation of this book. We are deeply indebted to all of them. We would like to mention specifically those without whose contribution it would not have been possible to bring out the book in this shape.

At the outset, we owe special thanks to Dr F. Ram, Director and Senior Professor, International Institute for Population Sciences (IIPS), Mumbai, for his constant encouragement and support to bring out the volume. This book is an outcome of the national seminar on Population, Health and Environment jointly organized by IIPS, Mumbai and the Indian Institute of Forest Management (IIFM), Bhopal. We express our deep sense of gratitude to Professor P.K. Biswas, then faculty of the Department of Sociology and Community Development and Coordinator of the Centre for Livelihood Management, IIFM, Bhopal. Dr Biswas has helped in necessary academic and logistic arrangements required for the seminar including a review of the abstracts of the papers.

We are also thankful to all the anonymous reviewers who have meticulously reviewed the papers submitted to them and timely provided their valuable comments and suggestions to improve the quality of papers appearing in this book. The authors of the papers appearing in this book deserve our special thanks for submitting and patiently revising their papers in agreement with the comments and suggestions received from anonymous reviewers.

Our special thanks to the Ministry of Health and Family Welfare, Government of India since it provides an annual research grant to IIPS, Mumbai for organising the national seminar and publication.

We acknowledge the contribution and support by Dr P. Murugesan, Senior Research Assistant, for his assiduous task of interacting with authors and reviewers and editing the draft papers before submitting the manuscript to the publisher.

Last but not the least, we owe special thanks to the publishing unit at Rawat Publications, Jaipur, who conducted a thorough professional and independent review and editing of this volume.

31 March 2016

– ***Editors***

Foreword

The International Institute for Population Sciences (IIPS) is a premier institution dedicated to high quality teaching and research in the field of Population, Health and Development. Since its establishment in 1956, IIPS has helped immensely in creating trained human resources in India and abroad. IIPS has regularly conducted studies that have provided key policy inputs to the Government of India and other national and international organizations. The National Family Health Surveys, the District Level Household Surveys, Youth in India Study, etc. conducted by the Institute have played a pivotal role in shaping different policies and programmes of the Government of India.

One of the missions of IIPS is to generate and disseminate scientific knowledge and evidence. To fulfil this mission, every year IIPS organizes a national seminar focusing on certain state(s) and themes. In 2013, we focused on developmental challenges, particularly population, health and environment. The seminar organized by the Institute in Bhopal received overwhelming response from researchers, students, policy makers and government officials. The Ministry of Health and Family Welfare, Government of India provided the required funds for organizing the seminar. This book is a collection of twenty selected papers presented at the national seminar. The papers address a wide range of issues in the context of India and Nepal. The papers have been grouped into four major sections: fertility and family planning, health and health care services, maternal health care, and population dynamics and environment. These papers provide excellent analysis and interpretation of the issues by making use of available data from various sources. I am sure that this volume will be of immense use to those interested in the population, health and environment issues in India and Nepal.

I appreciate the efforts of the seminar coordinators, Professor Sayeed Unisa, Professor T.V. Sekher, Professor Chander Sekhar, Dr Abhishek Singh,

Dr Laxmikant Dwivedi and Dr Manas Ranjan Pradhan for bringing out this edited book. I hope that this book will be a useful resource to researchers, students, policy makers, NGOs working in the fields of population, health and environment.

Professor F. Ram
Director & Senior Professor
International Institute for Population Sciences,
Mumbai

1

Population, Health and Environment

An Overview

The interconnectedness between people and their environment is a matter of discussion for long. Population size, components of growth, settlement patterns, and resource availability will certainly impact the environment. A better understanding of how and when these aspects of population growth impact the environment is required. It is also important to know how the environmental changes impact the health and well-being of population. There is a need for discussion based on scientific evidence on the linkages between population, health, and environment. In this perspective, it is important to promote exchange of knowledge and ideas from multiple perspectives across researchers. Therefore, the focus of this book is to examine these complex issues in detail, the interrelationships with supportive evidence and also to identify thrust areas of further research and action. From a multidisciplinary perspective, it highlights the issues relating to the environment and discusses its linkages with fertility, health and family planning.

This volume contains twenty papers dealing with issues of population, health and environment. These papers were presented at the national seminar of International Institute for Population Sciences held at Bhopal. Papers are categorized into four sections according to the main theme discussed in the papers. In this chapter, we provide a broad overview of the papers included in this volume.

Fertility and Family Planning

Researching on fertility is one of important focus of demographers in India for a long time. Levels, trends, causes and consequences of higher fertility and factors behind the contraceptive prevalence has attracted considerable research attention of population scientists and continue to do so. In this edited book, there are few papers dealing with different dimensions of fertility decline and contraceptive practices.

D.A. Nagdeve in his paper titled 'Fertility Trends and Differentials in Madhya Pradesh' has observed that the total fertility rate in the state declined from 5.6 in 1971 to 3.1 in 2011 according to sample registration system estimates. He argues that the fertility decline was mainly due to socio-economic development and the decrease in higher order births. The analysis indicates that education of women is contributing significantly to lower the fertility. As expected, the rural areas are lagging behind and need to be given more attention in order to achieve the replacement level fertility in Madhya Pradesh as soon as possible.

The paper by Sandhya Gupta addressing the contraceptive knowledge and practices among the slum women of Mumbai city provides some interesting observations. The awareness level about the modern contraceptive methods is quite high among the women working in both organized and unorganized sectors. Women of unorganized sectors showed more positive attitudes and willingness to use contraception. The common reasons for not using any contraception among the women in organized sector are fear of side effects; desire to have more children and disapproval of the husband. The author argues that despite good knowledge and favourable attitudes towards contraception, very few women are actually using. Better health education campaigns are necessary to counsel both men and women on the advantages of the small family norm and to motivate the eligible couples to regulate their fertility.

Using the three rounds of the data from the Demographic and Health Surveys, Manas Ranjan Pradhan assesses the trends and determinants of contraceptive prevalence rate (CPR) and its implications for policies and programmes in the selected South Asian countries. Bangladesh and Nepal are in a stage of contraceptive plateau while the CPR has slightly declined in Pakistan. Socio-demographic characteristics of women, exposure to family planning messages and household economic conditions are strong predictors of contraceptive use. To enhance the contraceptive use, it is necessary to broaden the method choices with quality services, strengthening of existing network and infrastructure, repositioning the spacing methods in family planning programmes and the increased role for private sectors.

Unmet need for family planning has been the major impediment in regulating fertility in developing countries. The unmet need arises out of knowledge, awareness about availability, accessibility and affordability of family planning methods for spacing and limiting. Utilizing the data of the District Level Household Survey, M.S.R. Murthy analyses the unmet need for family planning for the state of Uttar Pradesh. It was observed that some districts in the central part of Uttar Pradesh have a greater need for family planning services. Even some of the developed districts too have an unmet need for spacing methods. The state as a whole has a low unmet need (10%) for spacing methods whereas nearly one-fifth of the women reported as having an unmet need for limiting methods.

The increasing age at marriage among women in India and the decreasing age at sterilization indicate that the effective reproductive span of the women is contracting considerably. The paper by Abhishek Saraswat and Sayeed Unisa examines the reproductive span of Indian women by successive marriage cohorts by utilizing the available data from the last round of the National Family Health Survey (NFHS), which was undertaken in 2005-06. It was found that the effective reproductive span of women of successive marriage cohorts decreased from 11.5 to 2.8 years among those who married in 1970s and 2000-04 respectively, clearly indicating that younger women are opting to end their reproductive span faster than those women of the previous cohort. The authors suggest that couples should be encouraged to postpone child bearing and spacing of birth with reversible modern contraceptives. This can be achieved through better IEC campaigns and counseling of eligible couples.

Health and Health Care Services

Madhya Pradesh has the dubious distinction of having the second lowest expectation of life at births among the major states of India. The paper by Aalok Ranjan Chaurasia analyses the mortality and health transition in Madhya Pradesh during the 35 years between 1970–75 through 2006–10 and explores the factors that may have attributed to relatively low transition in mortality in the state. The analysis also suggests that substantial demographic, social class and regional differences in mortality and health situation continue to persist in the state. Persistence of poor health and mortality situation has implications for the social and economic development of the state and improvement in the quality of life of its people. What are the options available for Madhya Pradesh? There is a need to reinvigorate the health care delivery system through user perspective by promoting local level collective health action by building the capacity of the people to identify their health needs and to initiate sustainable action to address those needs.

The accurate knowledge of adult mortality levels and trends in many developing countries is not available due to the incomplete vital registration system. Even in India, very little research work has been carried out to study the levels, trends and differentials in adult mortality, mainly due to a shortage of reliable data. The paper by K.B. Gotpagar and P. Murugesan attempts to calculate the adult male mortality rates for Madhya Pradesh in comparison to other states of India through an application of widowhood method. The district level analysis of Madhya Pradesh showed that there is a difference of five years of life expectancy at the age of 20. The study illustrates that in the Madhya Pradesh, mortality levels are not equally distributed among the districts.

According to some estimates, about 366 million people are affected with diabetes worldwide. India is a major contributor to the disease burden due to diabetes. By systematically reviewing the available literature, A. Devarajan makes an effort to understand the burden of Type II diabetes in India. This growing burden of disease received various responses at national and international level. However, the responses are fragmented and may not address the multi-causal disorder in a comprehensive manner. According to the author, a multilevel inter-disciplinary inquiry is required to deal with the growing disease burden in India as a result of increasing incidences of diabetes across all age and social groups.

The public health infrastructure in India underwent considerable changes particularly after the initiation of the National Rural Health Mission (NRHM) in 2005. NRHM made a serious effort to improve the rural health care infrastructure by injecting a lot of money into our public health care system. We need to find out how far have the efforts made under NRHM helped in improving the availability of human resources, health infrastructures including the drugs and equipments, at the levels of the primary health centres (PHCs) and community health centres (CHCs). The authors (Chander Shekhar, Garima Dutta, and Sarang Pedgaonkar) used the District Level Household and Facility Survey (DLHS) (2007–08) data as well as Rural Health Statistics and Sample Registration System to analyse this. It was observed that most of the public health facilities still lack in critical equipment for newborn care and neonatal resuscitation. Combined scarcity of trained staff, equipment, poor outreach and essential service are much larger than their independent absence. In Madhya Pradesh, Vindhyanchal and South Western regions need special attention in improving the health infrastructure and manpower.

Affordable and quality health care is indispensable for a decent quality of life. The poorer section of our country continues to have less access to the health care services. Lack of affordability and accessibility of health care services to the marginalized sections of the society is a major challenge even now. The paper authored by Varun Sharma, Jyotsna Jha and Divya Krishnaswamy attempts to analyse the distribution of public health spending in Karnataka state by analysing the budgetary provisions and the available data from Reproductive and Child Health Surveys.

The public health care system offers subsidies targeting to poorer sections. However, two crucial questions arise – 'Who have the access to these health care subsidies?' and 'Who is reaping the benefits of subsidies?'. To answer these important questions, one needs to look at the access and utilization of government-run health facilities by people belonging to different income categories. Using the 60th round data of the National Sample Survey, Montu Bose examines the benefits enjoyed by different sections of the population. The study found that the poorest and the most vulnerable sections of the population receive the least benefits from the public health care services. According to the author, the benefits are mostly enjoyed by middle-income groups. The presence of strong distributive biases across income classes and regions highlights the need for a change in the policy design of our health programmes to better target the limited resources to the needy and marginalized groups.

Maternal Health Care

In the recent decades, considerable attention has been given to strengthening the maternal and child health services in most developing countries, including India and Nepal. The four papers included in this section deal with the extent of utilization of MCH services in India and Nepal. The paper by Dipika Subba aims to examine the maternal complication in the eastern states of India. The author has particularly focused on the situation in West Bengal by analysing the data from the third round of DLHS. West Bengal has the dubious distinction of achieving low fertility and mortality with high maternal complications. The utilization of ANC which is essential for safe motherhood is just above the national average.

The findings of the study highlight the need to create awareness among socially and economically disadvantaged groups about the benefits of utilizing the health care services. In order to achieve the targets set out in Millennium Development Goals (MDGs) regarding maternal health care services, more focus should be given to disadvantaged groups by implementing effective policies.

Another paper by Gunjan Gaurav and Suhas Kadam considers the involvement of men in maternal and newborn care, based on a household survey in Bihar. Most of the respondents are not aware of the complications and warning signs during pregnancy. Socio-economic and demographic factors like age, education, standard of living were influencing the involvement of men in maternal and child health care.

This volume also has two papers discussing the situation in Nepal. Komal Prasad Dulal emphasizes the role of women's education in facilitating maternal health care utilization. Various initiatives of the Government of Nepal such as establishment of new birthing centres, improvement in quality of services, training of manpower, and free maternity services must have improved the situation in the rural parts of the country. Using the Nepal Demographic Health Survey of 2011, the author observed that even after controlling some socio-economic and development variables, the effect of female education is considered as an important variable to enhance maternal health care utilization, which will ultimately contribute in the reduction of maternal and child mortality.

Ramesh Babu Kafle examines the relationships of modern contraceptive use and women's education in Nepal. He found that the net effect of women's education on modern use of contraception is insignificant after controlling for age, number of surviving children, number of living sons, place of residence, exposure to women's groups and family planning messages. These variables affect the modern contraceptive use more prominently among the less educated women in comparison to their counterparts having more education.

Population Dynamics and Environment

There are many studies that examine the complex interrelationships between population growth, economic development, and poverty reduction. M. Soundha Rajan and C. Satheesh Kumar in their paper attempt to test the well-known hypothesis – 'To increase the poverty reduction rate, the economic growth rate should be higher than the population growth rate'. The authors have compiled available secondary data on population growth, gross state domestic product (GSDP) and the population living under the below poverty line (BPL). According to them, those states that have lower BPL population have achieved a higher rate of GSDP growth than the states of higher BPL population. In other words, those states that have stabilized the population growth have the better chance of achieving high and sustaining human development by meeting the needs of the present generation without compromising the needs of future generations.

H.C. Srivastava and Palani Murugesan in their paper titled 'Population Dynamics and Environmental Degradation in India' review the levels and trends in population dynamics and its linkages with environmental degradation. According to them, the persisting high rate of population growth in our country continues to be a matter of concern which would have adverse implications on land use patterns, decrease in area under crops, and considerable increase in non-agricultural lands. Apart from developing infrastructure in cities and towns, it is also important that alternative employment is generated in villages as well. Public-private partnership may be enhanced for improving the environmental conditions. Rapid urbanization is another concern which may have an adverse impact on the environment and the living conditions of the people.

In India, nearly 7 per cent of child deaths are attributed to indoor air pollution. The study by Avijit Mistri and Nasrin Banu deals with the trends and patterns of cooking, fuel consumption and the kitchen environment in India with special emphasis on female-headed households. The study suggests that more than two-thirds of households used unclean fuels in 2011 where firewood, crop residue, and cow dung cake were the most common forms of everyday energy needs. The authors have effectively utilized the available data from the Census of India. While acute respiratory infections and low birth weight were recognized as priority health problems among children, the health hazards of cooking fuel consumption have not received the deserving attention, partly due to lack of awareness of health hazards and also due to lack of sufficient scientific data.

Though the Indian economy has recorded commendable growth over the last decade, one of the unresolved puzzles is the persisting malnutrition and food insecurity despite the 'apparent economic growth'. Balakrushna Padhi in his study examined the nature of changing food consumption of households and its implications on nutrient intake and undernutrition in India for the period 1993–2009. This study documents the paradoxical changes in food consumption both in rural and urban areas and depicts an increase in the prevalence of undernourishment during the last two decades. The main factors behind this shift are a decline in the essential food consumption items such as cereals leading to significant rise in calorie undernourishment. The author has observed a stark difference between money-metric and calorie-metric deprivation in rural and urban India. In order to better understand the changes in the living standards of the households, one needs to go beyond the standard expenditure based money-metric measures.

The twenty papers included in this volume provides multi-disciplinary perspectives on the inter-relationships between population, health and environment. These papers discuss the present scenario, highlight future implications, and suggest measures to be taken to address the emerging challenges.

Section I

Fertility and Family Planning

2

Fertility Trends and Differentials in Madhya Pradesh

D.A. Nagdeve

India has experienced substantial fertility decline but the rate of decline was different and it was slower in Madhya Pradesh as compared to other Indian states. The southern states achieved the total fertility rate (TFR) at below replacement level while northern states in India, still continued to be of high fertility level. Madhya Pradesh is one of these states with TFR of 3.1 births per woman. The National Population Policy, 2000 of India aimed to achieve the net replacement level fertility of TFR equal to 2.1 by 2010. Fertility has declined in Madhya Pradesh over the past several years and is in a state of fertility transition. However, there are wide variations in the fertility levels in rural and urban areas. With much reduced mortality levels, the potential for faster population growth exists in Madhya Pradesh unless their fertility declines rapidly in the years to come.

The analysis of age-patterns of fertility, based on district level estimates of aggregate measures of fertility data in Madhya Pradesh, revealed a clear zonal pattern in age-specific fertility rates in the state. These groups bring out high fertility rates in the north and north-western parts of the state, gradually declining toward the south-eastern zone. The author suggests that separate policies and programmes be evolved for each of the clusters of districts for the purpose of bringing about reduction in fertility and promoting family welfare in the state of Madhya Pradesh (1994). The present paper explains the fertility differentials among socio-cultural groups and regions in the central Indian state of Madhya Pradesh, and examines the role of such factors as general and female literacy, age at marriage and infant mortality in determining the fertility levels. The study indicates that no single factor is of overwhelming importance. Socio-cultural factors such as female literacy, age at marriage and infant mortality in combination, as revealed by multivariate analysis, account for about 29 per cent inter-district variation in fertility in the state (Gupta and Baghel, 1994).

The experiences of the European countries indicate that during the early stages of fertility transition of a country, urban fertility differs from rural fertility and usually urban fertility is lower than rural fertility (Mosk, 1980). Another study of rural-urban differentials in India, based on the Sample Registration System data of 1972–81, revealed that there was decline in the marital fertility at the older ages and marginal increase in fertility at the younger ages. Urban women were found to have lower fertility than rural women and voluntary fertility control was the main reason responsible for larger decline in marital fertility (Pathak and Murthy, 1987). In their study of fertility trends and differentials in Andhra Pradesh, Ramchandran and Ramesh showed the fertility differentials by individual characteristics, such as education, religion, caste and occupation. A strong negative association was observed between the educational level of women and fertility, both in rural and urban areas (Ramchandran and Ramesh, 2005).

Madhya Pradesh is located in the centre of the country with about 72 million population in 2011 and currently constitutes nearly six per cent of the total population. Madhya Pradesh is surrounded by five states of India, namely Uttar Pradesh, Rajasthan, Gujarat, Maharashtra and Chhattisgarh. Madhya Pradesh is the second largest state in the country in terms of area. This also reflects in the fact that the density of the state is about 230 which is much less than the national average. The state has a growth rate of about 20 per cent which is above the national average of about 17 and thus the population of the state is rising considerably given the progress in the state. The literacy rate in the state is about 70 per cent which is very close to the national average. One of the other aspects that the state will have to look at is the sex ratio that stands at 930 and below the national average.

The state of Madhya Pradesh has attracted the attention of demographers and development planners in recent years because fertility is the most important component of population growth, and fertility transition in Madhya Pradesh has proceeded more slowly than for India as a whole. Madhya Pradesh is the sixth most populous state in India trying to control its population growth by reducing fertility. Madhya Pradesh had experienced reduction in fertility but the levels and trends of fertility vary considerably in Madhya Pradesh. According to the recent report of the Sample Registration System (SRS) by the Office of the Registrar General and Census Commissioner of India (2013) the total fertility rate in Madhya Pradesh is observed to be 3.1 in the year 2011. In general, Madhya Pradesh has registered higher fertility in rural areas (3.3) as compared to urban areas (2.1). One of the main objectives of Madhya Pradesh Population Policy 2000 is to achieve TFR of 2.1 by the year 2011 (Government of Madhya Pradesh, 2000) but state could not achieve its objective. The underlying causes of differentials in levels and trends in fertility are, however, still a matter of debate among scholars and policymakers. The marked variations in fertility by residence and education in Madhya Pradesh provide the opportunity for systematic examination of the levels, trends and the factors contributing to fertility differentials. Therefore, the present paper is an attempt to study fertility trends and differentials in the Madhya Pradesh.

Data and Methodology

The data has been used from the Indian censuses and the Sample Registration System. An analysis of changes and trends has been conducted from 1981 to 2011.

Population Characteristics of Madhya Pradesh

Madhya Pradesh is the second largest state in the country in terms of area and the sixth most populous state in India after Uttar Pradesh, Maharashtra, Bihar, Madhya Pradesh and Andhra Pradesh. The population growth in the state varies from decade to decade. The selected population characteristics of Madhya Pradesh are presented in Table 1. According to the results of the Census of India 2011, the population of Madhya Pradesh is 73 million, compared to 42 million in 1971. Thus, the population of Madhya Pradesh has increased by 1.74 times during 1971 and 2011, an increase of 31 million in 40 years. About 57 per cent of this increase (24 million) took place after 1991. The decadal growth of population has decreased from 29.28 per cent in 1971 to 27.24 per cent in 1991 and it further decreased to 20.30 per cent in 2011. The percentage decadal growth rate witnessed a dramatic decline in the 2001–11 decade, around 20.30 per cent compared to 24.26 per cent during 1991–2001. The sex ratio in Madhya Pradesh has increased from 920 females per 1000 males in 1971 to 930 females per 1000 males in 2011. The density of population in Madhya Pradesh has increased from 94 persons per square kilometre in 1971 to 236 persons per square kilometre in 2011. The percentage of urban population has grown from 16.29 per cent to 27.63 per cent during 1971–2011.

Table 1 *Selected Population Characteristics of Madhya Pradesh, 1971–2011*

Year	*Population in million*	*Decadal population growth (%)*	*Sex ratio (females per 1000 males)*	*Density of population per sq km*	*% of urban population to total*	*Index of population*
1971	42	29.28	920	94	16.29	100
1981	52	27.16	921	118	20.29	124
1991	49	27.24	912	158	23.18	117
2001	60	24.26	919	196	26.46	143
2011	73	20.3	930	236	27.63	174

Source: Office of the Registrar General and Census Commissioner of India.

Vital Rates in Madhya Pradesh

The growth of population depends upon fertility, mortality and migration. The process of accelerated population growth in Madhya Pradesh till 1971 witnessed a marginal deceleration during 1981, as the decadal population growth was 27 per cent compared to 29 per cent in 1971. Further declines in fertility have been witnessed during 1991, 2001 and 2011. The trends in birth, death and infant mortality rate in Madhya Pradesh is presented in Table 2. It is revealed from the Table that birth rate in Madhya Pradesh has declined from 39.1 per thousand population in 1971 to 35.8 per thousand population in 1991 and it further declined to 31 per thousand population in 2001 and 26.9 per thousand population in 2011. At the same time, crude death rate has also declined from 15.6 per thousand population in 1971 to 13.8 per thousand population in 1991 and it further declined to 10.1 per thousand population in 2001 and 8.2 per thousand population in 2011. Infant mortality rate (IMR) per thousand live births in

Madhya Pradesh has steadily declined from 135 in 1971 to 117 in 1991 and it further declined to 86 in 2001 and 59 in 2011. Similarly, the birth rate, death rate and infant mortality rate have declined both in rural and urban areas but birth rate, death rate and infant mortality rate were higher in rural areas than urban areas during 1971–2011. The percentage change in average birth rate, death rate and infant mortality rate during 1971–2011 in Madhya Pradesh is 31.2 per cent, 47 per cent and 56 per cent respectively. Such decline in average birth rate, death rate and infant mortality rate in rural areas is 28 per cent, 48 per cent and 56 per cent as compared to 42 per cent, 38 per cent and 51 per cent in urban areas of Madhya Pradesh respectively.

Table 2 *Trends in Birth Rate, Death Rate and Infant Mortality Rate by Residence, Madhya Pradesh, 1971–2011*

Year	*Birth rate*			*Death rate*			*Infant mortality rate*		
	Total	*Rural*	*Urban*	*Total*	*Rural*	*Urban*	*Total*	*Rural*	*Urban*
1971	39.1	40	34.5	15.6	16.6	9.8	135	144	79
1976	39.8	41	33.2	16.5	17.7	10.2	138	145	88
1981	37.6	38.8	31.4	16.6	18	9.3	142	152	80
1986	37.2	39.0	30.1	13.6	14.8	8.8	118	124	82
1991	35.8	37.3	29.7	13.8	14.9	9.2	117	125	74
1996	32.3	34.2	23	11.1	11.8	7.6	97	102	61
2001*	31.0	32.9	23.1	10.1	10.8	7.2	86	93	54
2006*	29.1	31.2	21.9	8.9	9.6	6.3	74	79	52
2011	26.9	28.8	20.1	8.2	8.7	6.1	59	63	39
% change during 1971–2011	–31.20	–28.00	–41.74	–47.44	–47.59	–37.76	–56.3	–56.25	–50.63

Note: * excluded Chhattisgarh.

Source: India, Registrar General, Compendium of India's Fertility and Mortality Indicators 1971–2007.
India, Registrar General, Sample Registration System Statistical Report, 2011.

Fertility Trends in Madhya Pradesh

Trends in age-specific fertility rates per 1,000 women by residence in Madhya Pradesh are given in Table 3. The age-specific fertility rates are much higher in rural areas than in urban areas of Madhya Pradesh in all age groups. There is consistent fertility decline by residence among all age groups. The age-specific fertility rates declined from 1971 to 2011 in both urban and rural areas. The peak age of child bearing is 20–24, with steadily declining fertility rates thereafter. The high fertility is still concentrated in the prime child bearing age 20–29 years in both urban and rural areas. Fertility rates declined sharply in age group 15–19 and beyond the age of 25, reaching extremely low levels for women of age 40–44 and 45–49. Early child bearing is substantial in Madhya Pradesh, which accounted for 5.33 per cent of births in the age group 15–19. It was also observed that 80.53 per cent of births occur to women below the age 30. Surprisingly, the contribution of early child bearing (age 15–19) in Madhya Pradesh is higher 5.56 per cent in urban areas than 3.52 per cent in rural areas.

It is also found that the percentage of births occurring to women below the age 30 is 81.3 per cent in rural areas and 76.5 per cent in urban areas in 2011. The percentage change in age-specific fertility rate during 1971–2011 reveals that decline in fertility rates is more in urban areas compared to rural areas, except in the age group 30–34. The decline is perceptible for the higher age groups 40–49 in urban areas. During 1971–2011, the fertility declined by 91 per cent in the age groups 40–49 in urban areas as compared to 83 per cent in rural areas. It is slower in the middle age groups 20–29 for both the areas. The minimum decline of 8 per cent has been noticed in the age group 20–24 in Madhya Pradesh. The increase of 2 per cent in rural areas and decline of 39 per cent in urban areas has also been noticed in the same age group.

Table 3 *Trends in Age-specific Fertility Rate by Residence at Interval of 5 Years in Madhya Pradesh, 1971 to 2011*

(per 1,000 women)

Age Group	*1971*	*1981*	*1991*	*2001**	*2011**	*% change during 1971–2011*
				Total		
15–19	166.8	124.7	124.6	79	32.5	–80.52
20–24	295.4	287.9	287.6	278.5	273.1	–7.55
25–29	250.3	265.8	233.5	231.8	185.8	–25.77
30–34	212.6	188.7	143.8	108.7	77.2	–63.69
35–39	154.8	114	76.6	56.7	28.3	–81.72
40–44	73.7	44.3	32.6	23.5	9.3	–87.38
45–49	16.5	23	13.2	7.8	4	–75.76
				Rural		
15–19	181.4	132.4	137.9	92.1	37.1	–79.55
20–24	301.5	304.3	300.3	307.7	306.4	1.63
25–29	251.3	272.2	241.5	249	199	–20.81
30–34	220.9	201.1	155.2	116.4	78.4	–64.51
35–39	162	123.2	85.2	63.8	30.7	–81.05
40–44	79.6	48.7	36.7	28.3	10.8	–86.43
45–49	15.2	26.2	15.1	9.8	4.9	–67.76
				Urban		
15–19	97.4	88.8	68	30.9	14.9	–84.70
20–24	265.2	219.4	241.9	187	162.1	–38.88
25–29	242	239	203	170.9	146.9	–39.30
30–34	161.1	132.4	100.9	81.7	73.6	–54.31
35–39	108.9	66	41.6	30	20.1	–81.54
40–44	36.8	20.8	15.7	7.5	4.7	–87.23
45–49	27.2	5.5	4.1	0.7	1	–96.32

Note: * excluded Chhattisgarh.

Source: India, Registrar General, Compendium of India's Fertility and Mortality Indicators, 1971–2007.
India, Registrar General, Sample Registration System Statistical Report, 2011.

Table 4 *Trends in Total Fertility Rate by Residence at Interval of 5 Years in Madhya Pradesh, 1971 to 2011*

Year	*Total*	*Rural*	*Urban*
1971	5.6	6.1	4.7
1976	5.8	6.1	4.4
1981	5.2	5.5	3.9
1986	4.9	5.4	3.5
1991	4.6	4.9	3.4
1996	4.1	4.4	2.5
2001*	3.9	4.3	2.5
2006*	3.5	3.9	2.4
2011*	3.1	3.3	2.1
Index of TFR			
1971	100	100	100
1976	104	100	94
1981	93	90	83
1986	88	89	74
1991	82	80	72
1996	73	72	53
2001	70	70	53
2006	63	64	51
2011	55	54	45
% Decline in TFR			
1971–1981	–7.14	–9.84	–17.02
1981–1991	–11.54	–10.91	–12.82
1991–2001	–15.22	–12.24	–26.47
2001–2011	–20.51	–23.26	–16.00
1971–2011	–44.64	–45.90	–55.32
% Annual Decline in TFR			
1971–81	–071	–0.98	–1.70
1981–91	–1.15	–1.09	–1.28
1991–2001	–1.52	–1.22	–2.65
2001–2011	–2.05	–2.33	–1.60
1971–2011	–1.12	–1.15	–1.38

Note: * excluded Chhattisgarh.

Source: India, Registrar General, Compendium of India's Fertility and Mortality Indicators, 1971–2007.
India, Registrar General, Sample Registration System Statistical Report, 2011.

The total fertility rate declined considerably from 1971 to 2011 in Madhya Pradesh. The trends of total fertility rate by residence in Madhya Pradesh from 1971–2011 is presented in Table 4. From beginning, the TFR of Madhya Pradesh is found to be higher than the national level. But the rate of decline was different and it was slower in Madhya Pradesh as compared to all-India. During the period 1971–76, fertility seems to have increased slightly from a TFR of 5.6 per woman in 1971 to 5.8 in 1976. The pace of fertility decline is accelerated, with an estimated TFR of 5.2 in 1981 to 4.9 in 1986. Further, it declined to 4.6 in 1991,

3.9 in 2001 and to 3.1 in 2011. The fertility decline also shows a moderate fall through the 1980s and a steep drop during the 1990s and afterwards. The annual decline in fertility during the period 1971–2011 was 1.12 per cent for the state. The comparison of the TFR between 1971–81 and 1981–1991, shows that the rate of decline in the TFR is lower during 1971–1981 (0.71% per year) compared to 1.15 per cent during 1981–1991. Similarly, the comparison of the TFR between 1991–2001 and 2001–2011, indicates that the rate of decline in the TFR is lower during 1991–2001 (1.52% per year) compared to 2.05 during 2001–2011. On an average, women in Madhya Pradesh give birth to three children (3.1) as compared to six children (5.6) in 1971.

The TFR of rural Madhya Pradesh in 1971 was 6.1 and in the urban areas it was 4.7, thus having a difference of 23 per cent. It declined to 3.3 in rural areas and 2.1 in urban areas in 2011, difference of 36 per cent. The percentage of annual decline in the TFR was 1.15 in rural areas and in urban areas it was 1.38 during 1971–2011. In the recent decade (i.e. 2001–2011), the fertility decline in rural Madhya Pradesh has been faster (an average annual decline of 2.33% in the TFR) as compared to 1.60 per cent in urban areas. The difference between rural and urban TFRs has increased from 23 per cent in 1971 to 36 per cent in 2011.

Marital Fertility Trends in Madhya Pradesh

Age at marriage of females is a key factor that influences fertility. Based on the distribution of live births by age of married females, age-specific marital fertility rates (ASMFRs) are calculated. Trends in age-specific marital fertility rates per 1000 women by residence in Madhya Pradesh are given in Table 5. There is consistent marital fertility decline by residence among all age groups. The age-specific marital fertility rates declined from 1971 to 2011 in Madhya Pradesh. Marital fertility is much higher in rural areas than in urban areas in all the age groups and its peak is in the age group 20–24 years. A perceptible decline in marital fertility is seen for females in the age of 30 years and above both in rural areas and urban areas. The high marital fertility is still concentrated in the prime child-bearing age 20–29 years in both urban and rural areas. Marital fertility rates declined in age group 15–19 and it further declined sharply beyond the age of 25, reaching extremely low levels for women of age 40–44 and 45–49. Early marital fertility is substantial in Madhya Pradesh, which accounted for 26 per cent of births in the age group 15–19. It was also observed that 87 per cent of births occur to women below the age 30. Surprisingly, the contribution of early marital fertility (age 15–19) is higher: 29 per cent in urban areas of Madhya Pradesh and 25 per cent in rural areas of Madhya Pradesh, but 87 per cent of births occur to women below the age of 30 both in rural and urban areas in 2011. The percentage change in age-specific marital fertility rate during 1971–2011 reveals that decline in fertility rates is more in urban areas compared to rural areas. The decline is perceptible for the higher age group 40–49 in urban areas. During 1971–2011, the marital fertility declined by 82 per cent in the age groups 40–49 in urban areas as compared to 78 per cent in rural areas.

It is slower in the middle age groups 20–29 for both the areas. The increase in marital fertility of 12 per cent has been noticed in the age group 20–24 in Madhya Pradesh. The increase of 18 per cent in rural areas and decline of 16 per cent in urban areas has also been noticed in the same age group.

Table 5 *Trends in Age-specific Marital Fertility Rate at Interval of 5 Years by Residence in Madhya Pradesh, 1984–2011*

Age Group	*1984*	*1991*	*2001**	*2011**	*% change during 1984–2011*
		Total			
15–19	267.4	257.4	284.1	244.6	–8.53
20–24	342.3	326.9	355.9	382	11.60
25–29	273.9	244.4	246.5	200	–26.98
30–34	181.1	151.1	113.2	80.5	–55.55
35–39	108.3	81.2	60.2	30	–72.30
40–44	47.9	35.7	25.3	10.1	–78.91
45–49	24.4	15.4	8.9	4.5	–81.56
		Rural			
15–19	265	253.7	286.1	245.8	–7.25
20–24	337.2	325	358.1	397.2	17.79
25–29	285.2	250	258	208.8	–26.79
30–34	193.4	162.7	120.6	80.9	–58.17
35–39	120	90.3	67.6	32.5	–72.92
40–44	52.5	40.1	30.4	11.7	–77.71
45–49	27.6	17.5	11.1	5.6	–79.71
		Urban			
15–19	284.1	294.6	263.3	234.2	–17.56
20–24	365.2	335.8	345.1	307.9	–15.69
25–29	232.9	221.9	200.3	171	–26.58
30–34	133	106.8	86.7	79.2	–40.45
35–39	64.1	44.1	32	21.5	–66.46
40–44	26.5	17.4	8.1	5.2	–80.38
45–49	8.7	4.9	0.8	1.2	–86.21

Note: * excluded Chhattisgarh.

Source: India, Registrar General, Compendium of India's Fertility and Mortality Indicators, 1971–2007.
India, Registrar General, Sample Registration System Statistical Report, 2011.

The total marital fertility rate declined considerably from 1971 to 2011 in Madhya Pradesh. The trends of total marital fertility rate (TMFR) from 1971–2011 is depicted in Table 6. From the beginning, TMFR of Madhya Pradesh is found to be higher than the national level. But the rate of decline was different and it was slower in Madhya Pradesh as compared to all-India rate. During the period 1984–86, marital fertility seems to have decreased from a TMFR of 6.2 per woman in 1984 to 5.8 in 1986. It further decreased to 5.6 in

1991 and to 5.1 in 1996 but it increased to 5.5 in 2001. The pace of fertility decline is accelerated, with an estimated TFR of 4.9 in 2006 and further it declined to 4.8 in 2011. The marital fertility decline also shows a moderate fall through the 1990s, decelerated during 1991–2001 and a steep drop during the recent decade. The annual decline in marital fertility during the period 1971–2011 was 0.84 per cent for the state. The comparison of the TMFR between 1984–91 and 1991–2001, shows that the rate of decline in the TMFR is lower during 1991–2001 (0.18% per year) compared to 1.38 per cent during 1984–1991. Similarly, the comparison of the TMFR between 1991–2001 and 2001–2011, indicates that the rate of decline in the TMFR is higher in the recent decade (1.27% per year) compared to 0.18 during 1991–2001. On an average, married women in Madhya Pradesh give birth to five children (4.8) as compared to six children (6.2) in the early 1980s.

Table 6 *Trends in Total Marital Fertility Rate (TMFR) by Residence in Madhya Pradesh, 1984–2011*

Year	*Total*	*Rural*	*Urban*
1984	6.2	6.4	5.6
1986	5.8	6	4.9
1991	5.6	5.7	5.1
1996	5.1	5.3	4.1
2001*	5.5	5.7	4.7
2006*	4.9	5.2	4
2011*	4.8	4.9	4.1
Index of TMFR			
1984	100	100	100
1986	93.55	93.75	87.50
1991	90.32	89.06	91.07
1996	82.26	82.81	73.21
2001	88.71	89.06	83.93
2006	79.03	81.25	71.43
2011	77.42	76.56	73.21
% Decline in TMFR			
1984–91	–9.68	–10.94	–8.93
1991–2001	–1.79	0.00	–7.84
2001–2011	–12.73	–14.04	–12.77
1984–2011	–22.58	–23.44	–26.79
% Annual Decline in TMFR			
1984–91	–1.38	–1.56	–1.28
1991–2001	–0.18	0.00	–0.78
2001–2011	–1.27	–1.40	–1.28
1984–2011	–0.84	–0.87	–0.99

Note: * excluded Chhattisgarh.

Source: India, Registrar General, Compendium of India's Fertility and Mortality Indicators, 1971–2007.
India, Registrar General, Sample Registration System Statistical Report, 2011.

The TMFR of rural Madhya Pradesh in 1984 was 6.4 and in the urban areas it was 5.6, thus having a difference of 13 per cent. It declined to 4.9 in rural areas and 4.1 in urban areas in 2011, difference of 16 per cent. The percentage of annual decline in the TMFR was 0.87 and in urban areas it was 0.99 during 1984–2011. In the recent decade (i.e. 2001–2011), the marital fertility decline in rural Madhya Pradesh has been faster (an average annual decline of 1.40% in the TMFR) as compared to 1.28 per cent in urban areas. The difference between rural and urban TMFRs has increased from 13 per cent in 1984 to 16 per cent in 2011.

Fertility by Level of Education of the Women

Female education has a direct impact on fertility. To ascertain levels of fertility by educational status of the women age-specific fertility rate and total fertility rate by educational status of the women for rural and urban areas have been discussed in Table 7. The data reveals marked rural-urban differences with the rural areas generally reporting higher levels of fertility than the urban areas for all age groups. Fertility attains the peak in the age-group 20–24 years both in the rural and urban areas except for the women having education level 12th and above in urban areas. 'Illiterate' women have higher levels of age-specific fertility rates both in the rural and urban areas than the 'Literate'. Within the 'Literate' group there is a general decline in the fertility rates with the increase in the educational status both in the rural and urban areas, barring a few exceptions.

Table 7 *Age-specific Fertility Rates and Total Fertility Rates by Education and Residence in Madhya Pradesh, 2011*

					Literate				
Age Group	*Illiterate*	*Total Literate*	*Without any formal education*	*Below primary*	*Primary*	*Middle*	*Class X*	*Class XII*	*Graduate and above*
				Total					
15–19	91.4	26.6	278.7	176.7	43	12.5	3.5	4.7	0
20–24	325.7	258.3	315.6	390.8	323.7	228.3	138.6	97	92.6
25–29	194.2	180.7	195.6	204.2	201.9	181.2	157.3	135.9	118.8
30–34	83.8	71.2	96.7	83.5	61	60.9	67.9	43.6	97.5
35–39	32	23.3	39.6	36	19.2	3.4	19.9	38.8	12.7
40–44	12.3	4.6	0	9	4.9	6	0	0	0
45–49	4.9	2.2	0	1.4	4.8	4.3	0	0	0
TFR	3.7	2.8	4.6	4.5	3.3	2.5	1.9	1.6	1.6
				Rural					
15–19	95.1	30.6	295.9	186.2	45.9	12.7	4	0	0
20–24	336.3	296.1	299.9	405.8	345.9	244.9	152.2	139.3	88.2

Cont'd...

...Cont'd

25–29	201.2	197.2	187.6	214.5	210.4	188.5	162.7	134.7	178
30–34	85.7	69.3	96.4	86.2	54.8	63.6	56	53.7	56.7
35–39	33.7	25.1	29.1	38.7	19	3.8	15.6	38.7	19.3
40–44	13.4	4.9	0	10	0	7.4	0	0	0
45–49	5.7	2.5	0	0	5	8.2	0	0	0
TFR	3.9	3.1	4.5	4.7	3.4	2.6	2	1.8	1.7
				Urban					
15–19	66.2	11.9	161.3	94.1	25	11.2	2.3	8.6	0
20–24	235.2	154.1	397.6	282.9	220.6	178.3	113.9	67.3	93.9
25–29	138.8	148.3	247.1	153.3	174.6	166.4	151.2	136.6	103.3
30–34	69.8	74.8	98.7	71.2	79.2	56.5	82	38.1	107.7
35–39	19.6	20.3	126.3	24.9	19.8	2.8	23.6	38.9	11.6
40–44	5.3	4.3	0	5.2	14.6	4.2	0	0	0
45–49	0	1.7	0	5.8	4.4	0	0	0	0
TFR	2.7	2.1	5.2	3.2	2.7	2.1	1.9	1.4	1.6

Note: * excluded Chhattisgarh.

Source: India, Registrar General, Sample Registration System Statistical Report, 2011.

Pattern of Higher Order Births

The distribution of live births by order of birth gives an idea about the total number of children ever born to the eligible women and it gives a broad idea for the preference of small family. The examination of the trends in the pattern of higher order births (four and above) also indicates a decline in fertility of Madhya Pradesh. The change in the higher order births is a good indicator of fertility change and also helps to assess the overall fertility impact of contraceptive prevalence. Since the main focus of family planning programme in India is to reduce higher order births, changes in the proportion of higher order births over a period of time is expected to reflect changes in the fertility levels. The proportion of lower order births are expected to increase as a result of the reduction in higher order births when fertility declines from high to low levels. The distribution of live births by order of births in Madhya Pradesh is given in Table 8. From the table it may be observed that, the percentage of births of four children and above has declined from 27.9 per cent in 1991 to 13.4 per cent in 2011. As expected, the percentage of first order births and second order births has been increased from 26.4 per cent and 24.9 per cent in 1991, to 39.3 per cent and 31.9 per cent in 2011 respectively. The percentage of 3 order births has decreased from 20.8 per cent in 1991 to 15.6 per cent in 2011. It may also be noticed that the percentage of birth order up to 2 has increased from 51.3 per cent in 1991 to 71.2 per cent in 2011, whereas the percentage of birth order above 3 has declined from 48.7 per cent in 1991 to 29.0 per cent in 2011. This shows the evidence of fertility decline in Madhya Pradesh.

Table 8 *Percentage Distribution of Live Births by Order of Birth by Residence in Madhya Pradesh, 1991–2011*

Year	*Live Births by Order of Birth (Total)*				
	1	*2*	*3*	*4+*	*Total*
1991	26.4	24.9	20.8	27.9	100
1996	28.7	25.1	20.2	26	100
2001*	30	26.6	20.4	23	100
2006*	35.2	28.2	17.9	18.7	100
2011*	39.3	31.9	15.6	13.4	100
Live Births by Order of Birth (Rural)					
1991	25.7	24.9	21.1	28.3	100
1996	28	24.8	20.3	26.9	100
2001*	29.3	25.8	20.7	24.2	100
2006*	33.8	27.7	18.3	20.3	100
2011*	38.7	31.3	16	14	100
Live Births by Order of Birth (Urban)					
1991	29.9	25	19.3	25.8	100
1996	34.4	27.1	19.4	19.1	100
2001*	34.2	31.1	19.1	15.7	100
2006*	42.2	30.7	15.7	11.4	100
2011*	42.1	34.7	13.4	9.9	100

Note: * excluded Chhattisgarh.

Source: India, Registrar General, Compendium of India's Fertility and Mortality Indicators, 1971–2007.
India, Registrar General, Sample Registration System Statistical Report, 2011.

Summary and Conclusions

The analysis revealed that the total fertility rate was 5.6 children per woman in the 1971; it has since then reduced to 3.1 in 2011, according to Sample Registration System estimates. Madhya Pradesh had experienced reduction in fertility but the levels and trends of fertility vary considerably in Madhya Pradesh. It also shows a moderate fall through the 1980s and a steep drop during the 1990s and afterwards. The preliminary results of 2011 Census indicate the impact of fertility transition on population dynamics of Madhya Pradesh, where growth rates have decreased over a decade. Madhya Pradesh is still having higher fertility and it varies by residence and education. The pattern of fertility decline was not uniform in rural and urban areas and rural areas were lagging behind. A strong negative association was observed between the education level of women and fertility, both in rural and urban areas. The fertility decline was mainly due to the education, decrease in higher order births of three and above and decrease in fertility among older women in age group 30 and above. In spite of fertility differentials, the decline has been observed among all sections of the population, including the illiterate and poor. The causes of decline may be different among population of the state. There is need to analyse in greater detail the factors that have contributed to the rapid decline in fertility in the 1990s and recent decades. From the above analysis, it may be concluded that the fertility differentials exist in Madhya Pradesh because of variations in socio-economic development including education. There is a negative relationship between education and fertility. This indicates the education of women contributes to lower fertility. Therefore, education of the girls needs to be encouraged. There is a need to give more thrust on rural areas with high fertility for achieving below replacement fertility in Madhya Pradesh.

References

Gupta, H.S. and Baghel, A. 1994. Fertility Differentials in Madhya Pradesh, India. *Population Geography*, 16 (1–2): 49–58.

India, Registrar General and Census Commissioner of India. 2011. Final Population Totals. Census of India, Paper 1 of 2011, New Delhi: Controller of Publications.

——. 2013. *Sample Registration System Statistical Report 2013*. New Delhi: Registrar General and Census Commissioner.

India, Registrar General. 2009. *Compendium of India's Fertility and Mortality Indicators 1971–2007 Based on the Sample Registration System (SRS)*. New Delhi: Registrar General.

Mosk, C. 1980. Rural-Urban Fertility Differences and the Fertility Transition. *Population Studies*, 34 (1): 19.

Pathak, K.B. and Murthy, P.K. 1987. Rural-Urban Fertility Differential in India. *Janasamkhya*, 5 (1): 41–59.

Ramchandran, P. and Ramesh, P. 2005. Fertility Trends and Differentials in Andhra Pradesh. In Christophe Z. Guilmoto and S. Irudaya Rajan (eds), *Fertility Transition in South India*, New Delhi: Sage Publications, pp. 114–136.

Ranjan, A. 1994. Age Patterns of Fertility in Madhya Pradesh. *Population Geography*, 16 (1–2): 59–66.

3

Contraceptive Knowledge, Attitude and Practices among Slum Women

A Cross Sectional Study

Sandhya Gupta

Population of India is 1.21 billion (Census of India, 2011), which is on the rise with each passing year. India is the second most populous country in the world after China. It contributes about 20 per cent of births worldwide, with its annual population growth rate of 1.74 per cent. This uncontrolled population growth is one of the greatest threats to India's health, political, economic and social development. Increase in population size and fertility also places pressure on the environment and, in turn, these degraded natural resources impact the health and livelihoods of communities, and threatens long-term prospects of sustainable development.

India was the first country in the world to launch a National Family Planning Programme in 1952 with the aim to reduce the birth rate to stabilize its population. During the Third Five-Year Plan (1961–66), family planning was declared as the 'very centre of the planned development'. Since its inception, the family planning programme has experienced significant growth in terms of financial investment, type of services, and the range of contraceptive methods offered. As a result, India's TFR declined from six children per woman in the 1960s to just under three children (2.6) at present. But despite all the programmatic efforts, TFR for the country remained stationery at 2.6 during 2008 to 2009. This is due to low contraceptive prevalence rate for currently married women in India (56% as per NFHS–3). Female sterilization, with a prevalence of 37 per cent, and which accounts for 66 per cent of all contraceptive use in India is the most favoured method, while the male sterilization is the least common method of contraception all across the country (IIPS and Macro International, 2007). Moreover, use of other officially sponsored spacing methods (pills, IUD and condoms, injections) is comparatively low and their discontinuation rate is fairly high. Thus, family planning initiatives in India are usually stuck on only one thing – female sterilization and the demographic indicators points out that the female sterilization is not the correct solution to manage Indian population. Many factors contribute for this underutilization of contraceptives and this makes contraception as unfelt need of millions of women today.

According to NFHS–3 (2005–2006), the contraceptive use among married women varies markedly by education, religion, caste and wealth. Also, there is a clear gap between urban and rural areas regarding contraceptive knowledge and use, even differential exist within the urban areas between slum and non-slum population. This is because urban population of India is increasing rapidly due to continuous influx of people from rural areas. A major consequence of the surge in urban population is the rapid growth of slums inhabited by poor people. Slum residents have low socio-economic status, low literacy, poor access and availability of health services, including family planning services, which makes them most vulnerable and hence targeted group to deal with. Few slum-based studies have highlighted inadequate knowledge of contraceptive methods and incomplete or erroneous information about where to obtain methods and how to use them as the main reasons for not accepting family planning methods (Kumar et al., 2011; Reddy, 2011; Srivastava et al., 2005). Also the acceptance level and motivation for contraceptive usage is lower in slums than urban areas. This reveals that there is an unmet need for family planning among currently married women especially residing in slums, which demands more extensive efforts of family planning programmes. To improve the effectiveness of the programme, there is need to know about awareness, practice and various other factors affecting the use of spacing methods in the different segments of our population (Mahawar et al., 2011).

Keeping in view the above points, the present study was carried out to assess knowledge, attitude and practice of contraceptive methods among married women and to understand the reasons for using and not using various contraceptive methods in an urban slum of Mumbai.

Methodology

The present cross-sectional study was carried out in the organized and unorganized parts of B-sector of Cheetah camp slum in Mumbai from February to March 2012. A sample size of 130 married females of age group 16–40 years was decided, where 65 females from organized and 65 from unorganized parts were to be selected. A systematic random sampling was adopted to select eligible respondents. There was a total of 2,399 households in both organized and unorganized parts of B-sector, Cheetah camp. A household was considered as a unit of analysis. So, in order to obtain a sample size of 130 married females, first household was selected randomly in both organized and unorganized sector then every next household was selected at the 18th interval (2399/130= 18). If there were more than one eligible respondent in a single household, then the younger married female was selected and interviewed. Data was collected using a predesigned structured interview schedule and face-to-face interviews were conducted. The consent of all the respondents was taken prior to the study. A total of 122 married females, 64 in organized section and 58 in unorganized section gave consent and thus were interviewed. To assess knowledge regarding family planning methods a composite score was calculated on the basis of selected questions and knowledge was arbitrarily graded as Poor (0–5 score range), Moderate (6–11 score range) and Good (for 12–17 score range). The practice was defined as the usage of contraceptive methods by either partner. Data analysis was done using SPSS 20 and Chi square test was used to associate various findings.

Results

Socio-demographic Profile

The socio-demographic characteristics of women are shown in Table 1. The mean age of women in the study was 27.5 ± 4.95 years. Majority of the women were of age between 21–30 years in both organized and unorganized parts. Maximum women in the study were Muslim by religion in both the sections. More than 95 per cent women in both the sections were housewives. Women in organized sector were comparatively more literate, with 43.8 per cent women educated up to secondary school (8th class) and above. Unorganized section had more illiterate women (17%) compared to organized section (11%). In organized section women had higher monthly household income than unorganized section. Around 78 per cent women in organized section had monthly household income of ₹5,000 and above, compared to women in unorganized section (48.3%). The mean number of living children in unorganized part was higher (3 ±1.56) compared to organized section (2 ± 1.18). Around 34 per cent respondents in organized part had one child as compared to 15.5 per cent respondents in unorganized part of the slum.

Table 1 *Socio-Demographic Profile of the Women*

Socio-Demographic Variables	*Organized Part Frequency (%)*	*Unorganized Part Frequency (%)*
Age Group (years)		
15-20	3 (4.7%)	2 (3.4%)
21-25	24 (37.5%)	23 (39.7%)
26-30	23 (35.9%)	16 (27.6%)
31-35	9 (14.1%)	14 (24.1%)
36-40	5 (7.8%)	3 (5.2%)
Religion		
Hindu	4 (6.2%)	11 (19%)
Muslim	60 (93.8%)	47 (81)
Education		
Illiterate	7 (10.9%)	10 (17.2%)
Primary education	29 (45.3%)	32 (55.2%)
Secondary or higher	28 (43.8%)	16 (27.8 %)

Cont'd...

...Cont'd

Occupation		
Housewife	61 (95.3%)	57 (98.3%)
Self-employed	3 (4.7%)	1 (1.7%)
Total monthly Household Income (Rs)		
Less than 5,000	14 (21.9%)	30 (51.7%)
5,000-10,000	35 (54.7%)	25 (43.1%)
More than 10,000	15 (23.4%)	3 (5.2%)
Number of living children		
1	21 (33.8%)	9 (15.5%)
2-3	31 (50%)	35 (60.4%)
4 and above	10 (16.2%)	14 (24.1%)
Total	64 (100%)	58 (100%)

Knowledge

Around 43.8 per cent women in organized and 37.9 per cent women from unorganized parts knew the meaning of family planning. Majority of females from both sections explained family planning as having small family with less number of children and many mentioned it as keeping birth space between children. Majority of respondents in organized sector (68.8%) and 56.9 per cent respondents in unorganized section felt two children are ideal for a family. Most of the respondents (50% in organized and 48 per cent in unorganized sections) mentioned that ideal birth gap between children is 3 years.

Table 2 presents knowledge regarding various contraceptive methods among women of organised and unorganized sections. All the women from both organized and unorganized sections had heard of oral contraceptive pills and female sterilization. Majority of women in organized (94%) and unorganized (97%) sections were aware of male condom and Copper-T. Knowledge of emergency pills was more among women of organized section (60%) in comparison to unorganized section (32%). While more number of females in unorganized section had heard of injectables (79%) and male sterilization (60%) than in organized section. Around 56 per cent women knew about withdrawal method for contraception in both the sections. Only 1.6 per cent females knew about female condoms.

Maximum women in both organized (90.6%) and unorganized (86%) sections mentioned medical store as the place to obtain family planning methods. Most of women knew government hospitals (75% in organized and 86% in unorganized section) and private hospitals (64% in organized and 58.6% in unorganized section) as places to obtain contraceptives followed by Anganwadi centres.

The common sources of knowledge about family planning (FP) methods were friends/relatives (82%), television (69%) and health workers/doctors (57.8%) in organized section. In unorganized section, women mentioned friends (93%), health workers/doctors (81%) and television (70.7%) as the common sources of their knowledge about family planning methods.

Table 2 *Awareness Regarding Family Planning Methods*

Awareness regarding FP methods	*Organized sector (n=64) Frequency (%)*	*Unorganized sector (n=58) Frequency (%)*
Oral Contraceptive Pill (OCP)	64 (100)	58 (100)
Female sterilization	64 (100)	58 (100)
Male condom	60 (94)	56 (97)
Copper-T (IUCD)	60 (94)	56 (97)
Male sterilization	34 (53)	35 (60)
Withdrawal method	36 (56)	34 (58)
Emergency contraceptives	39 (60)	19 (32)
Injectables	44 (68)	46 (79)
Female condom	1 (1.6)	1 (1.7)

Note: Total exceeds more than 100 due to multiple responses.

Most of the women in organized section (53%) as well as unorganized section (57%) had moderate level of knowledge regarding family planning methods. Though there was no significant difference between the overall knowledge of women from both the sections.

Attitude

Majority of women in organized (89%) and unorganized (91%) had the opinion that having two children in a family is good. All women in unorganized section opined birth gap of 3 years or more as good compared to women of organized section (92%). Around 79 per cent women in unorganized section showed willingness to use FP methods in comparison to organized section (70%).

Practice

Around 77 per cent women in both organized and unorganized sections had used family planning method in the past. The current couple protection rate in the study population of unorganized section was 55.2 per cent compared to 43.8 per cent in organized section. Figure 1 shows that in organized section use of oral contraception pills (OCP) (35.7%), condoms (28.6%), tubectomy (25%) and

Figure 1 *Distribution of Women by the Type of Current Contraceptive Method Used in Organized and Unorganized Sectors*

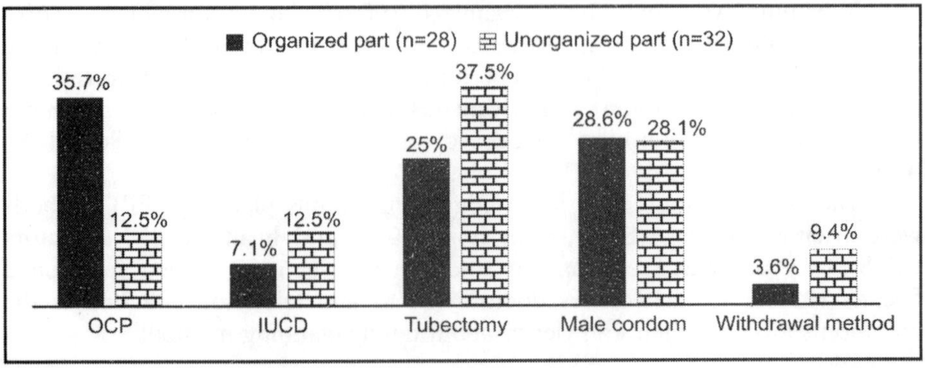

IUCD (7%) were more prevalent while in unorganized sector tubectomy (37.5%), condoms (28%), IUCD (13%) and OCP (13%) were more commonly used.

Reasons for Using Current Contraceptive Method

In both organized and unorganized sections the common reasons for using current contraceptive methods were convenience in usage (50% in organized and 41% in unorganized section), fear of side-effects of other methods (36% in organized and 44% in unorganized section), lack of proper knowledge of other methods, easy availability and affordability of current method. While females who underwent tubectomy cited no want more children as the reason for opting it.

Reasons for Not Using Any Contraceptive Method

Table 3 shows that fear of side-effects (27.7%), desire to have more children (27.7%) and husband's disapproval (22%) were the common reasons cited by women in organized section for not using any of the contraceptive methods. Other reasons mentioned by women were: husband stays away, religious barriers and lack of proper knowledge of contraceptives.

Table 3 *Reasons for Not Using Any of the Family Planning Methods*

Reasons for not using any of the family planning methods	*Organized sector (n=36) Frequency (%)*	*Unorganized sector (n=26) Frequency (%)*
Desire to have more children	10 (27.8)	2 (7.7)
Lack of proper knowledge about family planning methods	4 (11.1)	8 (30.7)
Not allowed in religion	7 (19.4)	2 (7.7)
Fear of side-effects	10 (27.8)	5 (19.2)
Husband disapproves	8 (22.2)	3 (11.5)
Do not feel the need of using any FP method	7 (19.4)	12 (46.2)
Husband stays away	8 (22.2)	4 (15.4)
Breast feeding (menses did not resume)	1 (2.8)	1 (3.8)
Currently pregnant	2 (5.7)	3 (11.5)

Note: Total exceeds more than 100 due to multiple responses.

Table 4 *Cross Table Between Level of Knowledge of Family Planning and Current Usage of Contraceptive Methods*

Level of Knowledge of Family planning	*Currently using FP method (Yes) Frequency (%)*	*Currently using FP method (No) Frequency (%)*	*Total Frequency (%)*
Poor	1 (14.3)	6 (85.7)	7 (100)
Moderate	27 (40.3)	40 (59.7)	67 (100)
Good	32 (66.7)	16 (33.3)	48 (100)
Total	62 (100)	60 (100)	122 (100)

χ^2=11.397, Degree of freedom= 2, p (0.003) < 0.01

In unorganized section the common reasons for not using any contraceptive method among non-users (n=36) were: no need felt for contraceptives (46.2%), lack of proper knowledge of family planning methods (30.7%), fear of side-effects (19.2%) and husband stays away. While other reasons mentioned by women included husband's disapproval, not allowed in religion and desire to have more children. Table 4 presents a highly significant positive association ($p < 0.01$, d.f=2) between knowledge of family planning methods and use of contraceptives through Chi-square test.

Discussion

Present study was conducted among women of 16–40 years of age in organized and unorganized section of B sector of Cheetah camp slum to assess their knowledge, attitude and practice of family planning methods. Results show that all the women from both organized and unorganized sections had heard of oral contraceptive pills, female sterilization; majority were aware of male condom and Cu-T in both sections. Knowledge of emergency pills and male sterilization was more among organized section respondents. Overall, both organized and unorganized sections have moderate to good knowledge score for family planning methods, with slightly better knowledge level of women of unorganized section than organized section. Common sources of knowledge for family planning (FP) methods were friends (83% or more) and media (69% or more) in both sections. The reason for better awareness of family planning methods among women might be higher exposure to media and social circle. Similar results were found by Srivastava et al. (2005) and Mustafa et al. (2008) in their study. Most of the female's attitude towards use of family planning method was satisfactory in both sections. While women of unorganized section showed more willingness to use FP methods than organized section.

Current contraceptive prevalence rate among women (55.2%) in unorganized section was higher as compared to organized sector (43.8%). According to National Family Health Survey (2005–2006), 56 per cent of ever married Indian women were using family planning. In organized sector use of OCP (35%), condoms (28.6%), Tubectomy (25%) and Copper-T (7%) were more prevalent while in unorganized sector Tubectomy (37.5%), condoms (28%), Copper-T (13%) and OCP (13%). The reason for lower prevalence of tubectomy in organized section may be comparatively higher proportion of younger women in organized section who wanted to conceive in future. Overall spacing methods were not much popular among women of the study population. User rate was significantly more in those having higher knowledge score regarding various family planning methods showing that the value of literacy is increasing the acceptance of contraceptive methods. This is in accordance with the study by Takkar et al. (2005).

In both the sectors main reasons for using current methods were convenience in its usage and fear of side-effects of other methods. The common reasons for not using any contraceptive method among non-users in organized sector were fear of side-effects (27.7%), desire to have more children (27.7%), husband's disapproval and religious barriers. In the unorganized sector common reasons for not using any contraceptives were: no want for contraceptives (46%), lack of proper knowledge about contraceptives (30%) and fear of side-effects (19%).

Conclusions and Recommendations

The study reveals high awareness and favourable attitude of slum women towards contraception. But contraceptive usage is low because of misinformation regarding contraceptive methods, fear of side-effects of contraceptive methods, husband's negative attitude and religious barriers. This highlights the need to impart correct knowledge regarding various contraceptive methods to clear off related misconceptions through media and health personnels. Involving husbands and motivating them is essential to achieve better outcomes of family planning efforts. So counselling and motivation of couples is needed to alleviate their fears and to increase usage of various contraceptive methods.

References

Census of India, 2011. http://www.censusindia. gov.in/2011-prov-results/data_files/india/final_ppt_2011_chapter3.pdf (accessed on 2 May 2012).

IIPS and Macro International, 2007. *National Family Health Survey (NFHS–3) 2005-6, India*. Mumbai: International Institute for Population Sciences.

Kumar, M., Meena, J., Sharma, S. et al., 2011. Contraceptive Use among Low-Income Urban Married Women in India. *Journal of Sex and Medicine*, 8 (2): 376–382.

Mahawar, P., Anand, S., Raghunath, D. and Dixit, S. 2011. Contraceptive Knowledge, Attitude and Practices in Mothers of Infants: A Cross-Sectional Study. *National Journal of Community Medicine*, 2 (1): 105–107.

Mustafa, R., Afreen, U. and Hashmi, H.A. 2008. Contraceptive Knowledge, Attitude and Practice among Rural Women. *Journal of the College of Physicians and Surgeons Pakistan*, 18 (9): 542–545.

Patel, M.G. et al., 2011. A Cross-Sectional Study on Knowledge, Attitude and Practice Regarding Spacing Methods among Married Women of the Reproductive Age Group in the Field Practice Area of UHTC in Surendranagar District. *Healthline*, 2 (2): 31–34.

Reddy, P.J. 1984. Differential Contraceptive Use among the Slum and Non-Slum Dwellers: A Study of Hyderabad City. *Health and Population: Perspectives and Issues*, 7 (2): 115–128.

Srivastava, R. et al., 2005. Contraceptive Knowledge, Attitude and Practice: KAP Study. *Journal of Obstetrics and Gynaecology of India*, 55: 546–550.

Takkar, N., Goel, P., Saha, P.K. and Dua, D. 2005. Contraceptive Practices and Awareness of Emergency Contraception in Educated Working Women. *Indian Journal of Medical Sciences*, 59 (4): 143–149.

4

Contraceptive Prevalence in South Asia

Trends, Determinants and Implications for Policy and Programmes

Manas Ranjan Pradhan

Population stabilization has been recognized as an issue requiring urgent attention, and has thus led to formulation of national population policies and programmes in South Asian countries of India, Pakistan, Bangladesh and Nepal (GoP, 2010; GoB, 2009; GoI, 2000; GoN, 1997). The limited success of the Family Welfare/Planning Programmes, however, may be due its direction, emphasis and strategies in India (Santhya, 2003), erosion in political will and certain systemic issues in Bangladesh (Barkat-e-Khuda and Barkat, 2010), neglect of family planning programmes due to historical political conflict and cultural restrictions on women in Pakistan (Hardee and Leahy, 2008), and socio-cultural and service delivery challenges in Nepal (Anand et al., 2010). Stalling in the upward course of contraceptive use questions the effectiveness of programme-related investments and implies failure to reduce unmet needs. By reducing the Total Fertility Rate (TFR), contraception significantly influences population stabilization, which is important for socio-economic development of the aforesaid countries; comprising 23 per cent of world's population (United Nations, 2011). The present study assesses the trends and determinants of contraceptive prevalence rate (CPR), and its implications for policy as well as programmes in India, Pakistan, Bangladesh and Nepal.

Data and Methods

The study used data from three rounds of Demographic and Health Survey (DHS) in each of the aforementioned countries. Specifically, the National Family Health Survey (NFHS) round 1 (1992–92), round 2 (1998–99) and round 3 (2005–06) of India; Pakistan Demographic and Health Survey (PDHS) in (2006–07), Status of Women, Reproductive Health and Family Planning Survey (SWRHFFPS) in (2001–03), and Pakistan Fertility and Family

Planning Survey (PFFPS) in (1996–97); Bangladesh Demographic Health Survey (BDHS) in 2007, BDHS (1999–2000), and BDHS (1993–94); and Nepal Demographic Health Survey (NDHS) 2011, NDHS (2006), and NDHS (2001) were used. The currently married women aged 15–49 years of the latest DHS were considered for detailed analysis; and the sample sizes were 93,089 for India, 10,192 for Bangladesh, 9,556 for Pakistan and 9,608 for Nepal. These surveys were approved by the Institutional Review Board of the institutions/organizations involved. The details of the DHSs are available elsewhere (MEASURE DHS, 2012).

Informed consent procedures were followed and only those respondents who voluntarily consented to participate in the surveys were included. Data was analysed through IBM-SPSS software (Version 20.0). Unmet need for contraception, if satisfied/met, has a significant impact on fertility. The same had been investigated using Bongaarts (1990) regression model (TFR= 7.178–0.0682 CPR + e). Logistic regressions were carried out to identify the factors associated with acceptance of any contraceptive method, any modern spacing method (IUD, pills, and condoms) and female sterilization. The explanatory variables used in the analysis were women's age, years of education, occupation, number of living son, frequency of watching television, final say on health care, religion, caste, number of household members, household wealth index (based on household assets and living conditions), type of place of residence and exposure to family planning messages. The significance level was set at 5 per cent.

Results

Trends in Contraceptive Use

The current contraceptive prevalence rate (CPR) of Nepal is 50 per cent, and the annual growth was 1.7 points between NDHS–1(2001) and NDHS–2 (2006), which was reduced to 0.3 points between NDHS–2 (2006) to NDHS–3 (2011) (Table 1). Further, female sterilization acceptance had declined (–0.6 point per year), while male sterilization had increased (0.3 points annually) during the last five years. Between NFHS-1 (1992–93) to NFHS–3 (2005–06), the CPR in India increased by 1.2 point annually, and currently 56 per cent of the women are using any contraception. Female sterilization acceptance increased at 0.8 point per year during the same period and, at present, 37 per cent women are sterilized. However, modern spacing method use increased at merely 0.4 point per year.

With an annual increase of 0.9 point between BDHS-1 (1993–94) to BDHS–3 (2007), the current CPR of Bangladesh is 56 per cent. The CPR increased at 0.3 point annually between BDHS–2 (1999–2000) to BDHS–3 (2007) as against 1.5 point between BDHS-1 (1993–94) to BDHS–2 (1999–2000). Female sterilization declined at 0.2 point between BDHS–1 (1993–94) to BDHS–3 (2007), while use of oral pills increased at 0.9 points annually. Contraceptive use in Pakistan increased at 0.6 point annually between PFFPS (1996–97) to PDHS (2006–07). The CPR increased steadily from 24 per cent in PFFPS (1996–97) to 32 per cent in SWRHFFPS (2001–03) at 1.3 points per year and declined thereafter to 30 per cent in PDHS (2006–07) at 0.6

Table 1 *Level and Trends of Contraceptive Prevalence Rate Among Currently Married Women Aged 15–49 Years in Selected South Asian Countries*

Country	*Indicators*	*Round–3*			*Round–2*				*Round–1*				*Annual growth*		
		2011	*2007*	*2006*	*2006*	*2003*	*2000*	*1999*	*2001*	*1997*	*1994*	*1993*	*R 3–R 2*	*R 2–R 1*	*R 3–R 1*
India	CPR			56.3				48.2				40.7	1.2	1.3	1.2
(last 13 years)	CPR_Urban			64				58.2				51.1	0.8	1.2	1.0
	CPR_Rural			53				44.7				37.1	1.2	1.3	1.2
	Any Modern Method			48.5				42.8				36.5	0.8	1.1	0.9
	Any Modern Spacing Method			10.1				6.8				5.5	0.5	0.2	0.4
	Female Sterilization			37.3				34.2				27.4	0.4	1.1	0.8
Bangladesh	CPR		55.8				53.8				44.6		0.3	1.5	0.9
(last 13 years)	CPR_Urban		62.0				60.0				54.0		0.3	1	0.6
	CPR_Rural		54.0				52.0				43.0		0.3	1.5	0.8
	Any Modern Method		47.5				43.4				36.2		0.6	1.2	0.9
	Any Modern Spacing Method		41.8				35.2				27.0		0.9	1.4	1.1
	Female Sterilization		5.0				6.7				8.1		–0.2	–0.2	–0.2
Nepal	CPR	49.7			48.0				39.3				0.3	1.7	1.0
(last 10 years)	CPR_Urban	59.6			60.0				62.2				–0.1	–0.4	–0.3
	CPR_Rural	48.2			45.9				36.9				0.5	1.8	1.1
	Any Modern Method	43.2			44.2				35.4				–0.2	1.8	0.8
	Any Modern Spacing Method	20.2			19.9				13.9				0.1	1.2	0.6
	Female Sterilization	15.2			18.0				15.0				–0.6	0.6	0.0
Pakistan	CPR		29.6			32.0				24.0			–0.6	1.3	0.6
(last 10 years)	CPR_Urban		41.1			NA				NA			NA	NA	NA
	CPR_Rural		23.9			NA				NA			NA	NA	NA
	Any Modern Method		21.7			24.0				16.0			–0.6	1.3	0.6
	Any Modern Spacing Method		13.4			16.0				10.0			–0.7	1.0	0.3
	Female Sterilization		8.2			8.0				6.0			0.0	0.3	0.2

point per year. Additionally, modern spacing method use declined at 0.7 point during 2003–07. Female sterilization continued to dominate the modern contraceptive methods used in India (77%), Pakistan (38%) and Nepal (35%). Majority (60%) of the modern contraceptive users in Bangladesh were using pills. Across the countries, the pace of CPR was faster in rural areas as against urban areas.

Determinants of Contraceptive Use

Table 2a and 2b presents the Odds Ratios (ORs) of logistic regression analysis on acceptance of any contraceptive method, any modern spacing method and female sterilization. Socio-demographic characteristics of women, exposure to family planning messages, household economic condition and place of residence were strong predictors of contraceptive use. As indicated by the adjusted ORs, compared with women aged 15–24 years, the women aged 30–49 years were more likely to use any contraception or female sterilization. The probability of using any contraception was high among literate women than those who were non-literates. However, the likelihood of female sterilization was less among women with 10 or more years of schooling, as against non-literates.

Working women were significantly more likely to accept any contraception than their non-working peers in India, Nepal and Bangladesh. However, Indian working women were less likely to use any modern spacing method [OR=0.89(0.85–0.93)] contrary to their counterparts in Nepal [OR=1.21(1.06–1.39)] and Bangladesh [OR=1.44(1.31–1.58)]. Nepali women with a surviving son were 7 times more likely to adopt female sterilization than those without a surviving son. The corresponding figure was 10 times, 5 times and 2 times respectively for women in Pakistan (statistically insignificant), India and Bangladesh. Across countries, women exposed to any family planning messages were more likely to use any contraception and modern spacing method. Exposure to family planning messages increases the chances of sterilization acceptance in Pakistan [OR=1.32(1.11–1.57)] contrary to India [OR=0.92(0.88–0.96)] and Nepal [OR=0.71(0.62–0.82)]. The likelihood of using any contraception was high among women reporting everyday television watching compared to 'women without television watching' in Nepal, India and Bangladesh. Higher health care autonomy enhances the likelihood of contraceptive use in India [OR=1.06(1.01–1.10)], but not in Nepal [OR=.59(.52–.68)] and Bangladesh [OR=.52(.45–.59)].

Indian Muslims compared to Hindus were more likely to use any modern spacing method [OR=1.38(1.29–1.47)] but less likely to use female sterilization [OR=0.44(0.42–0.47)]. Female sterilization was again less likely among non-Hindus than Hindus in Nepal [OR=0.39(0.31–0.50)], and more likely among non-Muslims compared to Muslims in Bangladesh [OR=1.91(1.48–2.48)]. General caste women in India were more likely to use any modern spacing method [OR=1.20(1.12–1.28)] and less likely to accept sterilization [OR=0.80(0.76–0.84)] compared to scheduled caste women. The probability of using any contraception and modern spacing methods was high

Table 2a *Adjusted Odds Ratios (With 95% Confidence Intervals) for Multivariate Logistic Regression Analysis of Contraceptive Use Among Currently Married Women Aged 15-49 Years in Selected South Asian Countries*

Background characteristics	*India (2005–06)*			*Bangladesh (2007)*		
	Any method	*Any modern spacing method*	*Female sterilization*	*Any method*	*Any modern spacing method*	*Female sterilization*
Current age of women						
15-24 years®	1.00	1.00	1.00	1.00	1.00	1.00
25-29 years	2.31[2.20-2.42][a]	1.14[1.07-1.21][a]	3.33[3.12-3.56][a]	1.37[1.21-1.56][a]	1.18[1.04-1.33][a]	8.06[4.20-15.45][a]
30-49 years	3.44 [3.30-3.59][a]	.56[.53-.60][a]	6.62[6.24-7.02][a]	1.24[1.11-1.38][a]	.65[.58-.72][a]	19.00[10.28-35.11][a]
Current education of women						
Non-literate®	1.00	1.00	1.00	1.00	1.00	1.00
< 10 years of schooling	1.28[1.23-1.33][a]	1.43[1.34-1.52][a]	1.15[1.01-1.09][a]	1.26[1.14-1.39][a]	1.40[1.26-1.55][a]	.50[.43-.62][a]
10 and above years of schooling	1.11[1.05-1.17][a]	2.57[2.39-2.76][a]	.45[.42-.47][a]	1.58[1.36-1.84][a]	1.61[1.39-1.86][a]	.32[.22-.48][a]
Current occupation of women						
Not-working/household work®	1.00	1.00	1.00	1.00	1.00	1.00
Work outside the household	1.32[1.27-1.36][a]	.89[.85-.93][a]	1.43[1.38-1.48][a]	1.57[1.43-1.73][a]	1.44[1.31-1.58][a]	1.11[.91-1.35]
Number of living son						
No living son®	1.00	1.00	1.00	1.00	1.00	1.00
At least one living son	4.34[4.17-4.51][a]	1.69[1.60-1.78][a]	5.42[5.14-5.72][a]	2.49[2.25-2.75][a]	2.19[1.97-2.43][a]	2.09[1.50-2.92][a]
Frequency of watching television						
Not at all®	1.00	1.00	1.00	1.00	1.00	1.00
Less than once/at least once a week	1.23[1.17-1.29][a]	1.11[1.02-1.20][a]	1.22[1.16-1.28][a]	1.28[1.14-1.44][a]	1.10[.98-1.23]	1.79[1.39-2.31][a]
Almost every day	1.58[1.51-1.67][a]	1.09[1.01-1.18][a]	1.79[1.69-1.89][a]	1.43[1.25-1.64][a]	1.37[1.17-1.54][a]	1.71[1.24-2.37][a]
Final say on health care						
Husband/partner/someone else®	1.00	1.00	1.00	1.00	1.00	1.00
Respondent alone	1.06[1.01-1.10][a]	1.13[1.07-1.20][a]	.99[.95-1.03]	.52[.45-.59][a]	.56[.49-.65][a]	.98[.74-1.29]
Respondent and husband/partner	1.02[.98-1.06]	1.17[1.11-1.23][a]	.87[.83-.90][a]	1.09[1.00-1.09][a]	1.08[.99-1.19]	.97[.79-1.20]

Cont'd...

...*Cont'd*

Religion						
Hindu®	1.00	1.00	1.00	—	—	—
Muslim$	.55[.52-.58][a]	1.38[1.29-1.47][a]	.44[.42-.47][a]	1.00	1.00	1.00
Others	.58[.55-.62][a]	1.22[1.13-1.30][a]	.56[.52-.59][a]	1.23[1.07-1.41][a]	1.00[.875-1.15]	1.91[1.48-2.48][a]
Caste						
Scheduled caste (SC)	1.00	1.00	1.00			
Scheduled tribe (ST)	.67[.63-.71][a]	.97[.88-1.07]	.68[.63-.72][a]	NA	NA	NA
Other backward class (OBC)	.89[.85-.93][a]	.80[.75-.86][a]	1.07[1.02-1.13][a]	NA	NA	NA
General caste	1.01[.97-1.07]	1.20[1.12-1.28]a	.80[.76-.84][a]	NA	NA	NA
Number of household members						
< 5 members®	1.00	1.00	1.00	1.00	1.00	1.00
>=5 members	1.09[1.05-1.13][a]	1.09[1.04-1.14][a]	1.01[.98-1.05]	1.04[.95-1.14]	1.13[1.03-1.23][a]	.71[.58-.87][a]
Wealth index						
Poorest®	1.00	1.00	1.00	1.00	1.00	1.00
Poorer	1.27[1.20-1.35][a]	1.31[1.16-1.49][a]	1.31[1.23-1.40][a]	1.02[.88-1.17]	1.07[.93-1.24]	.87[.64-1.19]
Middle	1.45[1.37-1.54][a]	1.49[1.32-1.67][a]	1.50[1.40-1.59][a]	.93[.81-1.07]	.99[.86-1.15]	.75[.55-1.04]
Richer	1.65[1.54-1.76][a]	1.78[1.58-2.01][a]	1.59[1.49-1.71][a]	.80[.69-.93][a]	.88[.75-1.02]	.79[.56-1.10]
Richest	1.72[1.60-1.85][a]	2.48[2.19-2.82][a]	1.30[1.21-1.41][a]	.80[.67-.95][a]	.86[.72-1.02]	.72[.49-1.07]
Type of place of residence						
Urban®	1.00	1.00	1.00	1.00	1.00	1.00
Rural	.93[.89-.96][a]	.84[.80-.89][a]	1.00[.96-1.04]	.73[.66-.81][a]	.77[.70-.85][a]	.90[.72-1.13]
Exposed to family planning messages						
No®	1.00	1.00	1.00	1.00	1.00	1.00
Yes	1.24[1.19-1.29][a]	1.51[1.42-1.61][a]	.92[.88-.96][a]	1.25[1.12-1.38][a]	1.18[1.07-1.31][a]	1.01[.79-1.28]

[a] P <0.05, Confidence intervals are given in square brackets, NA indicates data not available and not included in the model, ® Reference category, $ Reference category for Bangladesh.

Table 2b *Adjusted odds ratios (with 95% Confidence Intervals) for Multivariate Logistic Regression Analysis of Contraceptive Use Among Currently Married Women Aged 15–49 Years in Selected South Asian Countries*

Background characteristics	*Nepal (2011)*			*Pakistan (2006-07)*		
	Any method	*Any modern spacing method*	*Female sterilization*	*Any method*	*Any modern spacing method*	*Female sterilization*
Current age of women						
15-24 years®	1.00	1.00	1.00	1.00	1.00	1.00
25-29 years	1.74[1.51-2.00][a]	1.24[1.06-1.45][a]	3.67[2.53-5.33][a]	1.50[1.25-1.80][a]	1.38[1.12-1.71][a]	3.32[1.60-6.89][a]
30-49 years	2.98[2.61-3.39][a]	.95[.82-.1.10]	6.43[4.53-9.11][a]	2.44[2.08-2.87][a]	1.18[.97-1.43]	17.57[9.03-34.15][a]
Current education of women						
Non-literate®	1.00	1.00	1.00	1.00	1.00	1.00
< 10 years of schooling	1.00[.89-1.12]	1.31[1.15-1.48][a]	.50[.42-.58][a]	1.51[1.32-1.72][a]	1.51[1.29-1.78][a]	1.07[.87-1.13]
10 and above years of schooling	1.12[.95-1.32]	1.62[1.36-1.94][a]	.21[.15-.28][a]	1.40[1.18-1.65][a]	1.70[1.40-2.07][a]	.54[.40-.73]a
Current occupation of women						
Not-working/household work®	1.00	1.00	1.00	1.00	1.00	1.00
Work outside the household	1.35[1.20-1.53][a]	1.21[1.06-1.39][a]	.77[.65-.92]	1.10[.98-1.23]	1.05[.91-1.22]	1.14[.95-1.36]
Number of living son						
No living son®	1.00	1.00	1.00	1.00	1.00	1.00
At least one living son	3.03[2.69-3.42][a]	1.84[1.60-2.11][a]	6.99[4.79-10.19] a	4.87[4.10-5.77][a]	3.80[3.06-4.71][a]	10.93[5.79-20.65]
Frequency of watching television						
Not at all®	1.00	1.00	1.00			
Less than once/at least once a week	1.24[1.10-1.40][a]	1.06[.92-1.22]	1.20[.99-1.44]	NA	NA	NA
Almost every day	—	—	—	NA	NA	NA
Final say on health care						
Husband/partner/someone else ®	1.00	1.00	1.00			
Respondent alone	.59[.52-.68][a]	.75[.64-.88][a]	.86[.70-1.07]	NA	NA	NA

Cont'd...

…Cont'd

Respondent and husband/partner	1.41[1.25-1.59][a]	1.34[1.18-1.52][a]	.82[.68-.98][a]	NA	NA	NA
Religion						
Hindu®	1.00	1.00	1.00			
Muslim$	—	—	—	NA	NA	NA
Others	0.75[0.66-0.86][a]	1.43[1.24-1.65][a]	.39[.31-.50][a]	NA	NA	NA
Caste						
Scheduled caste (SC)						
Scheduled tribe (ST)	NA	NA	NA	NA	NA	NA
Other backward class (OBC)	NA	NA	NA	NA	NA	NA
General caste	NA	NA	NA	NA	NA	NA
Number of household members						
< 5 members®	1.00	1.00	1.00	1.00	1.00	1.00
>=5 members	1.28[1.16-1.41]	1.44[1.29-1.61][a]	1.07[.93-1.23]	1.66[1.38-2.00][a]	1.56[1.23-1.98][a]	1.31[.94-1.82]
Wealth index						
Poorest®	1.00	1.00	1.00	1.00	1.00	1.00
Poorer	1.38[1.19-1.60][a]	0.98[.82-1.16]	2.49[1.93-3.20][a]	1.39[1.16-1.68][a]	1.94[1.47-2.54][a]	.84[.63-1.11]
Middle	1.74[1.49-2.03][a]	0.98[.82-1.17]	3.67[2.85-4.74][a]	1.93[1.60-2.32][a]	2.36[1.80-3.10][a]	1.12[.85-1.47]
Richer	1.69[1.43-2.00][a]	0.86[.71-1.04]	4.04[3.08-5.29][a]	2.44[2.01-2.96][a]	2.70[2.04-3.57][a]	1.27[.95-1.70]
Richest	2.20[1.82-2.66][a]	1.05[.85-1.29]	4.46[3.30-6.02][a]	2.96[2.38-3.68][a]	3.24[2.39-4.39][a]	1.46[1.05-2.03][a]
Type of place of residence						
Urban®	1.00	1.00	1.00	1.00	1.00	1.00
Rural	.84[.75-.95][a]	.72[.63-.82][a]	1.02[.87-1.21]	.76[.67-.85][a]	.82[.71-.94][a]	.80[.66-.96][a]
Exposed to family planning messages						
No®	1.00	1.00	1.00	1.00	1.00	1.00
Yes	1.24[1.12-1.37][a]	1.34[1.19-1.51][a]	.71[.62-.82][a]	1.43[1.28-1.59][a]	1.27[1.11-1.46][a]	1.32[1.11-1.57][a]

[a] $P < 0.05$, Confidence intervals are given in square brackets, NA indicates data not available and not included in the model, ® Reference category, $ Reference category for Bangladesh.

among women from households comprising five or more members compared to women from households comprising less than five members. Better household wealth index signified higher likelihood of using any contraception, modern spacing method, and female sterilization in India, Pakistan and Nepal. Rural women in all four countries were less likely to use any contraception compared to urban women.

Need for Contraception

Figure 1 reveals that Nepal had higher demand for contraception (77%) followed by Bangladesh (73%), India (69%) and Pakistan (55%). India (82%) followed by Bangladesh (77%) lead the group in addressing the demand. Only 54 per cent of the total demand for contraception was satisfied in Pakistan and 25 per cent women had an unmet need for contraception. Again, 27 per cent women in Nepal, 17 per cent in Bangladesh and 13 per cent in India had unmet need.

Figure 1 *Total Demand for Contraception, Met and Unmet Need, in Selected South Asian Countries*

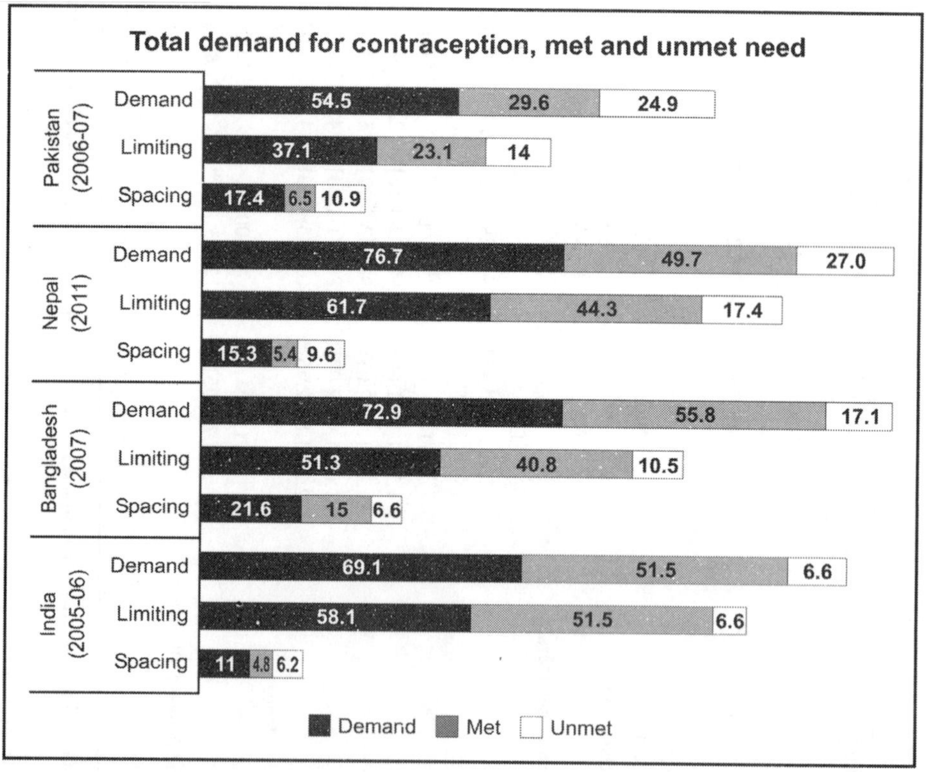

Demographic Impact of Unmet Need

Table 3 reveals that a significant demographic impact would follow for a majority of the countries studied if all women who wished to limit or postpone births became contraceptive users. For example, the TFR of Nepal, Bangladesh and Pakistan would be greatly reduced, from 2.6 to 1.9 births (25%), 2.7 to 2.2 births (18%) and 4.1 to 3.5 births (16%) respectively, if the unmet need for contraception was met. Only in the case of India would the corresponding decline be marginal: from 2.7 to 2.5 births (9%).

Table 3 *TFR If Total Demand for Contraception Satisfied*

Country	*Current TFR*	*Current CPR*	*Unmet Need*	*Total demand for contraception*	*Estimated TFR if total demand for contraception satisfied*	*% reduction in TFR if total demand for contraception satisfied*
India	2.7	56.3	12.8	69.1	2.5	8.7
Bangladesh	2.7	55.8	17.1	72.9	2.2	18.3
Nepal	2.6	49.7	27.0	76.7	1.9	25.1
Pakistan	4.1	29.6	24.9	54.5	3.5	15.6

Reasons for Not Intending to Use a Contraceptive Method in the Future

Many of those women not intending to use family planning in future (80% in Nepal, 74% in Bangladesh, 66% in India and 58% in Pakistan) cited fertility related reasons (Figure 2). About 23 per cent of Pakistani women revealed opposition to use contraception as the major reason. The corresponding figure was 15 per cent, 12 per cent and 5 per cent respectively in India, Bangladesh and Nepal. Additionally, 12 per cent women each in India and Pakistan, 10 per cent in Nepal, and 8 per cent in Bangladesh had cited method related reasons (health concerns, side effects, higher cost, inconvenient to use and perceived interference with body's normal processes) for negative future intention.

Figure 2 *Per cent Distribution of Currently Married Women Age 15–49 who are not Using Contraception and who do not Intend to use in the Future, by Main Reason for not Intending to Use in Selected South Asian Countries*

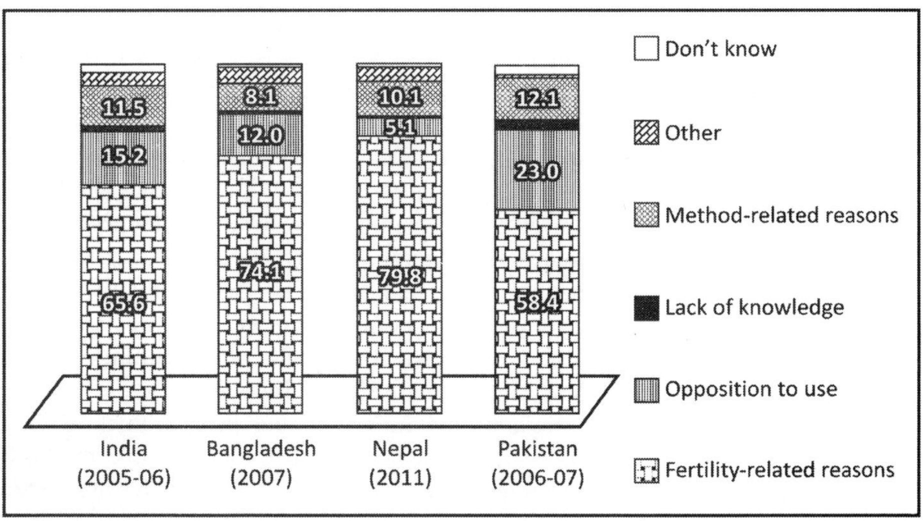

Discussion and Conclusion

The study found that the countries under study differ in CPR, trends, method mix and the determinants. Bangladesh and Nepal were in a stage of contraceptive plateau while the CPR in Pakistan was declining. Modern spacing method use in India was in a plateau as well. Various policy and programme issues along with socio-cultural norms had influenced the trends and method mix. These countries would become closer to replacement level fertility of 2.1 births per woman, if women with unmet need for contraception became contraceptive users. The plateau in contraceptive use questions the efficacy of family planning programme related investments. Moreover, in the given situation, it would be difficult for these countries to achieve their national population policy goals of replacement level fertility, and Millennium Development Goal (MDG) 5 of improving maternal health by 2015.

The CPR in India had increased during NFHS-1 (1992–93) to NFHS–3 (2005–06), however assuming 0.5 point average annual increase per year (Ross et al., 2004), there was a contraceptive plateau in modern spacing method use. This might be due to the continuing unofficial focus on female sterilization (Pradhan and Ram, 2009) inadequate accesses to these methods, poor counselling and follow-up services, method-related complications, couples preference to have the desired number of children in quick succession and opt for sterilization (JSK, 2012) and perceived side effects (Patel et al., 2011). The CPR in Nepal increased considerably during the NDHS–1 (2001) to NDHS–2 (2006); mainly because of higher use of female sterilization, pills, condoms and injectables (MOHP Nepal et al., 2007).

In Bangladesh, overall CPR had increased between BDHS-1 (1993–94) to BDHS–3 (2007). Nevertheless, data indicated an emerging contraceptive plateau between last two rounds of surveys; BDHS–2 (1999–2000) to BDHS–3 (2007). Shortage of injectables during 2006–07 and decline in use of traditional methods could be the probable reasons (NIPORT et al., 2009). Gradual changes in method mix during 1994–2007 might be another factor. For example, Sterilization, IUD, and Norplant accounted for 13 per cent of total contraceptive use in 2007 as against 26 per cent in 1994 (NIPORT et al. 2009). On the other hand; Pakistan had experienced a steady increase in CPR between PFFPS (1996–97) to SWRHFFPS (2001–03) and quick decline between SWRHFFPS (2001–03) to PDHS (2006–07). The increase was primarily due to the success of Lady Health Worker Programme (Sultan et al., 2002; Douthwaite and Ward, 2005) while the decline was attributed to the non-devolution of the programme from central control leading to lack of ownership at provincial and district levels, lack of support from the health sector especially its Lady Health Worker Program, and a disconnect between the community and facilities providing services caused by abolishing the Village Based Family Planning Worker component (NIPS Pakistan and Macro International Inc., 2008).

With the exception of Bangladesh, family planning programmes in other three countries had largely failed to encourage the use of reversible methods. Though provision of quality spacing methods had taken its place in government policies, promoting spacing methods had not been successful in the prevailing context of excessive preference for female sterilization. With a younger age pattern of fertility, sterilization usually after achieving desired family size in short interval, is not very beneficial for population stabilization. Similar concerns were found by Matthews et al. (2009). Female sterilization at an early age may further lead to low condom use, which is crucial for prevention of Reproductive Tract Infections (RTI)/Sexually Transmitted Infections (STIs) and Human Immunodeficiency Virus/Acquired Immunodeficiency Syndrome (HIV/AIDS), particularly among the young women who are more vulnerable in traditional settings, like in South Asia. It is rather difficult to motivate a sterilized couple to use condoms, which can prevent them from acquiring HIV/AIDS, as most couples view family planning primarily as a means for spacing/regulating fertility and not as an aid for protection against diseases/infections (Dhopeshwarkar, 2007; Deering et al., 2011).

The plateau or decline in male sterilization might be attributed to post-emergency resistances to vasectomy besides greater promotion of tubectomy in India (Basu, 1985); misconceptions, lack of information and lower priority accorded to the method in Nepal (MOHP Nepal et al., 2007); unwillingness to use before having desired family size, lack of institutional and logistic facilities, and inadequate motivational activities in Bangladesh (Jahid, 2003); and social norms, misconceptions, along with policy and programme issues in Pakistan (Agha, 2010).

Higher age, better education, exposure to family planning messages, regular television watching, better economic condition and urban residence found to enhance the contraceptive acceptance. This finding was in line with that from several previous studies (Satyavada and Adamchak, 2000; Kamal and Islam, 2010; Manna and Basu, 2011; Carton and Agha, 2012). As evident from past studies (Pradhan and Ram, 2009; Kamal and Islam, 2010; Manna and Basu, 2011), religious affiliations influenced the method choice; Muslim women were less likely to use sterilization. Caste continued to influence the contraceptive use and method mix in India; general caste women preferred spacing methods compared to their scheduled caste peers who accepted sterilization, probably because of higher literacy (Narzary, 2009) and better access to contraceptive methods (Mishra et al., 1999).

There was no uniformity in the magnitude and direction of association between women's occupation and modern spacing method use. Compared to their peers in other three countries, working women in India were less likely to use any modern spacing method than non-working women. A detailed investigation found that a majority of these working women had less than five years of schooling (70%); no exposure to any family planning message (53%); had at least one surviving son (78%), with poor health care autonomy (71%); and were aged above 30 years (61%). The result further confirmed past studies (Maleque, 1999; Saleem and Bobak, 2005; Kamal and Islam, 2010) showing son preference and poor health care autonomy of women as barriers to modern spacing method use. Importantly, these socio-cultural practices and poor health care autonomy often puts women at the risk of maternal morbidity and/or mortality due to repeated pregnancies/childbirths.

High unmet need questions the quality of family planning services in these countries. A similar concern was raised by (Chaudhury, 2001). Unmet need enhances women's vulnerability to unintended pregnancies, especially where they have limited control over their sexual and reproductive health. As apparent from a previous study (Hussain, 2003), inequalities in power often owing to the cultural beliefs about women's sexual roles and behaviours further acts as a barrier for women's ability to negotiate safe sex practices with their partners. Unmet need implied the need for enhanced communications on one hand and efficient service delivery on the other. Addressing unmet need and barriers to contraceptive use would undoubtedly facilitate early population stabilization and subsequent socio-economic development through better planning, resource allocation and programme management.

Results suggest broadening of method choices with quality service delivery, reconsideration/review of programme focus along with strengthening private sector, expansion of supply lines with increased infrastructure and strengthening existing network, repositioning spacing methods in national programmes, and demand assessment through monitoring age-sex distribution; all with country specific modifications are pertinent for enhanced contraceptive use. The strengths of the study are that it provides the trends and determinants of CPR, which are of extreme importance for ongoing and prospective family planning programmes and policies. Additionally, would be of use for understanding these countries' progress towards achieving national population policy goals and MDG 5. The limitation is that besides the variables included in the present analysis a number of other programmatic as well as non-programmatic variables might affect the contraceptive use and method mix. Further research with additional support from qualitative data might be required to understand the issue in a better way.

References

Agha, S. 2010. Intentions to Use Contraceptives in Pakistan: Implications for Behaviour Change Campaigns. *BMC Public Health*, 10: 450.

Anand, T., Subedi, G. et al., 2010. *The Status of Family Planning and Reproductive Health in Nepal*. Bangkok, Thailand: UNFPA and ICOMP Regional Consultation.

Barkat-e-Khuda and Barkat, S. 2010. *The Bangladesh Family Planning Programme: Achievements, Gaps and the Way Forward*. Bangkok, Thailand: UNFPA and ICOMP Regional Consultation.

Basu, A. 1985. Family Planning and Emergency: An Unanticipated Consequence. *Economic and Political Weekly*, 20 (10): 422–425.

Bongaarts, J. 1990. The Measurement of Wanted Fertility. *Population and Development Review*, 16 (3): 487–506.

Carton, T.W. and Agha, S. 2012. Changes in Contraceptive Use and Method Mix in Pakistan: 1990–91 to 2006–07. *Health Policy and Planning*, 27 (2): 166–174.

Chaudhury, H. 2001. Unmet Need for Contraception in South Asia: Levels, Trends and Determinants. *Asia-Pacific Population Journal*, 6 (3): 3–22.

Deering, K.N., Bhattacharjee, P. et al., 2011. Condom Use within Non-Commercial Partnerships of Female Sex Workers in Southern India. *BMC Public Health*, 11 (6): S11.

Dhopeshwarkar, R. 2007. *Factors Associated with Consistent Condom Use by Female Sex Workers with Their Non-Client Partners in Andhra Pradesh, India*. New Haven, CT: Yale School of Public Health and The Centre for Interdisciplinary Research on AIDS.

Douthwaite, M. and Ward, P. 2005. Increasing Contraceptive Use in Rural Pakistan: An Evaluation of the Lady Health Worker Programme. *Health Policy and Planning*, 20 (2): 117–123.

Government of India (GoI). 2000. *National Population Policy 2000*. National Commission on Population, Government of India.

Government of Nepal (GoN). 1997. *Second Long Term Health Plan, 1997–2017*. Ministry of Health and Promotion, Government of Nepal.

Government of Pakistan (GoP). 2010. *Draft National Population Policy 2010*. Ministry of Population Welfare, Government of Pakistan.

Government of the People's Republic of Bangladesh (GoB). 2009. *Bangladesh Population Policy*. Dhaka: Ministry of Health and Family Welfare, Government of the People's Republic of Bangladesh.

Hardee, K. and Leahy, E. 2008. *Population, Fertility and Family Planning in Pakistan: A Program in Stagnation*. Research Commentary 3, Washington, D.C.: Population Action International.

Hussain, S. 2003. Gender and Reproductive Behaviour: The Role of Men. *Indian Journal of Gender Studies*, 10 (1): 45–76.

International Institute for Population Sciences (IIPS) and Macro International. 2007. *National Family Health Survey (NFHS–3), 2005–06: India*. Mumbai: International Institute for Population Sciences (IIPS) and Macro International.

Jahid, H.K. 2003. *Male Involvement in Family Planning in Bangladesh: Factors Constraining Low Use and the Potential for Augmenting the CPR*. Centre for Policy Dialogue, Dhaka: UNFPA.

Janasankhya Sthirata Kosh (JSK). 2012. Population Concepts Simplified: Contraception and Population. Available from http://www.jsk.gov.in/contraception_and_population.asp (accessed on 18 May 2012).

Kamal, S.M. and Islam, M.A. 2010. Contraceptive Use: Socioeconomic Correlates and Method Choices in Rural Bangladesh. *Asia Pacific Journal of Public Health*, 22 (4): 436–450.

Maleque, M.A. 1999. The Trends of Contraceptives Use and Their Differentials in Bangladesh. *Health and Population: Perspectives and Issues*, 22 (3–4): 168–175.

Manna, N. and Basu, G. 2011. Contraceptive Methods in a Rural Area of West Bengal, India. *Sudanese Journal of Public Health*, 6 (4): 164–169.

Matthews, Z., Padmadas, S. et al., 2009. Does Early Childbearing and a Sterilization-Focused Family Planning Programme in India Fuel Population Growth? *Demographic Research*, 20 (28): 693–720.

MEASURE DHS. 2012. Available from http://www.measuredhs.com/what-we-do/survey-types/dhs.cfm (accessed on 18 May 2012).

Ministry of Health and Population (MOHP) Nepal, New ERA and Macro International. 2007. *Nepal Demographic and Health Survey 2006*. Kathmandu, Nepal: Ministry of Health and Population (MOHP) Nepal, New ERA and Macro International Inc.

Mishra, V.K., Retherford, R.D. et al., 1999. *Reasons for Discontinuing and Not Intending to Use Contraception in India*. Mumbai, India: International Institute for Population Sciences and Honolulu, Hawaii, USA: East-West Center, Population and Health Studies.

Narzary, P.K. 2009. Knowledge and Use of Contraception among Currently Married Adolescent Women in India. *Studies on Home Community and Science*, 3 (1): 43–49.

National Institute of Population Research and Training (NIPORT), Mitra and Associates and Macro International. 2009. *Bangladesh Demographic and Health Survey 2007*. Dhaka, Bangladesh and Calverton, Maryland, USA: National Institute of Population Research and Training (NIPORT), Mitra and Associates and Macro International.

National Institute of Population Studies (NIPS) Pakistan and Macro International Inc. 2008. *Pakistan Demographic and Health Survey 2006–07*. Islamabad, Pakistan: National Institute of Population Studies (NIPS) Pakistan and Macro International Inc.

Patel, M.G., Mahyavanshi, D.K. et al., 2011. A Cross-Sectional Study on Knowledge, Attitude and Practice Regarding Spacing Methods among Married Women of the Reproductive Age Group in the Field Practice Area of UHTC in Surendranagar District. *Healthline*, 2 (2): 31–34.

Pradhan, M.R. and Ram, U. 2009. Female Sterilization and Ethical Issues: Indian Experience. *Social Change*, 39 (3): 365–387.

Ross, John et al., 2004. Plateaus During the Rise of Contraceptive Prevalence. *International Family Planning Perspectives*, 30 (1): 39–44.

Saleem, S. and Bobak, M. 2005. Women's Autonomy, Education and Contraception Use in Pakistan: A National Study. *Reproductive Health*, 2: 8.

Santhya, K.G. 2003. *Changing Family Planning Scenario in India: An Overview of Recent Evidences*. New Delhi: Population Council.

Satyavada, A. and Adamchak, D.J. 2000. Determinants of Current Use of Contraception and Children Ever Born in Nepal. *Social Biology*, 47 (1–2): 51–60.

Sultan, M., Cleland, J. et al., 2002. Assessment of a New Approach to Family Planning Services in Rural Pakistan. *American Journal of Public Health*, 92 (7): 1168–1172.

United Nations. 2011. *World Population Prospects: The 2010 Revision*. United Nations: Department of Economic and Social Affairs, Population Division.

5

Differential Unmet Need for Family Planning

A Study of Uttar Pradesh

M.S.R. Murthy

Unmet need for family planning arises out of spacing and limiting methods. Spacing methods in developing country like India has been less in demand. Currently married women who are not using any method of contraception but who do not want any more children or want to wait two or more years before having another child are defined as having an unmet need for family planning. A society exhibiting norms of gender bias may show higher unmet need levels (Tauseef, 1993).

According to the report of the first phase of NFHS, 19.5 per cent of currently married women in India had an unmet need for both spacing and limiting births. This per cent had come down during the next phase of the survey to 15.8 and again to 12.8 in the recent third phase of the survey.

Laya (2012) has found that 12.8 per cent of the currently married women in India at present have an unmet need for family planning services; 6.2 per cent for spacing and 6.6 per cent for limiting based on National Family Health survey (2005). The percentage of women having unmet need are much higher among those in the rural areas, at the younger ages and women having less than three children. Educational and working status of women is found to be highly significant with respect to their unmet need in India. Policies and programmes should be implemented to reach out to the rural illiterate poor married women so that they can avail the services easily and effectively without any barriers. Radha Devi, Rastogi and Retherford (1996) found the unmet need for spacing was around 55 per cent while limiting around 89 per cent in Uttar Pradesh. Over the years, family planning acceptance has increased; however, development seems to be a major indicator of acceptance of family planning. The present study makes an attempt to study unmet need in Uttar Pradesh at district level.

Methodology

District Level Health Survey 3 has been taken for analysis. Correspondence analysis (a form of factor analysis) of unmet need for spacing and limiting methods of family planning has been considered. This analysis gives a contingent table and contribution of rowwise (district) and columnwise (unmet need for spacing and limiting) to each other. In addition, the influence of wealth index and education to the unmet need has been planned. Bivariate logistic regression at the state level and at district level Chandauli have been computed.

Results and Discussion

One-tenth (10.07) of the state as a whole has an unmet need for spacing method of family planning. Two districts viz., Kanpur (3.11%) and Gautam Buddha Nagar (4.45%) have lowest unmet need for family planning.

Sultanpur, Bahraich, Sharwasti, Balarampur, Gonda and Siddarthanagar districts have largest need for spacing. There are two peaks of unmet need in the state: one group: Shahjahanpur, Kheri, Sitapur and Hardoi and the other: Sultanpur, Bahraich, Sharwasti, Balarampur, Gonda and Siddarthanagar. Kanpur Nagar (3.11) has the lowest demand for spacing methods in the state (Table 1 and 2).

Table 1 *Broad Category of Districts for Unmet Need for Spacing Methods of Family Planning*

Proportion Spacing	*Districts*
Below 5 (2)	Kanpur Nagar (3.11), Gautam Buddha Nagar (4.45).
5–10 (38 districts)	Jalaun (5.04), Jhansi (5.21), Lalitpur (5.86), Ghaziabad (6.19), Banda (6.3), Hathras (6.49), Meerut (6.71), Mahoba (6.73), Kanpur Dehat (6.83), Saharanpur (6.89), Hamirpur (6.96), Chandauli (7.06), (Baghpet (7.37), Deoria (7.45), Mainpuri (7.46), Unnao (7.76), Bulandshahar (7.94), Ambedkar Nagar (8.23), Muzaffarnagar (8.24), Rampur (8.39), Kushinagar (8.45), Auria (8.46), Sonbadra (8.47), Bijnor (8.55), Maharajganj (8.55), Pilibhit (8.58), Bareilly (8.67), Jyotiba Phule Nagar (8.76), Varanasi (8.96), Mathura (8.97), Lucknow (9.14), Barabanki (9.33), Kannauj (9.45), Mirzapur (9.46), Gorakhpur (9.6), Aligarh (9.65), Agra (9.92), Ballia (9.58).
10+ (30)	Moradabad (10.08), Basti (10.1), Allahabad (10.13), Mau (10.16), Farrukhabad (10.23), Firozabad (10.24), Sant Kabir Nagar (10.27), Etah (10.42), Chitrakoot (10.44), Pratapgarh (10.44), Jaunpur (10.67), Etawah (10.97), Kaushambi (11.07), Hardoi (11.17), Faizabad (11.4), Rae Bareilly (11.53), Gazipur (11.67), Sant Ravidas Nagar (11.88), Sultanpur (12.38), Siddarthanagar (12.53), Fatehpur (12.6), Budaun (13.1), Kheri (13.32), Shahjahanpur (14.04), Azamgarh (14.11), Gonda (15.6), Sitapur (16.73), Bahraich (17.03), Shrawasti (19.39), Balrampur (20.29).

Unmet Need for Spacing

The total inertia (eigen values) has been 0.012*100=1.2 per cent only. The correspondence analysis reflects that the correlation between region/districts and unmet need, while significant, was weak. Of the total inertia mainly Sitapur (0.001), Kanpur Nagar (0.001), Bahraich (0.001), Shrawasti (0.002), Balarampur (0.002) have contributed to unmet need for spacing totalling 0.012.

Table 2 *Summary for Spacing Methods*

		Score in Dimension		*Contribution*		
Unmet Need of Spacing Method (as DLHS–2)				*Of Point to Inertia of Dimension*	*Of Dimension to Inertia of Point*	
	Mass	*1*	*Inertia*	*1*	*1*	*Total*
Yes	.101	.983	.011	.899	1.000	1.000
No	.899	–.110	.001	.101	1.000	1.000
Active Total	1.000		.012	1.000		

Table 3 *Overview Column Points*[a]

					Proportion of Inertia		*Confidence Singular Value*
Dimension	*Singular Value*	*Inertia*	*Chi Square*	*Sig.*	*Accounted for*	*Cumulative*	*Standard Deviation*
1	.108	.012			1.000	1.000	.004
Total		.012	1022.597	.000[a]	1.000	1.000	

a. 69 degrees of freedom

a. Symmetrical normalization

The total inertia for the columns was 0.011 and 0.001 for yes and no categories respectively

Transformed District Categories

There were several peaks of unmet need for spacing. The first small peak appears at Moradabad district. The low point starts from Saharanpur district, Muzaffarnagar, Bijnor and Moradabad and reaching Moradabad. The need

Figure 1 *Spacing Method*

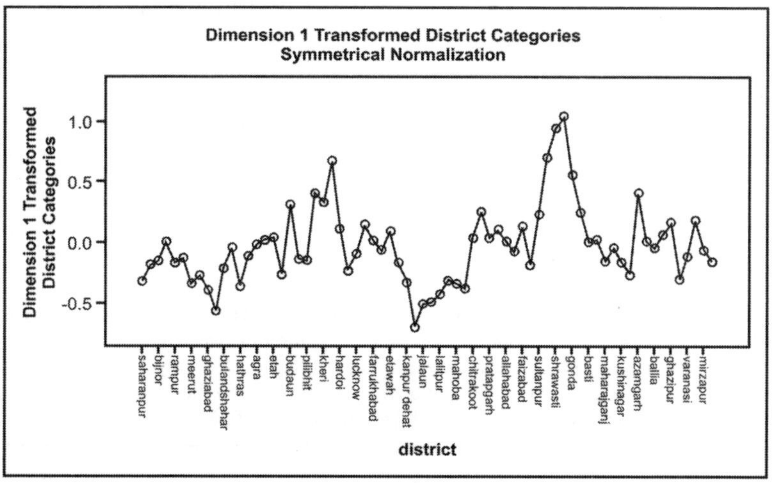

Figure 2 *Spacing Method Wise*

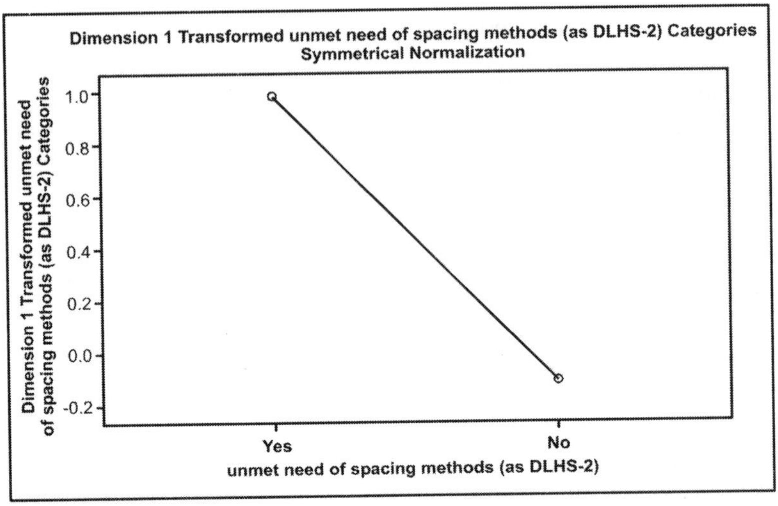

declines from Rampur, Jyotiba Phule Nagar, Meerut, Bhagpet, Ghaziabad, and Gautam Buddha Nagar. A part of Guatam Buddha Nagar includes NOIDA (New Okhla Industrial Development Area), a part of National Capital Region, New Delhi. Guatam Buddha Nagar district might have been benefitted by adjacent New Delhi. Similarly, Mathura and Hathras districts might have great influence from New Delhi with low unmet need for spacing. Another district worth mentioning is Mainpuri showing low unmet need. It is surrounded by high unmet need districts: Firozabad, Etah, Etawah, Farrukhabad, Hardoi, and Kannauj.

Unmet Need for Limiting Family Size

Unmet need for limiting family size has been given according to percentage of requirement. Only 3 districts have below 10 per cent of need. On the other extreme, Budaun (31.23%) and Firozabad (33.49%) have high unmet need for limiting methods (Table 4, 5).

Table 4 *Unmet Need for Limiting*

Value (%)	*Districts*
Below 10 (3 districts)	Jhansi (7.31), Varanasi (8.8) and Sonbhadra (9.7).
10–15 (7 districts)	Lalitpur (10.54), Meerut (11.28), Jalaun (11.66). Mahoba (13.56), Hamirpur (14.17),Gautam Buddha Nagar (14.89), Ghaziabad (14.96).
15–20 (19 districts)	Saharanpur (15.26), Banda (15.75), Allahabad (16.32), Chitrakoot (16.43), Faizabad (17.15), Kanpur Dehat (17.17), Kanpur Nagar (17.44), Ballia (17.52), Gorakhpur (17.77), Sant Ravidas Nagar (18.23), Maharajganj (18.32), Chandauli (18.71), Baghpet (18.82), Ambedkar Nagar (18.95), Barabanki (19.16), Kaushambi (19.55), Bijnor (19.85), Jaunpur (19.95).

Cont'd...

...Cont'd

20–25 (32 districts)	Kheri (20.11), Sultanpur (20.44), Bulandshahar (20.71), Siddarthanagar (20.72), Hathras (20.86), Rampur (20.88), Mau (21), Lucknow (21.03), Basti (21.03), Pilibhit (21.12), Jyotiba Phule Nagar (21.25), Ghazipur (21.8), Kushinagar (21.83), Azamgarh (21.92), Rae Bareli (22), Unnao (22.31), Sitapur (22.49), Pratapgarh (22.84), Shrawasti (23.1), Muzaffarnagar (23.23), Sant Kabir Nagar (23.29), Mainpuri (23.33), Bareilly (23.47), Kannauj (23.53), Moradabad (24.11), Farrukhabad (24.19), Shahjahanpur (24.25), Deoria (24.34), Bahraich (24.62), Gonda (24.74), Aligarh (24.75),Mathura (24.93).
25+ (9 districts)	Fatehpur (25.48), Hardoi (26.25), Auraiya (26.35), Balrampur (26.55), Etawah (27.08), Agra (28.63), Etah (29.5), Budaun (31.23), Ferozabad (33.49).

Unmet Need for Limiting

The total inertia (eigen values) has been 0.016*100=1.6 per cent only. The correspondence analysis reflects that the correlation between region/districts and unmet need, while significant, was weak. Meerut, Etah, Budaun, Jalaun, Jhansi, Lalitpur, Varanasi, Mirzapur and Sonbhadra each contributed (0.001) and Firozabad contributed (0.002) totalling 0.016 for limiting methods. The columnwise values reveal 1.3 per cent for unmet need and .03 per cent for no need (Table 6, 7).

Table 6 *Summary Table*

					Proportion of Inertia		*Confidence Singular Value*
Dimension	*Singular Value*	*Inertia*	*Chi Square*	*Sig.*	*Accounted for*	*Cumulative*	*Standard Deviation*
1	.127	.016			1.000	1.000	.003
Total		.016	1404.030	.000[a]	1.000	1.000	

a. 69 degrees of freedom

Table 7 *Overview Column Points*[a]

		Score in Dimension		*Contribution*		
				Of Point to Inertia of Dimension	*Of Dimension to Inertia of Point*	
Unmet Need of Limiting Method (as DLHS–2)	*Mass*	*1*	*Inertia*	*1*	*1*	*Total*
Yes	.206	.698	.013	.794	1.000	1.000
No	.794	–.181	.003	.206	1.000	1.000
Active Total	1.000		.016	1.000		

a. Symmetrical normalization

Transformed District Categories

The following graph shows the several peaks of unmet need for limiting:

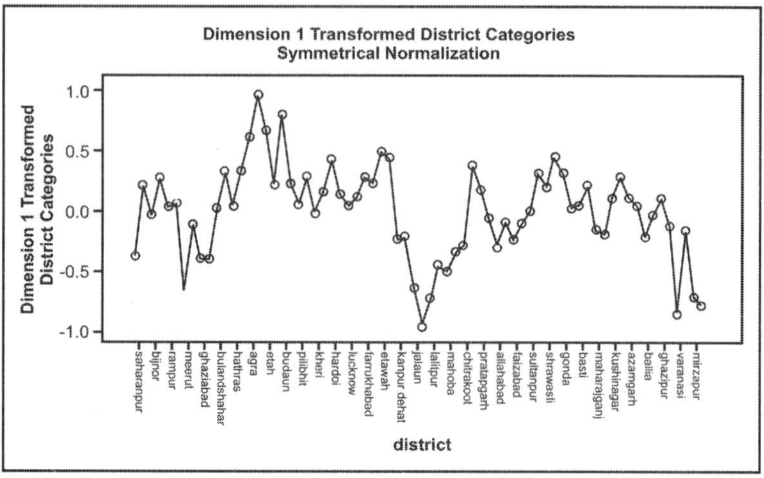

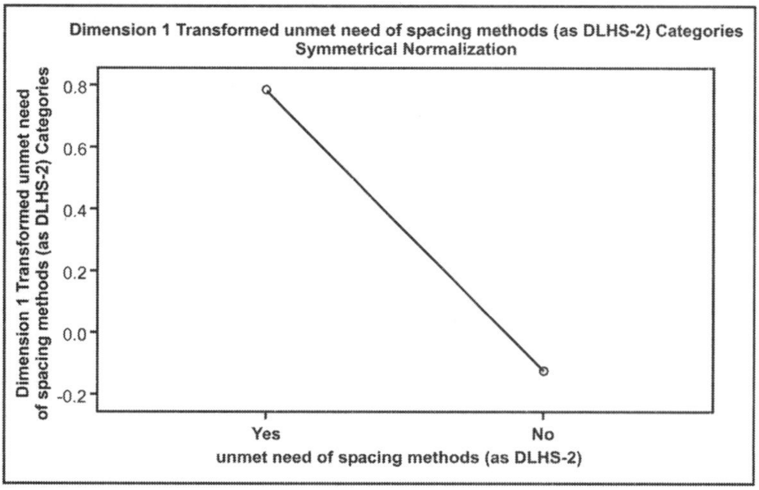

Of the total inertia, mainly Sitapur (0.001), Kanpur Nagar (0.001), Bahraich (0.001), Shrawasti (0.002), Balarampur (0.002) have contributed to unmet need for limiting, totalling 0.012. Whereas Meerut, Etah, Budaun, Jalaun, Jhansi, Lalitpur, Varanasi, Mirzapur and Sonbhadra each contributed (0.001) and Firozabad (0.002), totalling 0.016 for limiting methods.

Unmet need for spacing and limiting family size in relation to outcome for the last pregnancy as given in Table 8 reveals that 12.1 per cent (10555/87564*100) need spacing methods. Women with no loss children constitute major portion followed by spontaneous abortion, induced abortion and still births. Around 95 per cent who were in need of spacing methods of family planning desire spacing methods after having live births. A similar proportion of respondents (97.45%) with live births desired limiting methods of family planning. Around 2 per cent of respondents with the experience of induced/spontaneous abortion desired spacing methods. Around 1 per cent of respondents with spontaneous abortion desire to have limiting methods of family planning.

Table 8 *Outcome of Pregnancy in Relation to Unmet Need for Limiting and Spacing Methods of Family Planning*

Unmet Need for Limiting	*Outcome of Pregnancy*	*Unmet Need of Spacing*		*Total*
		Yes	*No*	
Yes	Live birth		95(10027)	10027
	Still birth		0.9(95)	95
	Induced abortion		1.99(210)	210
	Spontaneous abortion		2.11(223)	223
	Total		100(10555)	10555
No	Live birth	97.45(7265)	20394	27659
	Still birth	0.47(35)	403	438
	Induced abortion	0.46(34)	662	696
	Spontaneous abortion	1.62(121)	1405	1526
	Total	100(7455)	22864	30319

Type of Family Planning Method Used

Around two-fifths (36.5 per cent: 31943/87564*100) were using some method of family planning. Among them around half (45.9%) have underwent sterilization. Remaining half were using different methods of temporary contraception. Rhythm and condom/nirodh were the major ones. Sterilizations constitute only 16.75 per cent (14665/87564*100) for the total population.

Logistic Regression

This analysis has been made for the whole state. There were some differences when it came to the determinants of spacing and limiting methods. It may be due to two different age groups of women practising these methods. Spacing mostly has been followed by younger women and the limiting methods by older cohort of women or women who have completed their family size. Respondents' years of schooling, respondents' age at first birth (not significant) and number of live births were positively correlated with spacing methods, whereas it was negative in the case of limiting methods. However, wealth index was positively correlated with spacing and limiting (at rich level) methods. Semi-pucca house was correlation positively with spacing and negatively with spacing methods.

Table 9 *Logistic Regression*

Variable	*Spacing*	*Significance*	*Limiting*	*Significance*
Respondents' years of schooling	1.011	.048	.987	.008
Respondents' age at birth	1.008	.228	.997	.635
Live births	1.687	.000	.745	.000
Wealth Index (Poor)				
Moderate	1.261	.000	1.079	.130

Cont'd...

...Cont'd

Rich	1.537	.000	1.294	.000
Had BPL card (No)				
No	.962	.428	.852	.000
Type of house (kutcha)				
Semi-pucca	1.181	.000	.834	.000
Pucca	.919	.730	.975	.911
Constant	1.340	.009	15.517	.000
–2 log likelihood	21083.685		27491.158	

Logistic Regression for Chandauli District

Spacing methods was followed by women with number of children, not having a below poverty line (BPL) card, and high wealth index and limiting was otherwise.

Table 10 *Logistic Regression for Chandauli District*

Variable	*Spacing*	*Significance*	*Limiting*	*Significance*
Respondents' years of schooling	.959	.453	.955	.240
Respondents' age at birth	.902	.061	.998	.960
Live births	1.885	.000	.791	.000
Wealth Index (Poor)				
Moderate	3.123	.053	.840	.694
Rich	2.842	.026	.807	.593
Had BPL card (Yes)				
No	2.350	.041	.980	.950
Type of House (Kutcha)				
Semi-pucca	.908	.522	1.549	.138
Pucca	.000121	.999	.000269	.999
Constant	4.656	.094	9.575	.002
–2 log likelihood	247.322		442.564	

Conclusion and Recommendations

Unmet need for contraception varies from district to district based on development, namely wealth index. Some districts near to the national capital had more unmet need for spacing and limiting at rich category of wealth index and some districts with less development had shown at poor category. It means that most of the households in these districts either belonged to rich or poor category. Moderate level of wealth index was second highest either in the case of poor/rich highest. Meerut and Ghaziabad districts (spacing) and Ghaziabad (limiting) had highest (above 75%) unmet need in the state as a whole. We have 12 and 10 districts in the category of 50–75 per cent respectively for spacing and limiting. Highest proportion of districts were listed with 25–50 per cent category for spacing (39) and limiting (36), needs followed by below 25 per cent (see Table 11).

Table 11 *Wealth Index in Relation to Unmet Need for Spacing and Limiting Methods in the Districts of Uttar Pradesh*

		Spacing		*Limiting*
Wealth index (Rich)				
Above 75 per cent (2)	2	Meerut (83.3), Ghaziabad (81.8)	1	Ghaziabad (80.6),
50–75 per cent (12)	12	Jyotiba Phule nagar (52.5),Bulandshahar (53.3),Lucknow (53.4), Aligarh (55.7), Mathura (55.8), Agra (57.7), Kanpur Nagar (61.5), Bijnor (64.2), Saharanpur (64.3), Baghpat (66),Muzaffarnagar (70.5), Gautam Buddha Nagar (76.1)	10	Saharanpur (53.5),Bijnor (53.7),Varanasi (54.1), Agra (54.6), Mathura (56.4), Muzaffarnagar (61.8), Baghpat (66.7), Gautam Buddha Nagar (68.8), Meerut (72.1),
25–50 per cent (39)	39	Kaushambi (25.3), Maharajganj (27), Mahoba (27.5), Hamirpur (28.3), Philibhit (28.6), Banda (29.5), Sultanpur (30.3), Faizabad (30.6). Kushinagar (30.9), Basti (32.1), Ambedkar Nagar (32.3), Unnao (33.3), Sant Kabir nagar (33.3), Ghazipur (34.2), Auraiya (35.1), Etah (35.2), Kanpur Dehat (35.7), Azamgarh (36.7), Allahabad (37), Pratapgarh (37.6), Ballia (37.8), Mirzapur (37.3), Mainpuri (39.3), Sant Ravi Das Nagar (40.4), Bareilly (41.3),Etawah (42.2), Chandauli (43.4), Rampur (43.6),Gorakhpur (49.3), Firozabad (45.4), Varanasi (45.1), Jhansi (46.2),Hathras (46.7), Mau (47.5), Moradabad (47.6), Jalaun (48.1), Deoria (50), Jaunpur (50)	36	Kaushambi (26.5), Mainpuri (27.3), Rae Bareilly, Faizabad (28), Maharajganj (28.5), Etah (28.8), Pratapgarh (30.5), Ghazipur (31), Pilibhit (31.1), Sultanpur (32.2), Hamirpur (32.4), Azamgarh (32.5), Deoria (32.8), Bareilly (33.1), Basti (33.4), Ambedkar Nagar (33.9), Mau (35.5), Sant Ravidas Nagar (36.1),Rampur (37.1), Mirzapur (37.3), Chandauli (38.2), Jaunpur (38.3), Etawah (38.9), Gorakhpur (39.1), Allahabad (41.1), Firozabad (42.1), Moradabad, Jalaun (43.2), Hathras (46.6), Bulandshahar (47.9), Jyotiba Phule Nagar (49), Aligarh (49.5), Kanpur Nagar (56.2), Jhansi (57.5), Lucknow (59.5),
Below 25 per cent (18)	18	Bahraiach (8.2), Shrawasti (11.6), Hardoi (12.3),Sitapur (13.8), Kheri (14.4), Chitrakoot (14.9), Fatehpur (15.9), Sonbhadra (16.7), Balarampur (18.5), Budaun (19.4), Gonda (20.4), Shahjahanpur (20.8), Kannuj (21.5), Farrukhabad (21.7), Siddarthanagar (22), Barabanki (22.5), Lalitpur (23.2), Rae Bareilly (24.6)	26	Shrawasti (14.4), Sitapur (15.1), Kheri (17.7), Balarampur (18.2), Budaun (18.4), Banda (18.5), Bahraich (18.9), Chitrakoot (19), Hardoi, Siddarthanagar, (20.6), Shahjahnpur (20.9), Kanpur Dehat (21), Gonda (21.6), Kannauj (21.7), Lalitpur, Sonbhadra (21.8), Fatehpur (22.2), Unnao (22.7), Ballia (23.2), Sant Kabir nagar (23.6), Kushinagar (23.9), Barabanki (24.1), Farrukhabad (24.3), Mahoba (24.5), Auraiya (24.8),
Wealth Index (Poor)		Districts		Districts
Above 75 per cent		Bahraich (79.3)		

Cont'd...

...Cont'd

50–75 per cent	Basti (50), Barabanki (50.5), Kushinagar (52.1), Rae Bareilly (52.8), Siddarthnagar(53.3), Faizabad (53.7), Ambedkarnagar (54.2), Kaushambi (55.1), Shahjahanpur (57.4), Farrukhabad (58.6), Budaun (60.7), Chitrakoot (61.2), Gonda (61.9), Balarampur (62.3), Kheri (62.4), Sonbhadra (65.6), Fatehpur (65.9), Hardoi (67.5), Sitapur (71.7), Shrawasti (73.3),	Rae Bareilly (50.6), Kannauj (50.9), Mainpuri (51.6), Ballia (51.7), Etah (52), Maharajganj (53), Farrukhabad (53.1), Kanpur Dehat, Kaushambi, Ambedkarnagar (53.4), Unnao (53.6), Kushinagar (53.9), Fatehpur (54.1), Barabanki (54.8), Chitrakoot, Sant Kabir Nagar (55), Siddharthr.agar (55.1), Banda (55.4), Faizabad (56), Lalitpur (58.1), Shahjahnpur (58.5), Budaun (61.4), Gonda (62), Hardoi (62.7), Sonbhadra (63.6) Kheri (65.9), Balrampur (69.1), Sitapur (69.3), Bahraich (70.5), Shrawasti (72.6)

In general, respondents of some districts belonged equally to either poor or rich categories for *spacing* Chandauli (43.4 for both), Azamgarh (poor: 33.5 and rich: 36.7), Allahabad (poor: 40.3 and rich: 37) and Etah (poor: 36 and poor: 35.2)and *limiting* methods (Etawah (poor: 36.4 and rich: 38.9), Allahabad (poor: 39.1 and rich: 41.1), Gorakhpur (poor: 41.9 and rich: 39.1) and Chaundali (poor: 42.7 and rich: 38.2). Chandauli district, carved out of Varanasi division is an agriculturally developed district and aptly called 'Dhaan Ka Katora of Uttar Pradesh. All the other districts have their own importance having population of rich and poor alike.

Wealth index influences unmet need which invariably is linked to education. Unmet need depends on availability, affordability and acceptability of contraceptives. Hence, efforts were to be made in this direction. Unmet need exists due to several reasons. Spacing has been the main casualty. Women still are not still convinced about the efficacy of spacing methods and also difficult to maintain spacing methods. Terminal methods too are not properly favoured due to personal causes. Lot of persuasion is the need of the hour with benefits accruing out of following family planning methods.

References

Laya, K.S. 2012. Prevalence and Determinants of Unmet Need for Family Planning among Women in India. *Research and Social Practices in Social Sciences*, 7 (2): 59–70.

National Consultation of Civil Organizations on Family Planning: A Concept Note. 2012. New Delhi: India International Centre (IIC).

Radha Devi, D., Rastogi, S.R. and Retherford, R.D. 1996. Unmet Need for Family Planning in Uttar Pradesh. *National Family Health Survey Reports*, No. 1, Mumbai: International Institute for Population Sciences.

Tauseef, Ahmed. 1993. Unmet Need for Contraception in Pakistan: Pattern and Determinants. *Demography India*, 22 (1): 31–51.

6

Squeeze of Women's Effective Reproductive Span in India

Abhishek Saraswat and Sayeed Unisa

A woman's effective reproductive span is important in understanding the fertility levels of a society and a woman's or couple's reproductive planning, allocation of time for child-bearing and decision to end reproduction, as it is more closely related to a woman's life course. Reproductive spans of women depend upon family planning practices of women. Socio-cultural and demographic factors influence reproductive practices.[1] In developing countries like India child-bearing out of wedlock is forbidden and sexual union and child-bearing is expected after the marriage and sterilization was not common. This led to longer reproductive spans of Indian women.[2] Among various available family planning methods female sterilization is one of the most widely used, 20.3 per cent couples worldwide use female sterilization for spacing births; 8.1 per cent in developed to 22.3 per cent in developing regions. Share of sterilization in India is 37.3 per cent.[3] Many Indian couples never used temporary or reversible method for spacing births and often it is the only contraceptive method used by many couples to limit their family size.[4] The gradually increasing age at marriage of women and decreasing age at sterilization indicates that reproduction spans of women may be contracting.

Review of Literature

Sterilization is one of the most popular and widely used methods of contraception in the world and India too.[5] It was estimated that in India, about 30 per cent of all eligible couples seek family limitation by permanent methods. The average age of the acceptors of female sterilization was observed to have fallen during the 1981–91 decade from 30.3 years to 28.7 years; concomitantly, the percentage of acceptors below 30 years of age had increased from 48.7 per cent to 62.3 per cent of all female sterilization acceptors.[6] According to National Family Health Survey 3 (NFHS), 77 per cent of women in India had not used any reversible method of contraception before getting sterilized.[7,8,9]

A study done on Hooghly district of West Bengal found that the couple protection rate (CPR) among couples was 39.5 per cent of which 34.5 per cent had adopted a permanent method. Acceptance of sterilization was highest among women with more number of living children and religion did seem to have influenced use of sterilization, its acceptance being lower among Muslims as compared to Hindus. Over the years there have been marginal shifts in terms of younger and lower parity couples accepting a permanent method of contraception.[10] A study done on rural Maharashtra concluded that economic compulsion was the sole reason in 43 per cent users to opt for tubal sterilization followed by a desire for good upbringing of children (12%).[11] Another study stated that the incidence of childhood marriages has been on the decline while age at marriage and age at cohabitation have shown a slow and gradual increase over the years.[12] A study done on Andhra Pradesh found a gradual increase in the female age at marriage and a decreasing age at sterilization indicating possibilities of narrowing reproductive spans among women.[2]

Objectives

This paper attempts to analyse the length of effective reproductive spans of women along with its demographic and socio-economic correlates and the risk of contraction of reproductive span of women in India.

Data and Methods

Data from NFHS–3 were used to examine the effective reproductive span for this study. The reproductive span is defined as the duration between first marriage and menopause or sterilization of the women or her spouse. To account for right-censoring, we used life table to estimate the probability of infecundity at various times after first marriage and hence expected reproductive spans. To study trends in reproductive spans, we divided women according to their duration of marriage. We excluded from the analysis 30,661 never married women, women who had been sterilized before marriage. Around 4,688 women who married after 2004 were also excluded, because they were unlikely to have completed their reproductive span during short interval between marriage and the interview and 5,243 women who had no children at the time of survey were also excluded as they have little chances to be sterilized. Around 83,793 women were selected for analysis. Cox proportional hazards regression analysis was used to examine association between timing of marriage and risk of menopause or sterilization after first marriage. It also analyses effects of women's demographic and socio-economic characteristics, women's autonomy and reproductive attitudes.

Results

Table 1 shows the changes in total fertility rates, median age at first marriage and age at sterilization of women that have occurred from 1992–93 to 2005–06, i.e. during NFHS 1, 2 and 3. From 1992–93 to 2005–06 the Total Fertility Rate (TFR) of India has declined from 3.39 to 2.68 while the median age at which women married increased from 16.1 years to 16.8 years during 1992–93 to 2005–06 and the age at which they got sterilized declined from 26.6 years to 25.5 years.

Table 1 *Total Fertility Rates (TFR) and Median Ages at First Marriage and at Sterilization Among Indian Women Aged, National Family Health Surveys, 1992–93, 1998–99 and 2005–06*

	1992–93	*1998–99*	*2005–06*
Total Fertility Rate	3.39	2.85	2.68
Age at first marriage	16.1	16.4	16.8
Age at sterilization	26.6	25.7	25.5

Sterilization increased by 44 per cent among women aged above 30 years than other women (OR 1.4), and it decreased by 30 per cent among women who married prior to their twenties (OR 0.6). Sterilization was 42 per cent (OR 0.5) and 39 per cent (OR 0.6) less among women who experienced any child loss or an abortion respectively (Table 2). Women who had two or more children were twice more likely to get sterilized than women having one or no child (OR 2.1). As the ideal number of boys increased, sterilization decreased by 20–40 per cent.

Table 2 *Odds Ratio (OR) from Logistic Regression Analysis Assessing the Relationship Between Sterilization, According to Different Demographic Characteristics*

Demographic Characteristics	*Exp β*
Age	
Below 30®	
Above 30	1.448***
Age at marriage	
Below 20®	
Above 20	0.699***
Child death	
No®	
Yes	0.581***
Ever had abortion	
No®	
Yes	0.615***
Children ever born	
Below 2®	
Above 2	2.159***
Ideal number of boys	
0®	
1	0.801***
2	0.800***
3+	0.619***

® represents reference category; *** represents significance at 1%

Rural women were 11 per cent less likely to be sterilized as compared to urban women (OR 0.8), among Muslims and Christians likelihood of getting sterilized was around 50–60 per cent less (Table 3). In terms of sterilization Other Backward Classes (OBCs) outpaced women of other caste groups by 12–37 per cent. Educated women were 17–38 per cent more likely to get sterilized as compared to uneducated women (OR 0.5–1.3). Likelihood of sterilization was 10 per cent less among women living in joint families (OR 0.9). As compared to poorest, people of middle and rich class were 34–84 per cent more likely to become sterilized. Women exposed to media and working women were 30–35 per cent more likely to get sterilized.

Table 3 *Odds Ratio from Logistic Regression Analysis Assessing the Relationship Between Sterilization, According to Different Socio-economic Characteristics*

Socio-economic Characteristics	*Exp β*		*Exp β*
Place of residence			
Urban®		Higher	0.596***
Rural	0.894***	**Household structure**	
Religion		Nuclear®	
Hindu®		Joint	0.926***
Muslim	0.422***	**Wealth Index**	
Christian	0.506***	Poorest®	
Others	0.757***	Poor	1.348***
Caste		Middle	1.644***
SC®		Rich	2.018***
ST	0.752***	Richest	1.847***
OBC	1.126***	**Working status**	
None of them	0.862***	No®	
Respondent's education		Yes	1.355***
No education®		**Exposure to media**	
Primary	1.389***	No®	
Secondary	1.171***	Yes	1.309***

® represents reference category; *** represents significance at 1%

In 1970–79, half of the women completed their reproductive spans in-between 9–13 years of marriage (Table 4). Among women of marriage cohort 1980–89, 57 per cent completed their reproductive spans during 5–9 years of marriage and this span further reduced to 84.5 per cent and 100 per cent among women of marriage cohort of 1990–99 and 2000–04 respectively. Majority of couples ended their effective reproductive span within 9 years of marriage.

Table 4 *Cumulative Percentage of Ever-married Women Aged 15–49 Completing Effective Reproductive Spans, According to Durations Since Marriage, by Marriage Cohort, India, 2005–06*

Marriage Cohort	*Duration of Marriage*						
	<4	*<9*	*<14*	*<19*	*<24*	*25+*	*Total*
1970–1979	5.30	40.10	73.80	92.20	98.50	100.00	6174
1980–1989	12.70	56.90	86.80	98.30	99.80	100.00	14213
1990–1999	27.90	84.50	99.40	100.00	NA	NA	11976
2000–2004	83.60	100.00	NA	NA	NA	NA	1087
Total	19.10	65.10	89.40	97.80	99.60	100.00	33450

Figure 1 is showing the expected mean reproductive spans of women of different marriage cohort. It can be seen that women in cohort of 1970–79 had the longest reproductive span of 11.5 years, which has gradually shrunken to 9.2 years, 6.4 years and 3.0 years as we move on to marriage cohorts of 1980–89, 1990–99 and 2000–04 respectively. For Indian women as a whole mean length of reproductive span is 8.4 years.

Figure 1 *Mean Reproductive Spans Among Ever-married Women Aged 15–49*

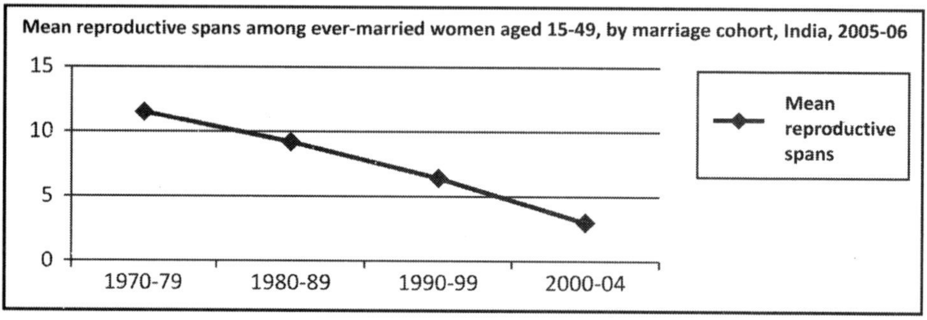

Pace of ending reproductive span was 26 per cent higher among women aged below 30 as compared to other women (hazard ratio 0.7), among those marrying in their 20s, the pace of accepting sterilization was 25 per cent more than those marrying before age 20 (hazard ratio 1.2), women of later marriage cohort viz., 1980–89, 1990–99 and 2000–04 ended their reproductive span faster than the women of reproductive cohort 1970–79 did (Table 5). Educated women completed their reproductive span faster than uneducated women. Among Muslims and Christians the pace of ending reproductive span was respectively 38 per cent and 13 per cent less than Hindus. With increasing wealth index pace of ending child-bearing increased among women. The pace of exit from the reproductive span was 30–40 per cent slow among those who experienced any child loss or abortion. As the number of ideal increased, the pace of ending child-bearing decreased (hazard ratio 0.9–0.6).

Table 5 *Hazard Ratio from Cox Regression Analysis Assessing the Relationship Between Pace of Squeeze of Effective Reproductive Span, According to Different Background Characteristics*

Background Characteristics	*Exp β*	Background Characteristics	*Exp β*
Age group		Christian	0.872***
Below 30®		Others	0.889***
Above 30	0.741***	**Caste**	
Age at marriage		SC®	
Below 20®		ST	0.915***
Above 20	1.258***	OBC	1.095***

Cont'd...

...Cont'd

Marriage cohort	
1970–79®	
1980–89	1.163***
1990–99	1.646***
2000–04	3.999***
Women's education	
No Education®	
Primary	1.207***
Secondary	1.143***
Higher	0.768***
Husband's education	
No education®	
Primary	1.030*
Secondary	0.913***
Higher	0.726***
Working status	
No®	
Yes	1.164***
Religion	
Hindu®	
Muslim	0.629***
None of them	0.926***
Wealth index	
Poorest®	
Poorer	1.116***
Middle	1.197***
Richer	1.290***
Richest	1.249***
Child death	
No®	
Yes	0.695***
Ever had terminated	
No®	
Yes	0.589***
Ideal number of son(s)	
0®	
1	0.916***
2	0.694***
3+	0.658***
Exposure to media	
No®	
Yes	1.078***

® represents reference category; *** represents significance at 1%, ** represents significance at 5%, * represents significance at 10% level.

Discussion

Present study aimed to analyse the reproductive spans of Indian women along with the factors that accelerate the completion of reproductive spans. During the course from NFHS 1 to NFHS 3 female sterilization has gained acceptance and its use has increased; on the contrary, male sterilization has decreased. Increasing age at first marriage and decreasing age at sterilization indicate that the effective reproductive spans of women have been squeezing. Findings from Cox regression show that demographic characteristics influence affect the decision to end child-bearing among women. Pace of sterilization is faster among women marrying in their 20s and women of younger marriage cohorts are ending their child-bearing span earlier than the women of older marriage cohorts did; as compared to the poor, decision of ending reproduction is faster among middle and upper financial groups because rich people are capable enough to afford costly family planning methods instead of sterilization which is cheaper. Among educated women and those who are working, pace of exit from reproductive span is quicker. Religion still continues to be affecting the pace of ending reproductive spans; exit from child-bearing is slower among Muslims and Christians as compared to Hindus. Muslim women have a lower acceptance of family planning methods as compared to women of other religious groups owing to religious norms. Among those who experienced child loss or abortion, the pace of sterilization is lower as compared to the others because of desire for having children; among those who have preference for sons, the pace for ending childbearing is slow. Exposure to media also speeds up the pace of ending reproductive span.

Conclusion

It can be concluded that there has been a squeeze of effective reproductive span of women in India resulting from increasing age at marriage and a trend of early acceptance of sterilization among women with little use of reversible methods of family planning or lack of method mix use of family planning methods. Family planning programme of India holds that people are able to choose a contraceptive method from a full range of methods with complete information about these methods. But people receive very meagre information pertaining to choice of contraceptive method from providers.[3] The most ideal contraceptive method as characterized by women all over the world should be highly effective, with prolonged active life, reversible, should not have side effects and complications, easily accessible and provide privacy of use and offer protection against HIV/AIDS and STI;[13] such a contraceptive method is yet to be developed. Squeeze of reproductive span is a matter of concern as it might have its implications on women's health and an early acceptance of sterilization among women can lead to morbid conditions at quite young ages.

Policy Recommendations

Providers need to be oriented about the client's right to exercise choice. Additionally, a variety of providers, including traditional medical practitioners, should be trained and engaged to promote detailed information on various contraceptive methods.

Information, Education and Communication (IEC) efforts to enable clients to exercise informed contraceptive choice have been increased, but inadequate collaboration between the health sector, IEC units and other stakeholders is rendering these efforts ineffective. Hence, inter-sectoral coordination needs to be promoted.

Method-mix use of contraceptives, awareness of reversible methods and the quality of services must be promoted. This clearly highlights the importance of state-specific interventions to improve family planning services.

Ways should be looked out to encourage women and couples to postpone childbearing and spacing of births with reversible modern contraceptives. So, spacing methods must be promoted among couples; this would help to lengthen the reproductive span of women.

Notes

1. Murthy, M.S.R. 2012. Determinants of Reproductive Duration among Women of Jharkhand State: A Study. *Journal of Human Ecology*, 37 (2): 111–117.
2. Padmadas, S.S., Hutter, L. and Willekens, F. 2004. Compression of Women's Reproductive Spans in Andhra Pradesh, India. *International Family Planning Perspectives*, 30 (4): 12–19.

3. World Contraceptives Use. 2009. United Nations: Department of Economic and Social Affairs, Population Division.
4. Xavier, F. and Padmadas, S.S. 2000. Use of a Spacing Method Before Sterilization among Couples in Kerala, India. *International Family Planning Perspectives*, 26 (1): 29–35.
5. Srinivasan, K. 1998. Population Policies and Programmes Since Independence: A Saga of Great Expectations and Poor Performances. *Demography*, 5 (1): 29–59.
6. Gupta, U., Kumar, P., Bansal, A. and Sood, M. 1996. Changing Trends in the Demographic Profile and Attitudes of Female Sterilization Acceptors. *Journal of Family Welfare*, 42 (3): 27–31.
7. International Institute for Population Sciences (IIPS). 1995. *National Family Health Survey-1: MCH and Family Planning*. Mumbai: IIPS.
8. International Institute for Population Sciences (IIPS). 1995a. *National Family Health Survey–2*. Mumbai: IIPS and Opinion Research Corporation Macro.
9. International Institute for Population Sciences (IIPS). 2007. *National Family Health Survey–3*. Mumbai: IIPS and Macro International.
10. Banerjee, B. 2004. Socio-economic and Cultural Determinants on Acceptance of Permanent Methods of Contraception. *Journal of Family Welfare*, 50 (1): 54–60.
11. Athavale, A.V. and Athavale, S.A. 2003. Factors Influencing the Decision to Undergo Tubectomy in a Rural Area of Maharashtra State. *Regional Health Forum WHO South-East Asia Region*, 7 (2): 42–47.
12. David, E.B. and Reddy, P.H. 1986. Age Patterns of Women at Marriage, Cohabitation, and First Birth in India. *Demography*, 23 (4): 509–523.
13. Mohan, P.V. and Nair, P.M. 2009. Correlates of Low Reproductive Span in Kerala: Evidence from NFHS–3. *Janasamkhya*, 26–27: 79–91.

Section II

Health and Health Care Services

7

Health and Mortality Transition in Madhya Pradesh

Aalok Ranjan Chaurasia

Madhya Pradesh has the dubious distinction of having the second lowest expectation of life at birth among the major states in India which reflects that health of the people of Madhya Pradesh is amongst the poorest in the country. According to the Sample Registration System, the expectation of life at birth in Madhya Pradesh was around 62 years during the period 2006–10 which was about 4 years less than the expectation of life at birth for India as a whole and almost 12 years less than the expectation of life at birth in Kerala (Government of India, 2012). Thirty-five years ago, during the period 1970–75, the expectation of life at birth in Madhya Pradesh was higher than that in Assam, Orissa (Odisha) and Uttar Pradesh (Government of India, 1984) but Assam is now the only state in India which has a lower expectation of life at birth than Madhya Pradesh. During the 35 years between 1970–75 through 2006–10, the annual average improvement in the expectation of life at birth in Madhya Pradesh has been slower than the improvement in the expectation of life at birth in Odisha, Uttar Pradesh and even Assam (Government of India, 2012). Obviously, poverty of longevity and health remains a major development challenge for Madhya Pradesh.

The present paper analyses mortality and health transition in Madhya Pradesh during the 35 years between 1970–75 through 2006–10 and explores factors that may be attributed to relatively slow transition in mortality in the state. The analysis is based on the life tables prepared for females and males on the basis of age and sex-specific death rates available through the Sample Registration System. The age and sex-specific death rates available through the Sample Registration System are known for year to year fluctuations of unknown origin. The standard practice, therefore is to construct life tables on the basis of five-year average age and sex-specific death rates, instead of annual age and sex-specific death rates. It is assumed that the life tables so prepared refer to the mid-year of the time interval used for the construction of the life table. Thus, life table for the period 1970–75 is assumed to refer to the year 1973. Similarly, life table for the period 2006–10 is assumed to refer to the year 2008.

The paper is divided into seven sections including this introduction. The next section of the paper analyses the trend in the expectation of life at birth in the state during the period under reference. The expectation of life at birth is the most commonly used indicator for analysing and comparing mortality transition across populations, population groups and over time. The expectation of life at birth, however, is a synthetic measure which gives the number of years, a new-born is expected to survive, given the prevailing age and sex schedule of mortality. The relationship between mortality transition and increase in the expectation of life at birth is essentially reciprocal but the exact connection is not straightforward (Vaupel and Canudas Romo, 2003). A deeper understanding of mortality transition, therefore, requires age-specific analysis. Such an attempt is made in the third section of the paper which analyses transition in the probability of survival at different ages and how survival probability in different ages contributes to the probability of survival up to a given age.

The fourth section of the paper analyses the disparity in the lifespan – variation among individuals in the age at death. There is generally a negative correlation between the expectation of life at birth and the lifespan disparity. Progress in preventing premature deaths reduces the lifespan disparity, whereas progress in reducing deaths at older ages increases this disparity.

Social class and within state, inter-district, variation in the expectation of life at birth that are so pervasive in Madhya Pradesh are discussed in section five of the paper. Information available through the Sample Registration System, however, does not permit analysis of transition in mortality by social class or across the districts of the state.

The sixth section of the paper discusses current levels and trends in key determinants of health and mortality. This section also discusses the state response to prevailing health and mortality situation and how state response has contributed to meeting the health needs of the people. The last, concluding section of the paper summarizes the findings of the analysis and discusses possible options for accelerating the pace of health and mortality transition in the state in terms of reinvigorating the health care delivery system.

Trends in Life Expectancy

Estimates available through the Sample Registration System suggest that the female expectation of life at birth in Madhya Pradesh increased from around 45.8 years during 1970–75 to 63.9 years during 2006–10. This means an average annual increase of around 0.52 years during the period under reference or an average increase of almost 2.6 years per quinquennials. The gain in the male life expectancy during this period, on the other hand, was 12.4 years which implies an average annual increase of 0.35 years or an increase of 1.8 years per quinquennials. Information available through the Sample Registration System thus suggests that the transition in female mortality in the state has been faster than the transition in male mortality. As a result, a female is expected to live, on average, 2.8 years longer than the male in the state during 2006–10 (Figure 1). This is in quite contrast to the period 1970–75 when a male was expected to live, on average, 2.9 years longer than a female. Increase in the female expectation of life at birth has been particularly sharp during 1970 through 1980 and again during the period 1991 through 2010. During the 15 years between 1991–95 and 2006–10, the female expectation of life at birth is estimated to have increased by more than 9 years at an average annual rate of increase of more than 0.6 years or more than 3 years per quinquennials. By contrast, this increase was only about 6.4 years in males which implies an average annual increase of less than 0.5 year or less than 2.5 years per quinquennials.

Increase in the expectation of life at birth in the state can be compared with global model mortality transition schedules developed on the basis of the empirical evidence about increase in the expectation of life at birth during the period 1950 to 2005 in countries where life expectancy ranged between 50 to 85 years (United Nations, 2004). These schedules represent average transition in mortality grouped according to 90th percentile (very fast increase), 75th percentile (fast increase), average (medium increase), 25th percentile (slow increase), and 10th percentile (very slow increase). They have been further extended to cover life expectancy ranging from 40 years to 92.5 years by fitting the Lee-Carter mortality model (United Nations, 2004a).

Figure 1 *Female and Male Expectation of Life at Birth in Madhya Pradesh*

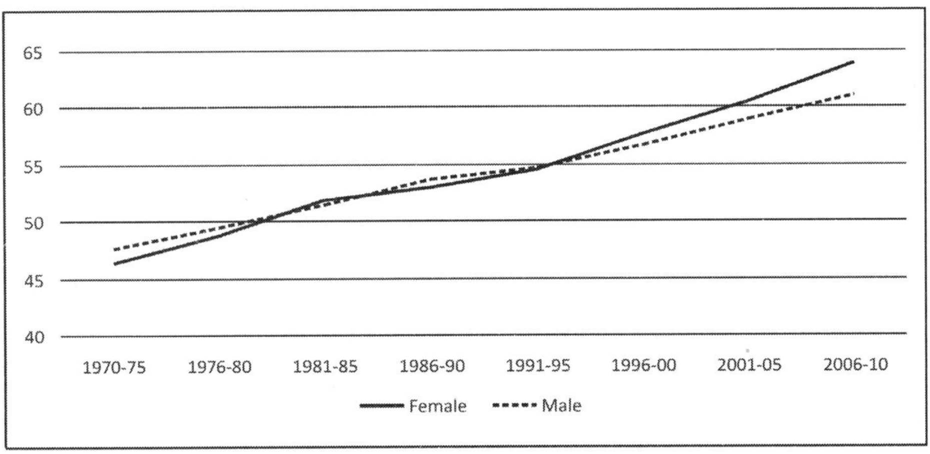

Figure 1 compares increase in the expectation of life at birth in Madhya Pradesh with the model mortality transition schedules separately for females and males. By global standards, male mortality transition in the state has been somewhere between very slow and slow model mortality transition schedules. By contrast, female mortality transition has been marginally faster than the average model mortality transition schedule. Transition in female mortality was quite fast during the period 1970–85 but slowed down considerably during 1985–95 and picked up the momentum again after 1995. On the other hand, male mortality transition was extremely slow during 1970–1980, although the pace of transition increased marginally after 1980.

The pace of mortality transition has been different in the rural areas of the state as compared to its urban areas. In rural females, the expectation of life at birth increased by more than 18 years during the period under reference compared to an increase of only around 13 years in the urban areas during the period under reference. Similarly, in rural males, the expectation of life at birth increased by more than 12 years during the period under reference compared to an increase of only 10 years in urban males. As a result, the urban rural gap in the expectation of life at birth in the state has narrowed down substantially over the years. During 1970–75 both urban females, and urban males, on average, lived around 10 years longer than their rural counterparts. This difference in the longevity of urban females and males decreased to around 7 years during the period 2006–10, although, in recent years, the urban-rural gap in male expectation of life at birth has widened again.

The expectation of life at birth depicts the combined mortality experience of population of different age groups. It is a synthetic measure which gives the number of years, a new born is expected to survive, given the prevailing age schedule of mortality. The relationship between mortality transition and increase in life expectancy is essentially reciprocal but the exact connection is not straightforward (Vaupel and Canudas Romo, 2003). Since, mortality transition varies by age, any analysis of mortality transition requires analysis of transition in age-specific mortality and how age-specific mortality transition contributes to transition in mortality of all ages combined. Such an analysis results in numerous comparative indexes which may be categorised as aggregative indexes and average of relative indexes (Schoen, 1970). Kittagawa (1966) has found that use of different indexes of mortality may provide different picture of mortality transition over time. It, therefore, seems reasonable to focus attention on differences in the pattern of death rates over the whole age spectrum (Schoen, 1970). A better understanding of mortality transition may be obtained by analysing transition in age-specific probability of death or, equivalently, age-specific probability of survival and analysing how mortality transition in different ages contributes to mortality transition in all ages combined. Results of such an analysis are presented in the next section.

Survival Probability

The age-specific probabilities of death derived from the age-specific death rates available through the Sample Registration System suggest that about 32 per cent of newborn females are expected to reach their 70th birthday given the age schedule of female mortality that prevailed in the state during 1970–75. On the other hand, given the age schedule of female mortality that prevailed in the state during 2006–10, around 55 per cent of newborn females are expected to reach their 70th birthday. Alternatively, given the 1970–75 age schedule of female mortality, about 68 per cent female newborn would fail to see their 70th birthday, whereas given the 2006–10 age schedule of female mortality, only 45

Figure 2 *Comparison of Female and Male Mortality Transition in Madhya Pradesh, 1970–2010 with Global Model Mortality Transition Schedules*

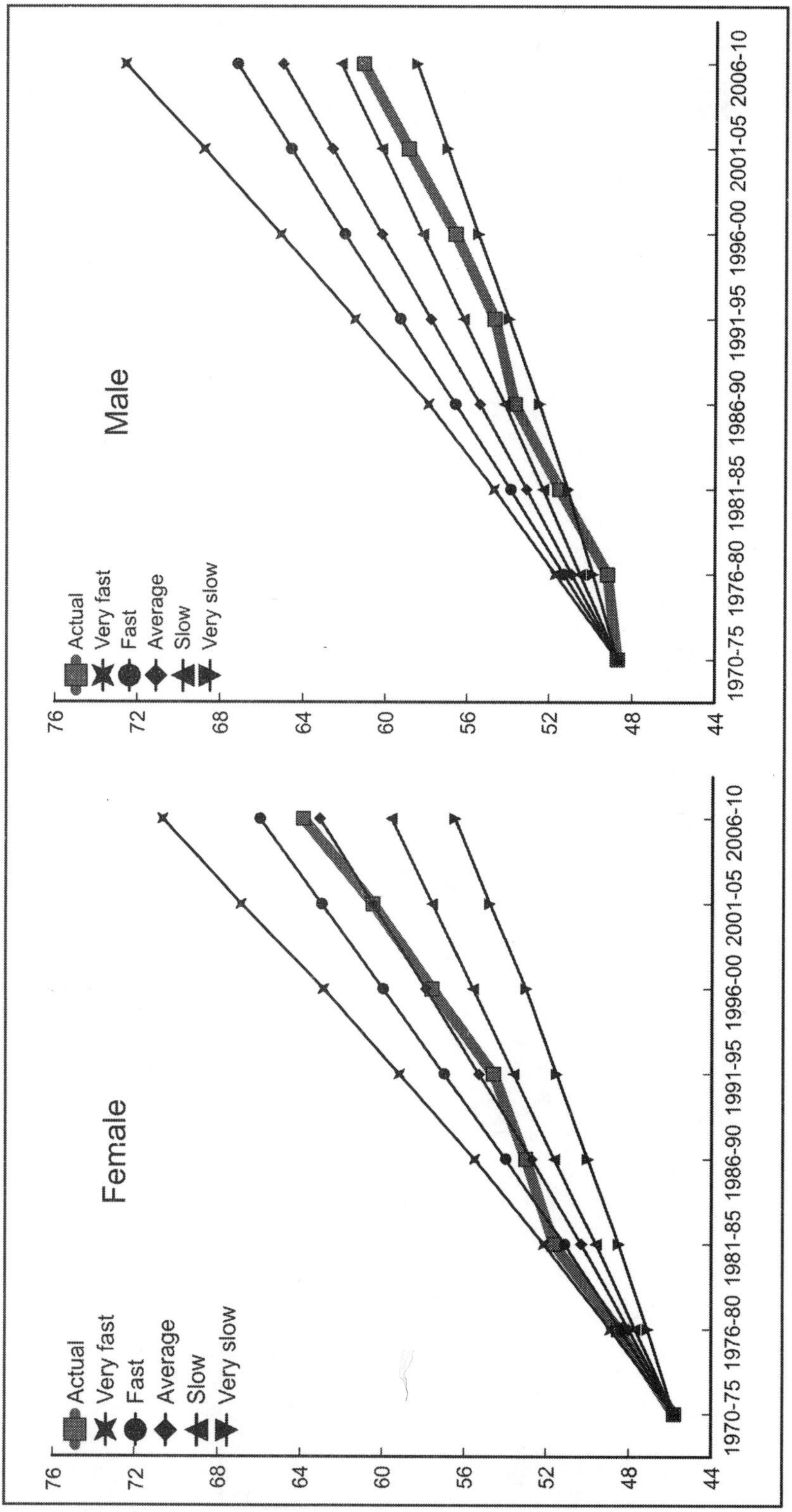

Figure 3 *Ratio of the Probability of Survival During 2006–10 and During 1970–75 in Different Age Intervals in Madhya Pradesh*

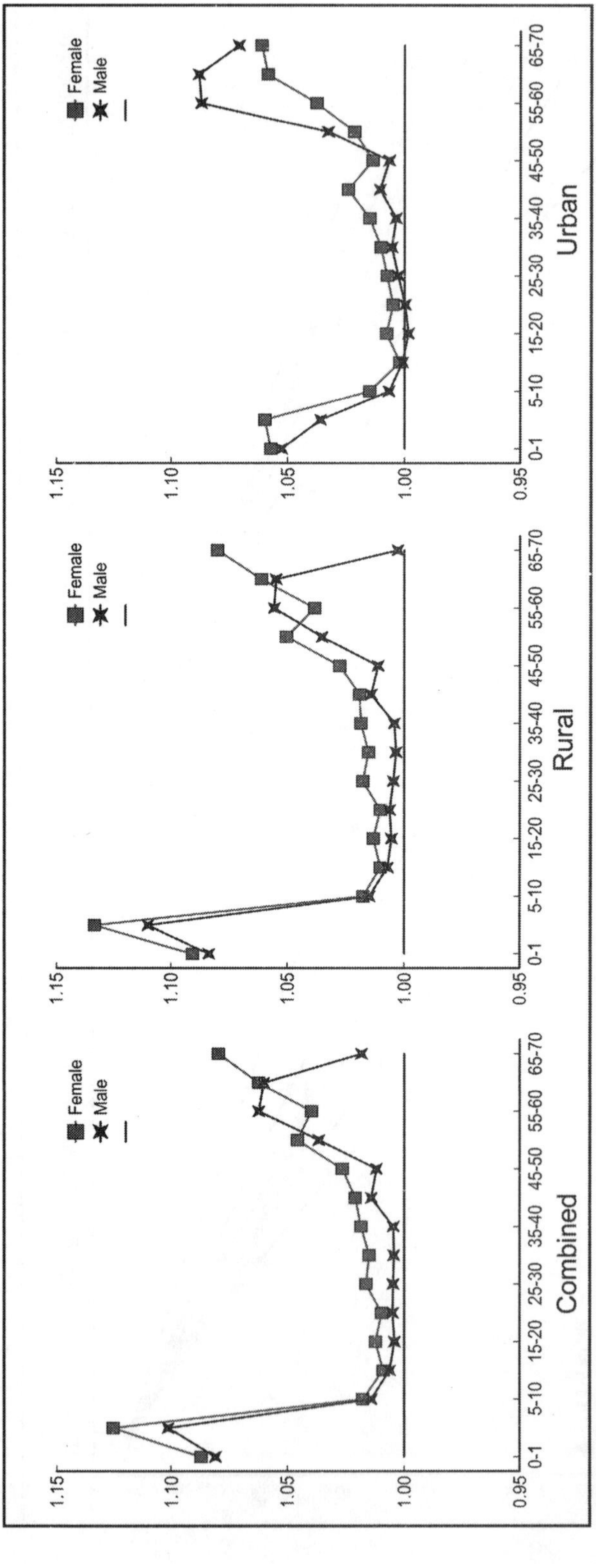

per cent of female newborn would not be able to see their 70th birthday. In case of males, 69 per cent of newborns would fail to survive up to their 70th birthday given the 1970–75 age schedule of male mortality, whereas this proportion would be 54 per cent given the 2006–10 age schedule of male mortality.

Table 1 breaks down the proportion of newborn dying before their 70th birthday under different age schedule of mortality. Given the 1970–75 age schedule of mortality, around 26 per cent of female newborns would die before reaching their fifth birthday; another about 3 per cent would die during 5–15 years of their life; about 5 per cent would die during 15–30 years of their life; about 9 per cent would die during 30–50 years of their life while about 25 per cent would die during 50–70 years of their life. The corresponding proportions, given the 2006–10 age schedule of mortality are 10 per cent; 1 per cent; 3 per cent; 6 per cent; and 24 per cent respectively.

Table 1 *Proportion of Females and Males Born During 1970–75 and During 2006–10 Expected to Die in Different Age Groups*

Age	*Female*		*Male*	
	1970–75	*2006–10*	*1970–75*	*2006–10*
	Combined population			
0–5	0.26	0.10	0.24	0.09
5–15	0.03	0.01	0.02	0.02
15–30	0.05	0.03	0.04	0.02
30–50	0.09	0.06	0.09	0.09
50–70	0.25	0.24	0.30	0.32
0–70	0.68	0.44	0.69	0.54
	Rural population			
0–5	0.28	0.11	0.25	0.10
5–15	0.03	0.01	0.03	0.01
15–30	0.05	0.03	0.04	0.03
30–50	0.09	0.06	0.09	0.10
50–70	0.25	0.25	0.29	0.32
0–70	0.70	0.46	0.70	0.56
	Urban population			
0–5	0.16	0.06	0.14	0.06
5–15	0.02	0.00	0.01	0.01
15–30	0.03	0.03	0.02	0.02
30–50	0.09	0.04	0.09	0.08
50–70	0.27	0.23	0.37	0.28
0–70	0.57	0.36	0.63	0.45

Source: Author's calculations

In case of males, on the other hand, given the 1970–75 age schedule of mortality, about 24 per cent of the newborns would be dying before reaching their fifth birthday; 2 per cent would die during 5–15 years of age; 4 per cent would die during 15–30 years of age; 9 per cent would die during 30–35 years of age while 30 per cent would die during 50–70 years of age. The corresponding proportions given the 2006–10 age schedule of mortality would be 9 per cent; 2 per cent; 2 per cent; 9 per cent; and 32 per cent respectively.

It is well known that the probability of survival up to age *a* is the product of the probability of survival up to age less than or equal to *a* (Shyrock and Siegel, 1976). In other words,

(1) ${}_{a}p_{0} = \prod_{i=1}^{a} {}_{1}p_{i-1}$

where *p* is the survival probability and *i* represents age. This implies that the change in the survival probability over time can be written as

(2) ${}_{a}\omega_{0} = {}_{a}p_{0}^{2}/{}_{a}p_{0}^{1} = \prod_{i=1}^{a}({}_{1}p_{i-1}^{2}/{}_{1}p_{i-1}^{1})$

where the superscript denotes the time. The ratio ω is a measure of transition in mortality. If ω = 1, there is no transition in mortality up to age *a*. On the other hand, larger is the value of ω, *the faster is the transition in mortality up to age a*. In this way, ω reflects the pace of mortality transition in a given age interval. Equation (2) suggests that mortality transition up to a given age can be decomposed into mortality transition in ages less than or equal to the given age.

The above argument suggests that, for females, the probability of survival up to 70 years of age in India is 77 per cent higher given 2006–10 age schedule of mortality as compared to 1970–75 age schedule of mortality. The corresponding proportion for males is only 52 per cent which shows that mortality transition in the age interval 0–70 years has been significantly faster in females than males in the state during the 35 years between 1970–75 through 2006–10. In the rural areas also, mortality transition has been significantly faster than males during the period under reference but in the urban areas, mortality transition in females and males has nearly been the same. In rural females, the probability of surviving up to 70 years of age given 2006–10 age schedule of mortality is more than 79 per cent higher than the corresponding probability given 1970–75 age schedule of mortality, whereas this increase was only about 49 per cent in rural males. However, in the urban areas, the corresponding proportions are 47 per cent in case of females and around 48 per cent in case of males. In other words, the pace of transition in male mortality has been more or less the same in rural and urban areas but female mortality transition has been faster in rural than in urban areas of the state.

Mortality transition in the age group 0–70 years is the combined result of mortality transition in different ages less than and equal to 70 years. Table 2 presents the increase in the probability of survival during 2006–10 over the probability of survival during 1970–75 in different age intervals less than 70 years of age while the ratio of the probability of survival during 2006–10 to the probability of survival during 1970–75 is presented in Figure 3 for different age intervals less than 70 years. It is apparent from the Table 2 as well as from the Figure 3 that nearly all the mortality transition in the age interval 0–70 years has been confined to age intervals 0–5 years and 50–70 years in both females and males as well as in the combined, rural and urban populations. By comparison, mortality transition in the age interval 5–50 years has been slow to very slow, although mortality transition in this age interval has been marginally faster in females as compared to males during the 35 years under reference. In fact, the probability of survival in urban males decreased and instead increased in the age interval 15–25 years during the period under reference. Among different age intervals, mortality transition has been the most rapid in the age interval 1–5 years followed by the age interval 0–1 years. In the age interval 50–70 years, the speed of transition in mortality increased in both females and males with a very rapid increase in the speed of transition in urban males in the age interval 55–60 years. At the same time, there has been little transition in male mortality in combined and rural populations whereas, in the urban population, the speed of mortality transition in the age interval 65–70 years has been substantially slower than the speed of transition in the age interval 60–65 years or in the age interval 55–60 years.

Table 2 *Increase (%) in Survival Probability in Different Age Groups Between 1970–75 and 2006–10*

Age	*Combined*		*Rural*		*Urban*	
	Female	*Male*	*Female*	*Male*	*Female*	*Male*
0–1	8.7	8.1	9.1	8.4	5.7	5.3
1–5	12.6	10.1	13.4	11.0	6.0	3.6
5–10	1.8	1.4	1.8	1.5	1.5	0.7
10–15	0.9	0.6	1.0	0.7	0.2	0.1
15–20	1.2	0.4	1.3	0.5	0.8	–0.2
20–25	1.0	0.5	1.0	0.6	0.5	–0.0
25–30	1.6	0.5	1.8	0.5	0.7	0.3
30–35	1.5	0.5	1.5	0.4	1.0	0.5
35–40	1.9	0.5	1.9	0.4	1.5	0.4
40–45	2.1	1.4	1.9	1.4	2.4	1.0
45–50	2.7	1.2	2.8	1.1	1.4	0.7
50–55	4.6	3.7	5.0	3.5	2.1	3.3
55–60	4.0	6.2	3.8	5.6	3.8	8.7
60–65	6.2	6.0	6.1	5.5	5.8	8.8
65–70	8.0	1.8	8.0	0.3	6.1	7.1
0–70	76.6	51.7	79.3	49.4	47.3	47.6

It may also be seen from Table 2 and Figure 3 that, in general, transition in female mortality has been more rapid than the transition in male mortality in the state. The only exceptions are the age interval 55–60 years in the combined and rural populations and the age interval 55–70 years in the urban population. Relatively slower female than male mortality transition in the age interval 55–70 years appears to be the reason behind relatively slow female mortality transition in the urban areas of the state in the age interval 0–70 years as compared to the rural areas.

It is now possible to summarize the basic features of mortality transition in Madhya Pradesh during the period under reference. First, except for urban males in the age interval 50–70 years, mortality transition in all age intervals has been faster in females than in males in the combined as well as rural and urban populations. Second, there has been virtually little transition in male mortality in the age interval 5–50 years. Third, there has been virtually no transition in rural male mortality in the age group 65–70 years. Fourth, mortality transition in rural females has been substantially faster than mortality transition in urban females.

Disparity in Lifespan

Another important aspect of mortality transition is the reduction in the variation among individuals in the age at death (Edwards and Tuljapurkar, 2005; Shkolnikov, Andreev and Begun, 2003; Smits and Monden, 2009; Wilmoth and Horiuchi, 1999). In general, there is a negative correlation between the expectation of life at birth and the variation among individuals in the age at death, although there may be discrepancies (Vaupel, Zhang and van Raalte, 2011). Progress in reducing premature deaths reduces variation among individuals in the age at death, whereas progress in reducing deaths at older ages increases variation among individuals in the age at death.

The variation in the age at death among individuals can be measured by the life disparity measure, eP†P (Vaupel and Canudas Romo, 2003). It is defined as the average remaining life expectancy at the age when death occurs. In other words, it is a measure of life years lost due to death. With the transition in mortality, deaths get increasingly concentrated at older ages resulting in the reduction in the variation in the age at which individuals die and the remaining lifespan of individuals who survive beyond this age.

The lifespan disparity does not decrease with the increase in the number of deaths prevented at any age as is the case with expectation of life at birth. Rather, it decreases or increases depending upon the balance between preventing deaths at early ages and saving lives at late ages. Generally, a fixed age, for example 65 years, is used to separate early deaths from late deaths. This approach is independent of the prevailing level of mortality. A more pragmatic approach is to define the age at death used for categorizing deaths as early or premature and late relative to the level of mortality. Separating the two is a unique threshold age, aP†P which is generally just below life expectancy. A recently developed demographic formula permits estimation of aP†P (Zhang and Vaupel, 2009) so that deaths occurring before the threshold age aP†P may be categorized as early or premature deaths while deaths occurring after this age are categorised as late deaths. In this approach premature deaths definition are defined relative to the level of mortality.

Results of the analysis are presented in Table 3. The average years of life lost due to death during 1970–75 was about 26 years in the state which reduced to around 18 years during 2006–10 which indicates that mortality transition in the state has been a result of reduction in the proportion of premature deaths. In fact, as may be seen from the table, the proportion of premature deaths in females decreased from around 49 per cent during 1970–75 to around 30 per cent during 2006–10 whereas in males, the proportion of premature deaths decreased from 40 per cent to around 29 per cent. Relatively slow reduction in the proportion of premature deaths indicates that mortality transition has been slower in males than in females during the period under reference. Reduction in the proportion of premature deaths has been the fastest in rural females but the slowest in urban males.

Table 3 *Reduction in Premature Deaths in Madhya Pradesh*

Population		*Average years of life lost due to death (e†)*		*Threshold age for premature deaths (a†)*		*Proportion of premature deaths (%)*	
		1970–75	*2006–10*	*1970–75*	*2006–10*	*1970–75*	*2006–10*
Total	Female	25.9	18.1	56.5	63.0	48.8	30.1
	Male	26.0	18.0	50.7	57.6	40.0	29.3
Rural	Female	26.4	18.7	56.4	62.6	50.7	31.7
	Male	25.1	18.3	53.3	57.0	42.0	29.8
Urban	Female	21.8	14.3	57.8	65.4	36.3	25.9
	Male	21.5	16.9	55.4	59.5	31.0	25.2

Source: Author's calculations

It may also be observed from the table that the age that separates early or premature deaths from late deaths has also increased over time. During 1970–75, a female death at age 56 and a male death at age 50 or below was an early or a premature death whereas during 2006–10, a female death at age less than 63 years and a male death at 57 years was a premature death according to our criteria.

Social Class and Regional Differentials

Estimates of expectation of life at birth by social class are not available from the Sample Registration System. However, estimates derived on the basis of 2001 population census suggest that the expectation of life at birth in the Scheduled Tribes of the state was very low, around 50 years only as compared to around 53 years in Scheduled Castes and more than 58 years in non-Scheduled Tribes/Castes (Chaurasia, 2011) (see Figure 4). There is, however, no evidence whether these differentials have narrowed or widened over time. The importance of social class differentials in mortality in the state lies in the fact that, according to the 2001 population census, around one-fifth of the state population was classified as Scheduled Tribes while another around 15 per cent was classified as Scheduled Castes.

District level estimates of the expectation of life at birth are also not available from the Sample Registration System. However, estimates based on 2001 population census suggest that mortality levels vary widely across the districts of the state (see Figure 5). The expectation of life at birth is estimated to be the highest in Indore district (64 years) which was the only district in the state having an expectation of life at birth of more than 60 years around the year 2001. On the other hand, the expectation of life at birth was estimated to be the lowest in district Katni of the state where an average individual was expected to live only 49 years around the year 2001 (Chaurasia, 2012). The wide inter-district variation in the expectation of life at births suggests that mortality transition varies widely across the districts of the state. Moreover, in 21 districts of the state, the expectation of life at birth was less than 55 years. It has been argued that a reduction in the inter-district disparity in mortality may contribute significantly in accelerating mortality transition in the state.

Figure 4 *Social Class Differentials in Expectation of Life at Birth in Madhya Pradesh*

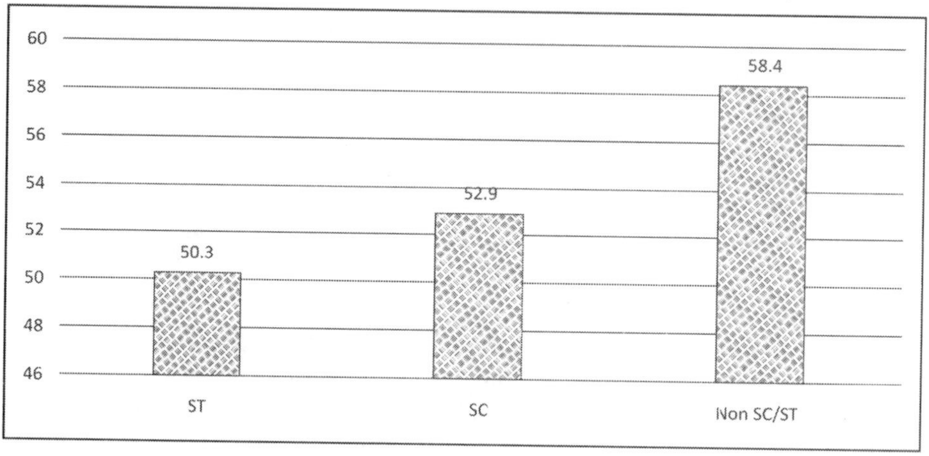

The State of Health

The foregoing analysis reflects the slow to very slow mortality transition in Madhya Pradesh during the 35 years between 1970–75 and 2006–10 by global standards. It also reflects poor transition in the health status of the people of the state. It appears that efforts to meeting the health needs of the people of the state have somewhere fallen short of the requirements and needs of the people. It also appears that a large proportion of the population of the state is still devoid of the basic minimum facilities that influence the key determinants of health and mortality – living conditions, nutritional status, especially of children, and an efficient and effective health care delivery system which are necessary for social, mental and physical well-being of the people of the state.

The straightforward ramification of the poor health status of the people is the high prevalence of morbidity – acute as well as chronic. Although, estimates of disease-specific prevalence rates are not available in the state and in its different population groups, yet information available through the annual health survey 2010–11 conducted by the Registrar General of India indicates that the prevalence of both acute and chronic mortality in the state is quite high, as close to 15 per cent of the state population is estimated to have been suffering from either acute or chronic morbidity at the time of the survey (Government of India, 2012). Moreover, there appears to be little difference in morbidity in rural and urban areas, although acute morbidity is higher in rural areas but chronic morbidity is higher in the urban areas of the state (Table 4). Moreover, both acute as well as chronic morbidity is estimated to be higher in females than in males in the combined as well as in rural and urban populations. It is worth pointing out here that the morbidity prevalence presented in Table 4 is based on acute and chronic conditions reported by the respondents and, therefore, may be biased by the knowledge and perception of the respondent about different disease conditions. In any case, it is very much clear from Table 4 that social, economic and environmental conditions in the state are not conducive to low levels of both acute as well as chronic morbidity in the state.

Figure 5 *Expectation of Life at Birth (years) in Districts of Madhya Pradesh, 2001*

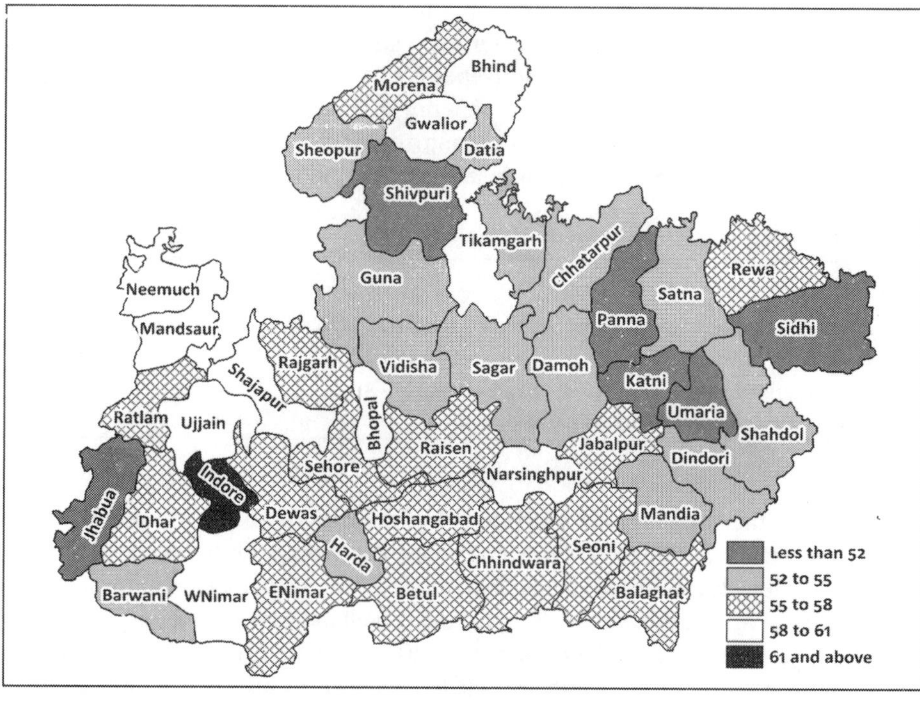

Table 4 *Acute and Chronic Morbidity in Madhya Pradesh*

Population		*Acute morbidity*	*Chronic morbidity*
Person	Combined	93.04	44.46
	Rural	100.87	39.97
	Urban	76.97	53.68
Male	Combined	88.41	40.77
	Rural	96.42	37.74
	Urban	72.10	46.94
Female	Combined	98.12	48.51
	Rural	105.73	42.40
	Urban	82.36	61.16

Source: Annual Health Survey 2010–11

Information related to some of the predisposing factors that contribute to acute and chronic morbidity and influence the health of individuals is presented in Table 5. The table suggests that the living environment of the people of the state needs to be improved substantially in order to have a telling impact on the health of the individuals. For example, almost one-third households in the state had none of the six household level assets – radio/transistor, television, phone (mobile or landline), computer (with or without internet), bicycle, two wheeler, and four wheeler – at the 2011 population census and this proportion was more than 40 per cent in the rural areas. A very high proportion of asset-less households suggests that poverty is still rampant especially in the rural areas of the state. Similarly, almost 48 per cent of the households did not have an improved drinking water source and this proportion was almost 55 per cent in the rural areas. Similarly, only one-fourth households in the state had access to improved sanitation facilities – only around 10 per cent in the rural areas. It is obvious that the prevailing living conditions of the majority of the population of the state is not conducive to an amenable health status of the people.

Table 5 *Living Conditions in Madhya Pradesh*

Indicator	*Combined population*	*Rural population*
Asset-less households	32.61	40.24
Households without access to improved drinking water facility	47.63	54.24
Households without access to improved sanitation	73.52	89.09

Source: Census 2011

One of the implications of poor living conditions in the state is the poor nutritional status of children. Information available through the National Family Health Survey 2005–06 suggests that more than 31 per cent children below three years of age in the state were stunted as well as wasted and this proportion was the highest in the country (Chaurasia, 2012). At the same time, about 27 per cent children were stunted but not wasted while around 14 per cent children were wasted but not stunted. This two-dimensional classification of the nutritional status of children suggests that more than 71 per cent children below three years of age in the state were undernourished either in one or both the dimensions of under nutrition.

Another reason that may be attributed to the unacceptably slow mortality and health transition in the state is the very unsatisfactory performance of the health care delivery system – public as well as private – in meeting the health care needs of the people. Although, it may be argued that the delivery of health care services is one of the many determinants of health and mortality, yet it is well known that health care in the form of life-saving and life-enhancing interventions plays a key role in health and mortality transition in terms of preventing majority of the premature deaths, especially deaths among young children and women who constitute the most vulnerable group of population and in terms of meeting the health care needs of the people. It is also well known that the medical technology that is currently available has the potential of preventing 90–95 per cent of the premature deaths but the challenge remains to reach those who are in need of health care. It is in this context that the performance of the health care delivery system in terms of meeting the health care needs of the people and in terms of preventing premature deaths matters in accelerating the pace of transition in both health status of the people and the mortality transition.

Using the information available through the district level household and facility survey, an attempt has been made to measure the performance of the health system in India at state and district levels (Chaurasia, 2013). The performance of the health system has been measured in two contexts – the coverage and the performance. The coverage index of the health system is based on coverage rate of 14 variables related to maternal health, child immunization and child health. On the other hand, the performance index is the coverage index adjusted for the prevailing levels of female literacy rate and the living conditions of the household. The health system performance index is zero when the composite coverage index based on the observed coverage rates of 14 public health interventions is less than the composite coverage index determined on the basis of the prevailing level of female literacy rate and the proportion of households with high standard of living index.

Results of the analysis, presented in Table 6 reflect the poor performance of the health care delivery system in the state in meeting the health care needs of the people. The performance of the health system of the state is found to be zero in the context of 14 interventions of public health importance in the combined population and in the rural population. For the combined population, the performance index is estimated to be zero in 26 of the 45 districts that existed in the state in 2007–08 and less than 20 per cent in the remaining districts. In the rural population, the health system performance is estimated to be zero in 29 districts (Chaurasia, 2013). Obviously, poor performance of the health system in the state has also been a dominating factor behind slow to very slow health and mortality transition in the state.

Table 6 *Nutritional Status of Children 0–3 Years of Age*

Indicator	*Combined Population*	*Rural Population*
Stunted as well as wasted	31.25	NA
Stunted but not wasted	26.63	NA
Wasted but not stunted	13.60	NA
Undernourished	71.47	NA
Stunted	57.87	NA
Wasted	44.85	NA

Source: Chaurasia (2012)

The coverage index and the performance index presented in Table 7 are constituted by three dimensions of health care – maternal health, child immunization and child health. The dimension of maternal health care reflects the performance of clinic-based services, the dimension of child immunization reflects the performance of extension services while the dimension of child health reflects the performance of behaviour change communication services. Table 7 suggests that the coverage index of the health care delivery system in the state is relatively the poorest in terms of behaviour change communication services but relatively the best in case of extension or child immunization services. However, when the coverage index is adjusted for the prevailing levels of female literacy and the standard of living index, the performance index turns zero in the maternal health and child immunization domains. Obviously, there is a very substantial scope of improving the performance of health care delivery system in the state to achieve the long cherished dream of universal health care and to accelerate the pace of health and mortality transition.

Table 7 *Coverage Index and Health System Performance Index in Madhya Pradesh*

Population	*Dimension of Health Care*	*Coverage Index*	*Performance Index*
Combined	All dimensions	46.35	0
	Maternal health	40.51	0
	Child Immunization	57.09	0
	Child health	34.60	6.47
Rural	All dimensions	42.37	0
	Maternal health	34.96	0
	Child Immunization	53.51	0
	Child health	33.31	6.36

Source: Chaurasia (2013)

The State response to addressing health and longevity issues facing the state is articulated in the state health policy which still remains a draft. This policy envisions that all people living in the state will have the knowledge and skills required to keep themselves healthy and will have equity in access to effective and affordable health care, as close to the family as possible, that enhances their quality of life, and enables them to lead a healthy productive life (Government of Madhya Pradesh, 2007). In order to realize this vision, the policy has aimed at:

1. Ensuring universal geographic and economic access to quality primary and secondary health care and family welfare services to all people of Madhya Pradesh within a span of five to seven years.
2. Prevention of disaster, to the extent possible, and preparedness for disaster management as and when necessary.
3. Reducing the risk of death due to complications of pregnancy and delivery – measured in terms of maternal mortality ratio – to 220 maternal deaths for every 1,00,000 live births by 2011 from the level of 498 (1997 level).
4. Reducing the risk of death during infancy – measured in terms of infant mortality rate – to 62 infant deaths for every 1,000 live births by 2011 from the level of 97 (1997 level).

Figure 6 *Progress in Selected Indicators of Mortality and Health in Madhya Pradesh, 1997–2011*

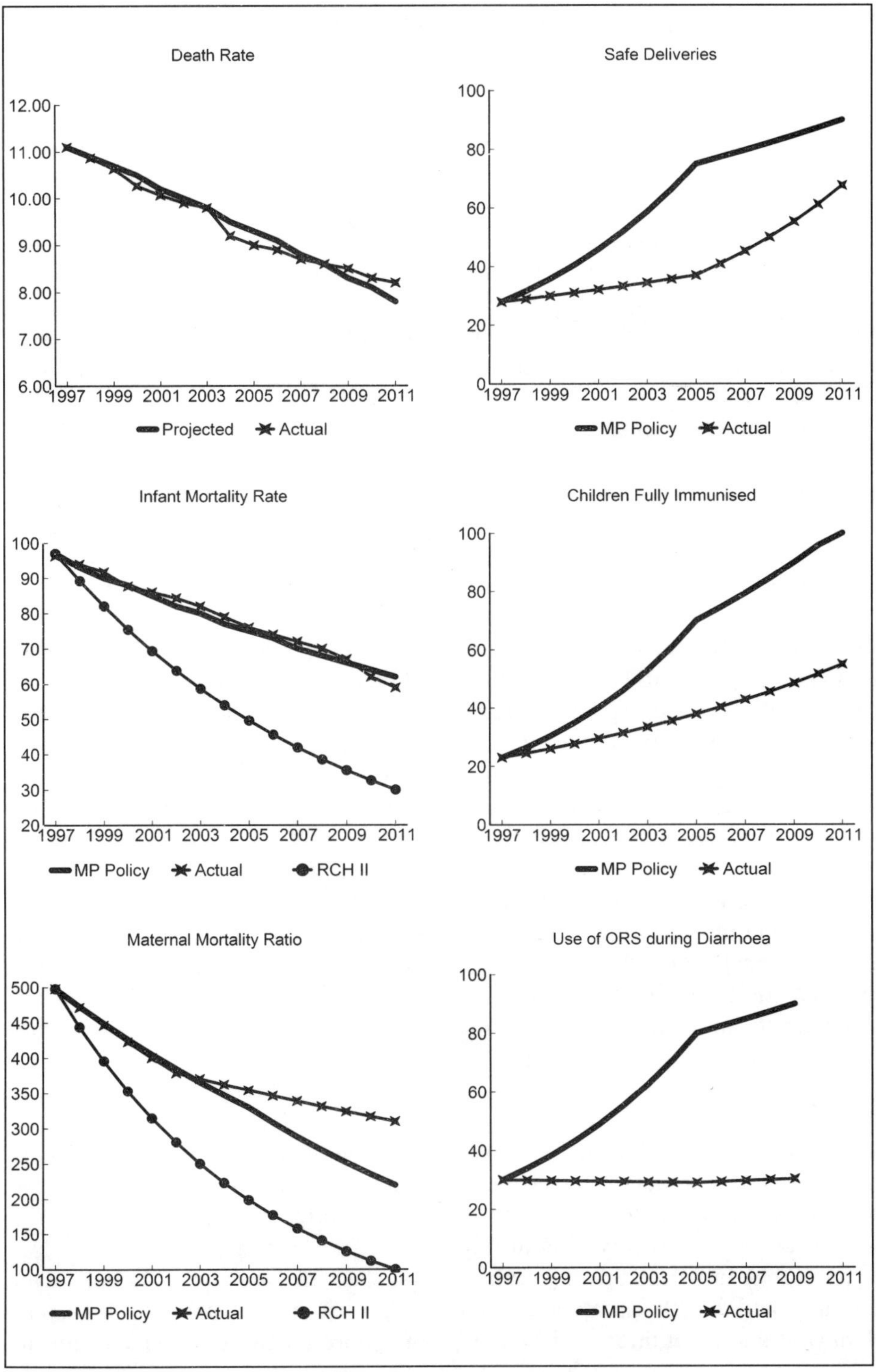

5. Reduction of the total fertility rate in a manner so as to reach the replacement level fertility (i.e. a TFR of 2.1) by the year 2011.
6. Stabilize the prevalence of HIV/AIDS at low level (present level) and further decrease it.
7. Address problems related to mental health care and initiate action to create information base and introduce preventive interventions for improved mental health situation in the state.

The state has also adopted the goals and objectives set under the National Rural Health Mission which was launched by the Government of India in 2005 and which aims at architectural corrections in the public health care delivery system and concomitant reduction in infant mortality rate, maternal mortality ratio and total fertility rate; prevention and control of communicable and non-communicable diseases; and revitalization of local health traditions. Madhya Pradesh was among the 18 priority states of the country under the Mission.

Interestingly, neither the draft state health policy nor the National Rural Health Mission focuses on health and mortality transition in the entire age spectrum. The analysis presented here indicates that mortality transition in males in the state has been substantially slower than the mortality transition in females. Moreover, mortality transition has been very slow in the age group 15–50 years, and in males, there has been virtually little transition over the last 35 years. However, these issues have not been addressed in the draft state health policy. Similarly, female mortality transition in the age group 50–70 years in the urban areas appears to have been slower than that in males and there are significant social class and regional differentials in mortality. The draft state health policy has, however, paid little attention to these issues.

Figure 6 presents the progress of the state against the stated goals and objectives of Madhya Pradesh Health Policy 2000 and the National Rural Health Mission. It is very much evident from the figure that the state lags behind in terms of the progress towards the goals and objectives of the National Rural Health Mission as well as in terms of universal access to health care. It is only in case of infant mortality rate that the progress conforms to what was visualized in the draft state health policy 2000, but this progress is significantly short of what has been envisaged in the National Rural Health Mission. Obviously, the reach of the health care delivery system in meeting the health care needs of the people is, at best, limited.

Conclusions

It is obvious from the analysis presented here that Madhya Pradesh has somehow not been able to meet the health needs of the people of the state – medical as well as non-medical – so that the transition in health and mortality has remained slow to very slow during the last 35–40 years. The analysis also suggests that substantial demographic, social class and regional differentials in mortality and health situation continue to persist in the state. As a result, Madhya Pradesh continues to be amongst the poorest states of India in terms of health and mortality. Persistence of poor health and mortality situation, incidentally, has implications for the social and economic development of the state and improvements in the quality of life of the people.

What are then the options for Madhya Pradesh? There is a need to reinvigorate the health care delivery system through user perspective and not through the provider perspective. Key initiatives that may be taken include but are not limited to:

- Evolve and institutionalize an information system that facilitates understanding the health needs of the people. This understanding should incorporate both medical and non-medical determinants of health and mortality.
- Promote local level collective health action by building the capacity of the people and their organizations to identify their health needs and initiate and sustain action to address these needs in an effective yet efficient manner.
- Support local level collective health action by creating and sustaining community partnerships for health care delivery especially by reaching out to non-traditional partners.
- Provide health system support to local collective health action by improving the availability, affordability and quality of specialized health care services either through the public or through the private health care delivery system.
- Develop policies and institutional capacity for regulating health care service delivery either through public or through private health care delivery system.
- Promote determinants of health research by establishing partnerships with research centres and academic institutions from within and outside the health sector directed towards increasing knowledge to support informed decision-making, especially at the local level.
- Create health disaster management network by involving the entire health care delivery system and the broadest possible inter-sectoral and inter-institutional collaboration and coordination to reduce the impact of emergencies and disasters on the health of the people.
- Revamp and expand the human resources development (education and training) network to develop a health workforce profile that is adequate in terms of knowledge and skills for the delivery of health care services necessary to meet the health needs of the people.
- Strengthen monitoring, evaluation and analysis of health status at the level of the individual and at the level of the community with especial emphasis on identifying inequalities or disparities in risks and threats to healthy lifestyle.

The key to accelerating health and mortality transition in Madhya Pradesh is an astute mix of substantive and formal health care. A focus on the formal, institution-based, health care alone has only limited potential in Madhya Pradesh.

References

Chaurasia, Aalok Ranjan. 2011. *Human Development and Population in India: The Case of Madhya Pradesh*. Bhopal: Shyam Institute.

——. 2012. The Challenge of Under-Nutrition in India. In Aalok Ranjan (ed.), *India 2011: Mortality, Health and Development*. Bhopal: MLC Foundation and Shyam Institute.

——. 2013. *India: Health System Performance Assessment*. Bhopal: MLC Foundation and Shyam Institute.

Edwards, R.D. and Tuljapurkar, S. 2005. Inequality in Life Spans and a New Perspective on Mortality Convergence across Industrialized Countries. *Population and Development Review*, 31 (4): 645–674.

Government of India. 1984. *SRS Based Abridged Life Tables 1970–75*. New Delhi: Registrar General and Census Commissioner.

——. 2012. *Annual Health Survey Fact Sheet 2010–11: Madhya Pradesh*. New Delhi: Registrar General and Census Commissioner of India.

Government of Madhya Pradesh. 2007. *Draft Health Policy*. Bhopal: Public Health and Family Welfare Department.

Kittagawa, E.M. 1966. Theoretical Considerations in the Selection of a Mortality Index and Some Empirical Comparisons. *Human Biology*, 38 (3): 293–308.

Schoen, R. 1970. The Geometric Mean of Age-Specific Death Rates as a Summary Index of Mortality. *Demography*, 7 (3): 317–324.

Shkolnikov, V., Andreev, E. and Begun, A.Z. 2003. Gini Coefficient as a Life Table Function: Computation from Discrete Data, Decomposition of Differences and Empirical Examples. *Demographic Research*, 8 (11): 305–358.

Shyrock, H.S. and Siegel, J.S. 1976. *The Methods and Materials of Demography*. New York: Academic Press.

Smits, J. and Monden, C. 2009. Length of Life Inequality around the Globe. *Social Science and Medicine*, 68 (6): 1114–1236.

United Nations. 2004. *World Population Projections: The 2004 Revision, Volume III: Analytical Report*. New York: United Nations.

——. 2004a. *World Population Prospects: The 2002 Revision, Volume III: Analytical Report*. New York: United Nations.

Vaupel, J.W. and Canudas Romo, V. 2003. Decomposing Change in Life Expectancy: A Bouquet of Formulas in Honour of Nathan Keyfitz's 90th Birthday. *Demography*, 40 (2): 201–216.

Vaupel, J.W., Zhang, Z. and van Raalte, A.A. 2011. Life Expectancy and Disparity: An International Comparison of Life Table Data. *British Medical Journal Open*, 1 (1).

Wilmoth, J.R. and Horiuchi, S. 1999. Rectangularization Revisited: Variability of Age at Death within Human Populations. *Demography*, 36 (4): 475–495.

Zhang, Z. and Vaupel, J.W. 2009. The Age Separating Early Deaths from Late Deaths. *Demographic Research*, 20 (29): 721–730.

8

Adult Male Mortality in Madhya Pradesh and Selected States of India

An Application of Widowhood Method

K.B. Gotpagar and Palani Murugesan

India still focuses largely on infant and child mortality (Arokiasamy, 2004; Bang, Reddy and Deshmukh, 2002; Claeson et al., 2000; Singh, et al., 2007; Singh, Mahapatra and Dutta, 2008; Whitworth and Stephenson, 2002). This focus is obviously due to considerably high levels of overall mortality during infancy and childhood. The infant mortality rate in India is 57 per 1,000 live births with huge variations across the different states from 73 per 1,000 live births in Uttar Pradesh to 15 per 1,000 live births in Kerala. Similarly, under-five mortality within India ranges between 96 per 1,000 live births in Uttar Pradesh and 16 per 1,000 live births in Kerala (IIPS and ORC Macro, 2007).

Unlike infant and child mortality, adult mortality has not received appropriate attention in India, but there is an urgent need for research in this area for numerous reasons. Firstly, the adult population aged, 15–59 in India is very large in both its absolute as well as its relative size. According to the 2001 Indian Census, with a population of 585 million, the adult population aged 15–59 years constitutes 57 per cent of India's total population. Calculations based on life tables derived from the Sample Registration System for the most recent period suggest that 89 per cent of newborns are likely to survive to age 15, but only 72 per cent of children aged 15 years are likely to survive to age 65 (Registrar General of India, 2008). In addition, the maternal mortality rate is very high in India at 212 maternal deaths per 100,000 live births for the period 2007–09 (Registrar General of India, 2011).

Estimation of premature adult deaths for small geographical units in a diverse country like India can be particularly beneficial for monitoring the achievement of different population and health-related policies such as the

National Population Policy of 2000, the National Health Policy of 2003 and the Millennium Development Goals. Such analysis gains special significance in the light of Millennium Development Goals 5 and 6, which attempt to reduce maternal mortality and mortality due to HIV/AIDS, tuberculosis, and malaria (District Level Household Survey round 3). This evidence clearly underscores the need for mortality estimation at local levels to correctly estimate the impact of infections that are at times highly localized in nature. Such an exercise is also likely to help local policymakers and programme managers formulate evidence-based interventions.

Need for the Study

A small of amount of research has been undertaken about the adult mortality in India. While a great deal has now been discovered about infant and child mortality, about their causes and underlying determinants and about the ways to prevent child death, not much is known about level, trend and differences in adult mortality. Hence, an attempt is made to find out the level and trend of adult mortality in India and some selected states.

Objectives of the Paper

(i) To examine the changes in adult mortality level summarized by the probability of dying between the ages 15 and 60 or ${}_{45}q_{15}$ in a standard life table notation using the recent Sample Registration System (SRS) abridged life table (i.e. from the period 1995–99 to 2006–10).

(ii) To examine the level and trend in adult mortality using the census marital status data in Madhya Pradesh, all-India and some selected states of India.

(iii) To compare the level and trend obtained by widowhood data with SRS based estimates.

(iv) To examine at the district level variation for adult mortality in Madhya Pradesh.

Methodology

The widowhood method for estimating adult mortality from information about the death of husbands and wives was first proposed by Hill and Truessell in 1977. Techniques were derived from estimating male adult mortality from reports of female respondents and vice-versa. The original method was subsequently revised by Hill and Truessell (1977) in order to remove the confounding effects of remarriage. Information used here is the survival of the first spouse, as it is an indicator of the adult mortality since the exposure to the risk of the target person begins in adulthood i.e. at the marriage of the respondent. The exact question in any survey should be 'is your first husband still alive?' This method seeks to estimate probabilities of survival of males from the age 20 to age n (n=25, 30, ..., 55, 60). Experience suggests that the most reliable information about the survival of the first spouse is provided by women and also remarriage rate is lower among widows than that of widowers in India, a fairly good means of estimating male mortality.

Data Required

The proportion of ever-married women in each five-year age group whose first husband was alive at the time of census (interview)

Proportion of ever-married males and females in each five year age group to compute singulate mean age at marriage for men ($SMAM_m$) and women ($SMAM_f$).

Steps of the Computational Procedure

Step-I

The proportion of female respondents not widowed in the age group from age n to n+5, denoted by NW_f (n), is equal to the ratio of the female respondents aged from n to n+5 whose first husbands were alive at the time of interview and the total number of ever-married female respondents aged from n to n+5 who declared survivorship status of their first husband.

Step-II

Calculation of Singulate Mean Age at Marriage (SMAM) for both males and females with the Hajnal method

$$SMAM_m = \frac{15 + 5\Sigma_5 S_x - k * s_k}{1 - S_k},$$

where ${}_5S_x$ is the proportion single in the age group x to x+5

K is the maximum age up to which marriage occurs (in the present study k is taken as 50)

$$\text{where } S_k = \frac{{}_5S_{k-5} + {}_5S_k}{2}.$$

Step-III

Calculation of survivorship probabilities. The regression model proposed for calculating survivorship probability is:

$$l_m^{(n)}/l_m^{(20)} = a(n) + b(n) * SMAM_f + c(n)*SMAM_m + d(n) * NW_f(n-5)$$

where a(n), b(n), c(n), and d(n) are coefficients and NW* (n–5), the proportion of ever-married females aged n to n+4 not widowed.

$NW_f(n-5)$ is considered because it has been mentioned that wives are five years younger to husbands.

Step-IV

Calculation of number of years before the census/survey to which survivorship probabilities refer; in case where mortality has been changing regularly during the 15 or 20 years proceedings, the survey estimates of time, t(n) will be;

$$t_m(n) = (n - 2.5\ SMAM_f)\ (1.0 - u_m(n))/2.0$$

where $u_m(n) = 0.33333\ln NW_f(n\text{–}5) + Z(SMAM_m + n - 2.5 - SMSM_f) + 0.0037 * (27.0 - SMAM_m)$

where Z values are given in Table 88 in UN Manual X.

Step-V

Calculation of expectation of life at age 20, corresponding to $l_m^{(n)}/l_m^{(20)}$ using South Asian Life Table Pattern and 'West' model life table system (Coale and Demeny, 1966; UNs, 1982).

The estimated regression coefficients a(n), b(n), c(n) and d(n) in step-III have been estimated by regression of simulated data. The details of the computational procedure are given in United Nations Manual X(UN, 1983).

Model Life Tables are the tabular representations of the age patterns of mortality and present all the life table functions for populations at a particular 'level' of mortality (Preston, et al., 2000). Studies have shown that the UN South Asian Model Life Table System and West Model Life Table System are most suitable for examining levels and trends in India (Bhat, 1998; Parsuraman, 1990; Ram, 1984). It is to be mentioned here that,

(i) The estimation of adult mortality using information on widowhood is applicable in populations in which marriage is almost universal,

  (i) Marriage is a clearly defined event.

  (ii) Mortality does not vary significantly by marital status. In developed countries, a high risk of mortality among unmarried compared to married women was found by Humer et al. (1998).

Since there is no systematic and scientific evidence on differential mortality experience in India, we assume that the third assumption should not induce bias in the estimates presented here.

Levels and Trends of Adult Mortality

Table 1 presents the adult mortality level summarized by ${}_{45}q_{15}$ using the SRS abridged life table for the recent period (2006–10) by sex and selected Indian states. The range of values is wide, from a minimum of 176 per 1,000 males in the state of Kerala to a maximum of 292 for Assam, which as not only highest male mortality but it has also had highest female mortality (224). In general ${}_{45}q^f_{15} < {}_{45}q^m_{15}$.

Table 1 *Probabilities of Dying Between Ages 15 and 60 (${}_{45}q_{15}$) by Sex for Sixteen Major States of India, 2006–10*

Name of the States	*Male*	*Female*
Andhra Pradesh	0.265	0.163
Assam	0.292	0.224
Bihar	0.198	0.172

Cont'd...

...Cont'd

Gujarat	0.232	0.140
Haryana	0.190	0.124
Himachal Pradesh	0.214	0.114
Karnataka	0.252	0.150
Kerala	0.176	0.077
Maharashtra	0.217	0.125
Madhya Pradesh	0.248	0.168
Orissa (now Odisha)	0.240	0.189
Punjab	0.233	0.131
Rajasthan	0.203	0.121
Tamil Nadu	0.227	0.137
Uttar Pradesh	0.244	0.176
West Bengal	0.195	0.135
India	0.229	0.152

Source: SRS Based Abridged Life Tables 2003–07 to 2006–10.
SRS Analytical Studies, Report No.1 of 2012.

Table 2 shows the trend in adult mortality by sex rural, urban and total for Madhya Pradesh, Kerala and India. Madhya Pradesh reveals a considerably higher adult male mortality in rural as well as in urban areas, in both the time period (i.e. in 1995–99 and 2006–10). Even though adult mortality has declined during 1995–99 to 2006–10, but the decline is not much significant (both for male and female). The percentage of decline for male and female in case of Madhya Pradesh being 12.1 and 28.8 percentage respectively, as compared to corresponding figure of 10.7 and 18.08 for Kerala.

Table 2 *Probabilities of Dying Between Ages 15 and 60 ${}_{45}q_{15}$ by Sex, Rural, Urban and Total for the State of Kerala, Madhya Pradesh and India, 2001*

States		*1995–99*		*2006–10*	
		Male	*Female*	*Male*	*Female*
Madhya Pradesh	T	0.282	0.236	0.248	0.168
	R	0.285	0.239	0.238	0.162
	U	0.226	0.222	0.207	0.106
Kerala	T	0.197	0.094	0.176	0.077
	R	0.202	0.099	0.180	0.080
	U	0.182	0.079	0.162	0.068
India	T	0.256	0.200	0.229	0.152
	R	0.266	0.212	0.238	0.162
	U	0.182	0.161	0.207	0.125

To assess the quality of NFHS–2 data on adult mortality for India and its major states, Saikia (2006) constructed life table for male and female separately using NFHS–2 data. The adult age-specific death rates for the life table have been calculated by applying the technique of Lexis diagram to back project usual resident age-sex structure for two years ago to the date of survey. Table 3 (borrowed from Saikia and Ram 2010) presents ${}_{45}q_{15}$ obtained from NFHS–2 and SRS, indicates a high level of concordance of adult mortality between these two sources. The main findings from the above table is given below:

(i) At the national level, ${}_{45}q_{15}$ (NFHS) > ${}_{45}q_{15}$ (SRS), both for males (12%) and females (20%).

(ii) Coverage of female deaths in NFHS seems to be better in almost all states.

(iii) Coverage of adult male mortality i.e. ${}_{45}q^{m}{}_{15}$ in Assam, Haryana, Kerala and Orissa (Odisha) in SRS is better than the NFHS.

Table 3 *Comparison of ${}_{45}q_{15}$ from NFHS–2 and SRS at National and Sub-national Level, India*

State/Country	*1998 Male*			*1998 Female*		
	NFHS–2	*SRS*	*Ratio = NFHS–2/SRS*	*NFHS–2*	*SRS*	*Ratio = NFHS–2/SRS*
Andhra Pradesh	0.32	0.28	1.11	0.25	0.20	1.23
Assam	0.28	0.32	0.89	0.31	0.29	1.06
Bihar	0.31	0.25	1.25	0.31	0.25	1.23
Gujarat	0.27	0.25	1.09	0.23	0.17	1.34
Haryana	0.19	0.24	0.79	0.17	0.16	1.07
Karnataka	0.30	0.27	1.09	0.20	0.18	1.10
Kerala	0.14	0.20	0.71	0.09	0.09	0.96
Madhya Pradesh	0.31	0.29	1.05	0.29	0.74	1.20
Maharashtra	0.25	0.24	1.02	0.22	0.16	1.35
Orissa (Odisha)	0.26	0.29	0.91	0.29	0.25	1.14
Punjab	0.23	0.24	0.95	0.17	0.17	0.98
Rajasthan	0.27	0.25	1.12	0.20	0.16	1.28
Tamil Nadu	0.35	0.26	1.31	0.20	0.18	1.08
Uttar Pradesh	0.32	0.27	1.25	0.24	0.22	1.07
West Bengal	0.24	0.23	1.04	0.19	0.19	0.97
India	0.29	0.26	1.12	0.24	0.20	1.19

Source: Nandita Saikia and Ram F., Determinants of Adult Mortality in India, *Asian Population Studies*, Vol. 6, No. 2, July 2010, p. 159.

One of the assumption of the widowhood method is that the information should be collected from the first spouse, but due to increasing rate of remarriage the estimate might be affected. As regards to adjustment for remarriages, some researchers such as Malaker (1986) and Bhat (1998) have made earlier attempt to estimate adult mortality in India. Malakar (1986) first attempted to estimate adult mortality in India using the 1971 and 1981 Census data. He further extended his study to examine district level variation in adult mortality in West Bengal (Malakar and Crook, 1989). It was found that the widowhood method gives consistent estimates of adult mortality for males. However, the female adult mortality were severely underestimated. There is a general agreement supported by social surveys that the incidence of remarriage among the widowed is higher among the Muslim population and generally higher for men than for women, men usually remarrying younger women. Bhat (1998) further found that the estimates of male adult mortality using widowhood data from women below age 40 were less acceptable than those obtained from widowhood data from women over age 40, which is simply because of high rates of remarriage among young widows. Bhat and Kanbargi (1984) estimated proportion of ever married population using adult mortality and age at marriage information by inverting the widowhood method. The difference between the estimated proportion of ever-married and currently widowed directly obtained from the census demonstrates that the percentage of ever married among ever widowed in India was 34 in 1971. During the recent periods, the widow remarriage rates must have gone up significantly. Even though we do not have a clear evidence, the widow remarriages are likely to go up.

Table 4 presents the percentages of women married more than once by age group during the three rounds of NFHS for Madhya Pradesh, Kerala, Punjab and India. The state level trend in remarriage rates among women show very negligible fluctuations over time. The table clearly shows a slight variation in remarriages among women in India and selected states. The maximum change for all women aged 15–49 among states under study is in Punjab with an increase of 1.3 per cent (from 0.90 to 2.21%).

Table 4 *Percentage of Women Aged 45–49 who Married more than Once from NFHS-1, 2 and 3, Madhya Pradesh and Selected States of India*

Age Group	*Madhya Pradesh*			*Kerala*			*Punjab*			*India*		
	NFHS			*NFHS*			*NFHS*			*NFHS*		
	1	*2*	*3*	*1*	*2*	*3*	*1*	*2*	*3*	*1*	*2*	*3*
15–19	0.90	0.67	0.34	0.60	1.18	0.00	0.00	0.00	0.00	0.63	0.64	0.65
20–24	2.26	2.17	1.02	2.18	0.55	0.66	0.76	0.00	0.46	1.24	1.25	1.24
25–29	3.60	2.26	1.68	2.63	1.45	1.22	0.82	1.06	0.92	1.83	1.65	2.10
30–34	2.94	2.81	2.84	2.88	2.07	1.17	0.54	0.36	3.04	2.12	1.92	2.48
35–39	3.13	3.14	1.85	3.15	3.26	3.28	1.33	1.46	3.70	2.16	2.42	2.72
40–44	2.45	2.73	2.29	3.40	3.79	3.52	1.07	1.78	3.29	2.27	2.29	2.52
45–49	1.75	1.99	1.42	4.62	4.45	4.51	1.45	0.00	2.33	2.20	2.18	2.83
Total	2.54	2.28	1.77	2.95	2.53	2.38	0.90	0.00	2.21			

Levels and Trends of Male Adult Mortality

Table 5 shows the estimated probabilities from age 20 to age n. These probabilities are further converted into life expectancy at age 20 by using 'South Asian Model Life Table System' (UN, 1983). Studies have shown that the UN South Asian Model Life Table System and Coale and Demeny (1966) West Model Life Table Systems are most suitable for examining mortality levels and trends (Bhat, 1998; Parasuraman, 1990; Ram, 1984). We present the survivorship probabilities ($l_m^{(n)}/l_m^{(20)}$) as well as life expectancy at age 20 in Table 5. However in Table 6 and 7 we give only $e^0_{20}(m)$ instead of male survivorship probabilities ($l_m^{(20)}/l_m^{(n)}$) for better understanding as life expectancy is a more often used indicator of mortality than the survivorship function. Estimates obtained from

Table 5 *Estimation of Male Survivorship Probabilities and $e^0_{20}{}^{(m)}$ Derived from First Husband, Madhya Pradesh, 2001*

Age Group	Age i	Total			Rural			Urban		
		$l_m^{(n)}/l_m^{(20)}$	$e^0_{20}{}^{(m)}$	Reference date	$l_m^{(n)}/l_m^{(20)}$	$e^0_{20}{}^{(m)}$	Reference date	$l_m^{(n)}/l_m^{(20)}$	$e^0_{20}{}^{(m)}$	Reference date
20–24	25	0.9911	48.4	September 99	0.9921	49.1	April 99	0.9983	46.5	July 2000
25–29	30	0.9866	50.8	June 97	0.9883	51.7	February 97	0.9816	48.9	April 98
30–34	35	0.9783	51.1	March 95	0.9807	51.8	November 94	0.9714	49.3	Jan 96
35–39	40	0.9628	50.5	January 93	0.9648	50.9	September 92	0.9558	49.4	November 93
40–44	45	0.9374	49.9	March 91	0.9399	50.2	November 90	0.9290	49.0	December 91
45–49	50	0.9129	50.6	September 89	0.9163	50.9	June 89	0.9011	49.6	June 90
50–54	55	0.8353	48.8	May 88	0.8377	48.9	January 88	0.8234	48.1	December 88
55–59	60	0.8482	LT20.0	January 88	0.8541	LT20.0	October 870	0.8201	LT20.0	May 88
		$SMAM_m$		23.00	$SMAM_m$		21.90	$SMAM_m$		25.40
		$SMAM_f$		19.10	$SMAM_f$		18.30	$SMAM_f$		21.10

Note: Estimates are obtained using South Asian Model Life Table Pattern of Model Life Table.

young widows aged 20–24 were close to recent periods. Estimates of life expectancy at age 20 (e^0_{20}(m)) obtained from young widows were much higher than those obtained from old widows. For example, in Rural Madhya Pradesh, e_{20} obtained from widows aged 25–29 was 51.7 in 1997, whereas the same from widows aged 50–54 was 48.9.

While estimating the proportion of widowed in 1991 by fitting regression on proportion widowed in 1961, 1971, 1981 and 2001 data, Saikia (2010) found that the new estimate from the estimated 1991 Census are consistent with e^0_{20} from other censuses, and the trends obtained from age group 30–34, 35–39 and 40–44 show very close patterns to the SRS trend of e^0_{20}. The trend obtained from 45–49 concurs with the SRS trend of e^0_{20} during 1970–75 to 1986–90. Mortality estimates derived from age group 45–49 and 50–54 appear to be best for application of widowhood method. In view of this, we present estimate of e^0_{20} from age groups 45–49 for rest of the two tables (i.e. Table 6 and 7).

Table 6 *Estimates of Male e^{20} from Widowhood Method * and their Comparison with the SRS Estimates, India, 1990*

Name of the States	*Widowhood 1990*	*SRS 1993*	*Difference*
	1	*2*	*3 = (1) – (2)*
Andhra Pradesh	47.7	47.1	0.6
Assan	46.6	45.4	1.2
Bihar	53.0	48.0	5.0
Gujarat	49.0	47.1	1.9
Kerala	49.1	50.9	–1.8
Maharashtra	48.8	48.8	0.0
Madhya Pradesh	50.6	47.2	3.4
Orissa (Odisha)	48.9	47.7	1.2
Rajasthan	50.7	47.2	3.5
Tamil Nadu	47.1	47.6	–0.5
Uttar Pradesh	52.0	47.3	4.7
West Bengal	47.9	48.7	–0.8
India	49.3	47.6	1.7

Note: *Widowhood estimates calculated from 45–49 age groups using South Asian Model Life Table and refers to 1990.

SRS estimates are obtained averaging SRS Abridged Life Tables for the period 1986–90 and 1991–95.

Tables 6 and 7 presents the male e^0_{20} from widowhood method and their comparison with the SRS estimates for India and major states. The SRS estimates refer to 1983 and 1993, whereas widowhood estimate refer to 1978 and 1990. It is evident from Table 6 that the widowhood estimates e^0_{20} for male were higher than the official SRS estimates of e^0_{20} and the maximum difference was found in Bihar (5.0) followed by Uttar Pradesh (4.7), and Rajasthan (3.5). In these states, there may be various reasons for a different patterns, such as possibility of under-enumeration of widows beyond age 45–49 in censuses, high digit preference at age 50 among the widows and choice of remarriage rate among the widows. The actual widow remarriage rates in these states may be higher than the marriage rates assumed. In Maharashtra, both the sources are close to each other. Except Bihar, Madhya Pradesh, Rajasthan and Uttar Pradesh, widowhood estimates of e^0_{20} either coincides or are very close to SRS for the recent periods. These are the states which are marked by highest levels of remarriages. Agarwala (1967) in a study of Rural Northern India found that the widow remarriage is about 80 to 90 per cent among widows under age 19 and the remarriage rates ranged between 19 per cent in Mathura district of Uttar Pradesh to 38 per cent in Delhi in early Sixties. Driver's (1963) study reveals that among the states, the remarriage rate varied between 9 per cent in Orissa (Odisha) to 38 per cent in Central India.

Table 7 *Estimates of Male Adult Mortality Measured by $e^0_{20}{}^{(m)}$ with and Without Adjustment for Remarriage Data, India, 1980–1990*

Name of the States	*$e^0_{20}{}^{(m)*}$ 1990*		*$e^0_{20}{}^{(m)}$ 1978*	
	With Adjustment for Remarriage⁺	*Without Adjustment for Remarriage**	*With Adjustment for Remarriage⁺*	*SRS Without Adjustment for Remarriage**
Andhra Pradesh	47.5	47.7	45.4	44.9
Assan	45.9	46.6	45.0	43.1
Bihar	51.8	53.0	49.2	NA
Gujarat	46.0	49.0	44.9	45.5
Kerala**	49.4	49.1	47.8	49.2
Maharashtra	47.3	48.8	45.7	46.1
Madhya Pradesh	49.1	50.6	46.3	45.8
Orissa (Odisha)	47.6	48.9	45.6	44.1
Rajasthan	50.0	50.7	49.1	46.3
Tamil Nadu	46.6	47.1	44.6	46.0
Uttar Pradesh	50.6	52.0	49.7	46.0
West Bengal	46.2	47.9	43.8	NA
India	47.8	49.3	46.3	45.8

Note: * Calculated from age group 45–49 using South Asian Model Life Table
** For Kerala, remarriage data has not adjusted
+ Nandita Saikia, 2010 'Adult Mortality in India: Levels, Trends, Determinants and Causes', unpublished Ph.D. Thesis submitted to IIPS, 2010, p. 180.

In Table 7 we have compared the estimates of male adult mortality with and without adjustment for remarriage. Columns 1 and 2 refers to 1990 whereas in column 3 and 4 we have compared SRS estimates of 1978 to those of widowhood estimates derived after adjusting for remarriage and which refers to 1983. The table clearly shows that in general, the life expectancy at age 20 i.e. e^0_{20} is generally lower for population where there is adjustment for remarriage than e^0_{20} when the data is not adjusted for remarriage. When we compare the e^0_{20} values at two points of time (refer to column 1 and 3), we found that at national level male life expectancy at age 20 increased by 1.5 years during 1980–90, the maximum gain in e^0_{20} was found in Gujarat (3 years) and the least among Andhra Pradesh followed by Kerala.

Table 8 *Estimates of Mortality Levels ($e^0_{20}{}^{(m)}$) from Widowhood Method* for Districts of Madhya Pradesh, 2001*

Name of the District	*($e^0_{20}(m)$)*	*Reference Date*	$_5q_0$**
Sheopur	51.0	April 1989	136
Morena	52.1	June 1989	108
Bhind	52.6	July 1989	84
Gwalior	50.3	February 1990	83
Datia	51.2	July 1989	134
Shivpuri	51.6	May 1989	143
Guna	52.5	July1989	151
Tikamgarh	52.8	April 1989	132
Chhatarpur	48.8	January 1989	141
Panna	51.9	July 1989	172
Sagar	50.8	October 1989	136
Damoh	50.4	August 1989	151
Satna	51.1	June 1989	158
Rewa	52.5	January 1989	131
Umaria	50.2	May 1989	160
Shahdol	49.2	May 1989	146
Sidhi	51.9	March 1989	128
Neemuch	50.3	May 1989	107
Mandsaur	50.6	April 1989	114
Ratlam	49.1	June 1989	140
Ujjain	50.0	June 1989	114
Shajapur	51.1	February 1989	111
Dewas	51.6	June 1989	131
Jhabua	50.3	September 1989	149
Dhar	50.3	August 1989	113
Indore	50.4	February 1990	66
West Nimar	50.9	September 1989	115
Barwani	50.8	July 1989	138
East Nimar	49.3	November 1989	130
Rajgarh	52.2	March 1989	134
Vidisha	51.4	October 1989	158
Bhopal	50.3	July 1990	90
Seore	51.7	August 1989	126
Raisen	52.5	December 1989	121
Betul	50.6	June 1990	127
Harda	49.4	March 1990	153
Houshangabad	50.0	March 1990	146
Katni	49.5	June 1989	187
Jabalpur	49.3	July 1990	116
Narsimhapur	51.1	December 1989	115
Dindori	48.7	July 1989	150
Mandla	48.0	October 1989	157
Chhindwara	48.9	April 1989	121
Seoni	48.6	January 1990	116
Balaghat	47.5	March 1990	131
Madhya Pradesh	50.6	September 1989	128

Note: * Calculated from age group 45–49 using South Asian Model Life Table
** District Level Estimates of Child Mortality in India based on 2001 Census data, RG India, New Delhi.

Results from Districts of Madhya Pradesh

District level analysis shows that there is a range of five years (Max-Min = 52.8–47.5) of life expectancy at age 20. The same value of all over Madhya Pradesh is 50.6 taking September 1989 as the reference date, which leads to the conclusion that the mortality pattern of Madhya Pradesh is not equally distributed among different districts but this may not be true because if we closely examine the geographical position, then it is possible to see that more equal level of mortality estimates are obtained for geographically and culturally adjacent districts.

In order to see whether child mortality is an indicator of adult mortality, we calculated Pearsonian Correlation Coefficient between $q^m{}_5$ and $e^0{}_{20}(m)$, and the same is found to be negative (–0.115) and insignificant. Existing literature proves that child mortality and adult mortality can vary independently so that $e^0{}_0$ and infant mortality rate (IMR) may not be significant indicator of adult mortality since the determinants of these two types of mortality are different. For example, in determinants of child mortality, where infections and parasitic diseases are predominant, the impact of environmental contamination is very high. But in case of adult mortality where chronic diseases predominate, the likelihood of death from environmental contamination is minimal. While medical innovations may lead to lower levels of adult mortality, their influence on infant and child mortality will be limited in the absence of significant socio-economic development, especially rising living standards and adult literacy.

Summary and Conclusions

According to World Health Organization (WHO) report that orders adult death rate in 2001, India ranked third highest among all South Asian countries, next only to Myanmar and Nepal. The probability of survival from exact age 15 to 60 in India is for lower than that of developed countries like United States, Japan and also well below that of Sri Lanka. Research in adult mortality in India is scarce than those of infant and child mortality due to paucity of data. The present paper presents in the first section, the estimates of adult mortality level summarized by the probability of dying between the exact ages 15 and 60, i.e. ${}_{45}q_{15}$ during 1995–99 to 2006–10 by sex and residence of Madhya Pradesh and selected states of India. The range of values is wide, from a minimum of 77 per 1,000 for females in Kerala in 2006–10 to a maximum of 292 per 1,000 for males in Assam. The corresponding expectation of life at age 10, i.e. e_{10} are 68.1 and 59.5 respectively (SRS, 2010).

In the second section, the paper describes the application of widowhood method of estimation of male adult mortality only to 1991 Census data for Madhya Pradesh and selected states of India with and without adjustment for remarriage data. Mortality rates derived from data on women of age 45–49 and also 50–54 appear to be better than those based on other age groups, but these too underestimates adult mortality in comparison to the SRS estimates of $e^0{}_{20}$ which indicates considerably high rates of widow remarriage. It was observed that except for a few states such as Bihar, Rajasthan, Uttar Pradesh and West Bengal, the difference in e^0_{20}(m) between widowhood and SRS is even less than one year. According to widowhood estimate, Assam experiences highest adult mortality (e^0_{20} is 45.9 years), whereas Bihar experiences least adult mortality (i.e. e^0_{20} $^{(m)}$ is 51.8 years). Estimates obtained from this method reliably depict the changes in mortality differential over time and place.

In the last part, an attempt is made to study the district-wise variation of adult mortality in Madhya Pradesh, which shows that there is a range of five years of life expectancy at age 20. The same value of all over Madhya Pradesh is 50.6 taking September 1989 as the reference data which leads to the conclusion that the mortality level of Madhya Pradesh is not equally distributed among districts. The Pearsonian Correlation Coefficient between $q^m{}_5$ and e^0_{20}(m) was found to be negative (–0.115) and insignificant.

It is worthwhile considering quantification effect on our estimate using the widowhood method for degree of remarriage. Remarriage imparts an upward bias on survival if the respondent reports her widowhood status in relation to the most recent marriage. For the sake of illustration let us assume that in the age group 30–34, 20 per cent of the widowed women have remarried and reported as 'married' rather than as 'widowed'. As a result, suppose 97 per cent of the women in this age group are recorded as not widowed, rather than the true 96 per cent. Using the Princeton West Model Life Tables (Coale and Demeny, 1966) we would estimate the survival level to be 19.7, when in fact the true level is 18.5. That is to say, we overestimate the male survival level by 1.2 levels. If, however, remarriage rates were 10 per cent in this age group at this level of mortality, the overestimation would be 0.6 level. This type of simulation, is however, sensitive to the model life table used. The details of the simulation exercise have been presented in the Appendix.

It has been shown in some Western countries, mortality among the widowed is higher than that of the general population. If this is so, we will again overestimate the survival level. We have, unfortunately no evidence in India to help us with this problem.

Appendix

Effect of Remarriage on Survival Levels and Life Expectancy in Estimation of Adult Mortality by Widowhood Method

Let T and R be the true and reported proportions never-widowed out of ever-married (considering the survival of the first spouse) in an age group; P = proportion of the widowed who remarry. Thus,

$R = 1 - (1-T)\ (1-P)$

$\therefore T = (R-P)/(1-P)$

In the following table calculations have been shown on widowhood for females from the 1981 Census of Kerala with three different values of P namely, .1, .2 and .3.

← *Proportion Not Widowed: NW_f (n–5)*

Age Group	*R*	*T*		
		P = 0.1	*P = 0.2*	*P = 0.3*
30–34	.9653	.9614	.9566	.9504
35–39	.9350	.9278	.9188	.9071
40–44	.8838	.8709	.8548	.8340

Mortality Levels (West Model)

Age n	*T*			
	R	*P = 0.1*	*P = 0.2*	*P = 0.3*
35	19.7	19.1	18.5	17.7
40	18.8	18.1	17.3	16.4
45	17.7	16.8	14.9	14.5
Average	18.7	18.0	16.9	16.2
e^0_0(m)	60.5	58.8	56.2	54.6

Note: 1. The mortality levels are based on $l_m(n)/l_m(20)$ values.
2. If we allow for 10 to 20 per cent of remarriage among widowhood females, the range of life expectancy at birth will be 56.2 to 58.8 years for the decade 1971–81.

References

Agarwala, S.N. 1967. Widow Remarriages in Some Rural Areas of Northern India. *Demography*, 4(1): 126–134.

Arokiasamy, P. 2004. Regional Patterns of Sex Bias and Excess Female Child Mortality in India. *Population*, 59 (6): 831–863.

Bang, A., Reddy, M.H. and Deshmukh, M.D. 2002. Child Mortality in Maharashtra. *Economic and Political Weekly*, 37 (49): 4947–4965.

Bhat, P.N.M. and Kanbargi, R. 1984. Estimating Incidence of Widow and Widower Remarriages in India from Census Data. *Population Studies*, 38 (1): 89–103.

Bhat, P.N.M. 1998. Demographic Estimates of Post-Independence India: A New Integration. *Demography India*, 27 (1): 23–37.

Claeson, M., Bos, E.R., Mawji, T., and Pathmanathan, I. 2000. Reducing Child Mortality in India in the New Millennium. *Bulletin of the World Health Organization*, 78 (10): 1192–1199.

Coale, A.J. and Demeny, P. 1966. *Regional Model Life Tables and Stable Populations*. Princeton: Princeton University Press.

Driver, E.D. 1963. *Differential Fertility in Central India*. Princeton: Princeton University Press.

Hill, K. and Trussell, J. 1977. Further Development in Indirect Mortality Estimation. *Population Studies*, 31 (2): 313–333.

Hummer, R.A., Rogers, R.G., and Eberstein, I.W. 1998. Socio-economic Differentials in Adult Mortality: A Review of Analytic Approaches. *Population and Development Review*, 24 (3): 553–579.

IIPS and ORC Macro. 2007. National Family Health Survey 2005–2006, India. Mumbai: International Institute for Population Sciences.

Malaker, C.R. 1986. Estimation of Adult Mortality in India: 1971–81. *Demography in India,* 15 (1): 126–135.

Malaker, C.R. and Crook, N.R. 1989. Use of Widowhood Data for Investigation of Mortality Differentials in West Bengal: A District Level Analysis. *Demography India,* 18, 121–129.

Parasuraman, S. 1990. Age Patterns of Mortality in India. In: Srinivasan, K. and Pathak, K.B. (ed.) *Dynamics of Population and Family Welfare,* Mumbai: Himalaya Publishing House.

Preston, S. Heuveline, P. and Guillot, M. 2000. *Demography: Measuring and Modeling Population Processes,* Wiley-Blackwell.

Ram, F. 1984. Some Contribution Onwards the Estimation of Vital Rates from Incomplete Data (PhD thesis). Bombay University, Mumbai.

Register General of India. 2008. SRS Abridged Life Tables 2002–2006. New Delhi: Registrar Government of India. [electronic resources]. Page 25 http://cghr.org/publication/causes_of_death_2001-03_20 RGI_CGHR.pdf.

Register General of India. 2010. Special Bulletin on Maternal Mortality in India 2007–2009. http://www.censusindia.gove.in/vital_statistics/SRS_Bulletins/Final-MR%20Bulletin-2007-09_070711.pdf.

Registrar General of India. 2009. Report on Causes of Death in India, 2001–2003: Sample Registration System, New Delhi: Registrar General of India.

Registrar General of India. 2011. Special Bulletin on Maternal Mortality in India 2007–2009. New Delhi: Registrar General of India.

Registrar General of India. 2012. SRS Based Abridged Life Tables 2003–07 to 2006–10, SRS Analytical Studies, Report No. 1 of 2012, New Delhi: Registrar General of India.

Saikia, N. 2006. Level and Trend of Adult Male Mortality: Application of Widowhood Method of India and Sixteen Major States and Districts of Assam (Term Paper, Master of Population Studies), International Institute for Population Sciences, Mumbai, 2006.

Saikia, N. and Ram, F. 2010. Determinants of Adult Mortality in India, *Asian Population Studies*. 6 (2): 159–171.

Singh, A., Mahapatra, B. and Dutta, S. 2008. Spousal Violence and Infant and Child Mortality in India. *Asia Pacific Population Journal*. 23 (2): 33–54.

Singh, A., Hazra, A., and Ram, F. 2007. Women's Autonomy and Sex Differential in Child Mortality in India. *Genus*. LXIII (3–4): 55–75.

Whitworth, A. and Stephenson, R. 2002. Birth Spacing, Sibling Rivalry and Child Mortality in India. *Social Science and Medicine.* 55 (12): 2107–19.

United Nations (UN). 1983. *Manual X Indirect Techniques for Demographic Estimation*. New York. NY: United Nations Publications.

9

Type II Diabetes

Trends in Prevalence, Popular Response and Level of Care in India

Arutselvi Devarajan

Non-Communicable Diseases (NCDs) account for approximately 53 per cent of the deaths in the country.[1] One of the major growing diseases among non-communicable disease is Type II diabetes. It is noted that 85 per cent to 95 per cent of all diabetes in high-income countries is Type II diabetes. It contributes for an even higher percentage in low and middle-income countries. The worldwide prevalence of Type II diabetes is estimated to be 8.5 per cent in 2011, affecting 366 million people and is expected to increase to 8.9 per cent in 2030, affecting 522 million people. Next to China in Western Pacific Region, India has ranked second in the prevalence of diabetes, affecting 61.3 (9.16%) million people and it accounts for 85 per cent of people with diabetes in South-East Asia Region. It is likely to increase to 101.1(9.57%) million in 2030. This information is pertaining to the people who are in the age group of 20 to 79 years. About half (56.5%) of the people living with diabetes are in the age group of 40 to 59 years.[2]

But in India there is a wider variation across the regions and across states and districts too in terms of demography, health, economic indicators.[3] With increasing urbanization in India, combined with nutrition transition, increasing life expectancy, physical inactivity and consumption of unhealthy and unbalanced diet, the environmental factors have played an important role in the occurrence of non-communicable diseases like diabetes. India's economic growth also indirectly paves the way to promote increase in number of diabetes cases, through increase of middle classes, unequal distribution of resources, mechanization and sedentary nature of work.[4] There is also call for action by the United Nations to combat NCDs at larger levels.[5] With understanding of this broader picture, it is important to look into the continuous process from the onset to management of chronic disease like diabetes from individual to population level to policy level for better insights to understand the subject in a comprehensive manner. Hence with this background, I intend to explore the answers for the following broad research objectives:

Objectives

- To understand the prevalence of Type II diabetes and its trends in India.
- To study the popular responses towards Type II diabetes by different stakeholders.
- To study the level of diabetes care in India.

Method

This is an exploratory research done through systematic review of available literature. The review papers on epidemiology of diabetes in India are considered important to understand the history of diabetes, its prevalence and its trends. Some of the papers cited in these review articles are also considered for better understanding. The key words (concepts) – epidemiology, prevalence, trends, complications, patterns of treatment, co-morbidity, cost of illness, accessibility, availability and affordability with diabetes and India as conjunctions are interchangeably used to search literature in the search engine, Pub Med and other publishing houses like Springer link, Science Direct. The national and international data base and other publishing houses are also used for the search to address the second and third research objectives. The key words like intervention, care, policies, programmes, treatment guidelines, cost of illness, clinical trials along with India and Type II diabetes are interchangeably used to gather information. The important national and international data sources like Indian Council for Medical Research (ICMR), National Institute of Health and Family Welfare (NIHFW), World Health Organization (WHO), International Diabetes Federation (IDF), World Diabetes Foundation (WDF), India Census, Associations of Physicians of India (API) are used. The information on clinical trials is taken from the National Institutes of Health data source as our Clinical trials of India registry was established in the year 2007. To understand the major community based projects for diabetes in India, the two major international agencies like IDF and WDF data sources are used. The level of care is explored through aspects of cost of illness, patterns of treatment and availability, accessibility and affordability towards diabetes care.

Results and Discussion

This section is divided further into three as per the objectives: (1) Prevalence of diabetes and its trend in India, (2) Responses by the different stakeholders, and (3) Level of Diabetes Care in India.

Prevalence of Diabetes and Its Trend in India

The evolution of diabetes as an epidemic in India has a vast history. There was evidence that diabetes had been prevalent in the ancient period around 1600 BC.[6] In the early 20th century, most of the studies were based on the clinic or hospital records. Early in 1938, Kolkata had shown the diabetes prevalence of one per cent. The diagnosis of diabetes was done with glycosuria i.e. testing urine for the presence of glucose. In 1963, Bombay (now Mumbai) had shown the prevalence of 2.2 per cent based on hospital data. Later on in 1964, WHO had organized for an Expert Committee and suggested the member countries to conduct mass screening camps for diabetes at community level to build the data on burden of diabetes. It also provided the basic information, for further planning, in dealing with the disease. The diagnostic criteria to define diabetes was also evolved during the same committee meet by the experts.

Similar detection programmes were also carried out in other parts of the country in 1966. The participants for testing were from large gatherings for other purposes or those who volunteered for the tests at detection camps. In 1966, a study conducted in Chennai had shown the prevalence of 5 per cent and 4.1 per cent in Hyderabad, followed by Chandigarh (2.7%) and Varanasi (2.9%) using the urine sample in urban areas in the age group of 20 years and above. But there was no systematic sampling and reporting system. In the early 1970s, a multi-centric study was conducted in 6 different parts of India by ICMR. It had shown the prevalence of about 2.1 per cent in urban and 1.5 per cent in rural areas. The same study had reported that the prevalence of 5 per cent in urban and 2.8 per cent in rural areas among those who were aged above 40 years.[7, 8]

It was observed that only the southern part, especially in and around Chennai, the population-based studies had taken place at regular point of time, which includes the major studies like Chennai Urban Rural Epidemiology Study (CURES). Several studies from different parts of southern region were showing the steady progress in the prevalence and at present, the figure is about 19 per cent in urban areas and 13.2 per cent in rural areas. There was also clear demarcation in the increasing trend in the prevalence of diabetes with the level of urbanization from the peri-urban (9.2%) to town (16.4%) and then city (18.6%) respectively.[8, 9, 10]

There were very few studies conducted to assess the prevalence of diabetes in the northern states. With the available studies, it would be conveyed that there is also a marked increase in the prevalence. There were studies conducted in urban areas of Jaipur which shows an increase from 12.3 per cent in 2003 to 20.3 per cent in 2007. In Delhi, the urban slum population had shown 10 per cent prevalence in 2001 and meanwhile, national survey had shown the prevalence of 11.3 per cent among the general population. There were very few studies conducted in eastern and western parts of India. Recent study conducted in 2008 in Kolkata has shown the prevalence of 11.3 per cent (urban) and 9.3 per cent (rural) respectively. Another study conducted at Sindhudurg in 2006 had shown the prevalence rate of 9.3 per cent in the rural population.[11] While looking into the multi-centric studies, the National Urban Diabetes Survey (NUDS) which was conducted in 2001 in six metro cities had shown the prevalence of diabetes range from 9.3 per cent in Mumbai to 16.6 per cent in Hyderabad. The prevalence in other regions was 13.5 per cent in Chennai, 12.4 per cent in Bangalore (now Bengaluru), 11.5 per cent and 11.6 per cent in Kolkata and New Delhi respectively.

In 2004 was started the Prevalence of Diabetes in India Survey (PODIS) in which 108 centres were included representing both urban and rural areas. This had shown the national prevalence of 5.6 per cent for urban and 2.7 per cent for rural areas, which revealed the 2:1 ratio of urban versus rural prevalence.[8] Followed by the study conducted as a part of national surveillance by ICMR between the period 2008 and 2010 in three major states and one union territory – Tamil Nadu, Maharashtra, Jharkhand and Chandigarh had shown the prevalence of urban-rural as 13.7 per cent : 7.8 per cent, 10.9 per cent : 6.5 per cent, 13.5 per cent : 3 per cent and 14.2 per cent : 8.3 per cent respectively. This had depicted the increasing trend in the prevalence of diabetes and impaired glucose tolerance (pre-diabetes) in both urban and rural areas.[12] Table 1 would give a better understanding on the trends in prevalence of diabetes in India. The previous studies, which were conducted in Chennai (CURES) had shown the decrease in Impaired Glucose Tolerance (IGT) and increase in diabetes prevalence. It is clearly indicated that there is a progress in the conversion of IGT into diabetes. It is also observed that age at onset of diabetes had decreased from NUDS to CURES.[8]

Another study from Delhi had reported a high prevalence of insulin resistance in post pubertal children which was associated with excess body fat and abdominal obesity.[13] The study which was done among the people aged 15–39 years had given a different picture. Despite low prevalence of the multiple risk factors like diabetes, impaired glucose tolerance, high levels of lipids among adolescents, there was a sudden rise of all the risk factors among the younger age adults.[14] Here the previous study informs us the earlier onset and the later, a picture of sudden onset, but both will be a threat to a health nation.

Risk factors: The factors such as family history, increasing body mass index (BMI), waist circumference, decreased physical activity, unbalanced diet (increased intake of sugar and fat i.e. High calorie dense foods), tobacco and alcohol intake could be predicted as major risk factors from the literature available.[8, 15]

Complications: A Chennai-based study in the year 2012 had shown that nearly one-third of the newly diagnosed Type II diabetes subjects were affected with some form of microvascular complications. The neuropathy and nephropathy was found to be microvascular (10.7%) than retinopathy (4.8%).[8, 16] It was also found that the complications were increasing with increase in age and duration of diabetes.

There were also studies showing the prevalence of retinopathy (17.6% to 26.8% in population-based study and 23.7% to 34% in clinic based study), Nephropathy, in which proteinuria varied from 6.9 per cent to 18.7 per cent and Microalbuminuria – 19.7 per cent to 36.3 per cent. All the studies were clinic based. Coronary artery diseases among diabetics accounted from 8.2 per cent to 21.4 per cent, whereas Neuropathy was seen in 9 per cent to 64 per cent (clinic based) and a population-based survey in 2008 had shown the prevalence of 26.1 per cent. This would show the brief picture of burden of complications due to diabetes.[11, 17]

Rural-urban difference could be observed in the presence of complications and further intensity of the same. A study was conducted among both urban

Table 1 *Type 2 Diabetes – Trends in Prevalence in India*

Period	*Prevalence*
1600 BC	Text books of Susruta and Ayurveda (Mention about evolution of diabetes)
1938 and 50	Kolkata and Mumbai – 1%
1964	WHO expert meet
1966	Chennai – 5%, Hyderabad (4.1%), Chandigarh (2.7%), Varanasi (2.9%)
1972–1975	ICMR – 6 different parts of the country – 2.1% (U) and 1.5%(R) > 40 years – 5% (U) and 2.8% (R)

	North	*South*	*East*	*West*
1980s	Delhi – 2.1%	Chennai – 5%	–	–
1990s	Delhi – 4.1% Punjab – 4.6%(R)>40yrs	Chennai – 8.2% – 11.2% Chennai – 12%, 15.5% and19.5%	Kolkata – 8.2(U) Guwahati – 11.7% U)	Ahmedabad – 3.1%
2000s	Delhi – 10.3% and 11.6% (2001) Srinagar – 4% (R) Jaipur U– 12.3%(2003) and 20% (2007), Rajasthan R – 1.2% (2004) Nagpur R–3.7%	TN rural – 8% Bangalore – 12.4% Trivandrum – 2.1% Kochi – 19.5% Godavari – 13.2(rural)	Kolkata – 12%(U) Manipur – 4%	Mumbai – 9.3%(U) Sindhudurg – 9.3 (R)

Multi-centric studies (NUDS – 2001, PODIS – 2004, ICMR – INDIAB – 2010)

National Urban Diabetes Survey (NUDS)	*Prevalence of Diabetes in India Study (PODIS)*	*Indian Council for Medical Research – India Diabetes Study (ICMR – INDIAB)*
6 Regions Hyderabad – 16.6% Chennai – 13.5% Bangalore – 12.4% Kolkata – 11.5% New Delhi – 11.6% Mumbai – 9.3%	108 Centres National prevalence Urban – 5.6% Rural – 2.7%	Tamil Nadu U – 13.7%, R – 7.8% Maharashtra U – 10.9%, R – 6.5% Jharkand U – 13.5%, R – 3.0 Chandigarh U – 14.2%, R – 8.3%

(n=1377) and rural(n=1265) diabetes patients who were having the similar duration of diabetes and peripheral vascular diseases at a foot clinic. From this study, it was observed that the rate of foot infection and amputation, recurrence of infection were high among rural diabetes patients than their urban counterparts.[18]

Recent evidence shows that there is an emerging relationship between diabetes and tuberculosis, which may act as the joint burden and further will complicate the control of tuberculosis as well. The study conducted in 3 districts in Tamil Nadu has shown the prevalence of 25.3 per cent (95% CI 22.6%–28.5%) diabetes and 24.5 per cent (95% CI 20.4% to 27.6%) pre-diabetes among the TB patients.[19, 20]

Popular Responses by Different Stakeholders

During Seventh Five-Year Plan (1987), there was an attempt made by Government of India to implement the national diabetes control programme, but due to paucity of funds, the programme could not be further expanded. Again in 2004, there was an inclusive agenda for the survey of NCD risk factors along with surveillance on communicable diseases under Integrated Disease Surveillance Project. But there was no emphasis on intervention. Prevention and control of diabetes is also one of the goals under National Rural Health Mission. In 2008, the pilot phase of National Programme for Prevention and Control of Diabetes, Cardiovascular Diseases and Stroke was launched. It is continuing with the initiation of the screening programmes in few districts in few states. Apart from planned 100 districts in Eleventh Five-Year Plan, 12th Five-Year Plan has given the plan to upscale the implementation to all the districts before 2017.[21, 22, 23]

Treatment Guidelines: In order to decrease the morbidity and mortality, there were several guidelines and consensus developed at national and international levels for the better management of the diabetes. Based on American Diabetic Association (ADA) and European Association for Study of Diabetes (EASD) consensus, experts from India in 2002 had reframed the guidelines suitable to our country for the provision of optimum diabetes care. International Diabetes Federation – Clinical Task Force Guidelines had framed three levels of care based on the availability and affordability of resources in the country – standard care, comprehensive care and minimal care. In 2003, ICMR had framed the guidelines for the management of the diabetes with emphasis on maintaining optimum glycaemic levels and prevention of complications. Later again in 2007, API had framed the guidelines for the clinical management of diabetes with complications.[24, 25, 26]

If we focus the treatment guidelines that how far it is practised by the practitioners, it is too minimal as described in the community-based study done in Chennai urban areas. It was shown that the patients who had attended public health facility were prescribed only with oral hypoglycaemic drugs irrespective of their age and duration of disease, severity of the disease. About 31 per cent patients who attended specialty hospital were asked to do HbA1c test, the clinical monitoring indicator for maintaining the normal blood sugar level.

There were no standard guidelines followed in treating the diabetic patients especially by the general practitioners.[27]

On other hand, it was seen that the majority of the patients were also depending on the Complementary and Alternative Medicine (CAM) and also modern medicine. A clinic based cross sectional study was conducted among 493 diabetic patients who had attended that clinic for the first time in UP. The results had shown that 24.2 per cent use only CAM, whereas combination of CAM and allopathy usage was found in 22.4 per cent, CAM, diet control and exercise was seen in 6.3 per cent and use of all CAM, allopathy, diet control and exercise was found among 47.0 per cent of the diabetic patients. The perception for the use of CAM given by the patients was quick and additional relief of the disease.[28] This actually raises the thought about the efficacy of the treatment and also cohesion between different systems of medicine. This may further drive the need for the standard consensus for the treatment guidelines across different systems of medicine.

Interventions at individual and community level are piloted and demonstrated in the prevention and control of the disease among Indian subjects.

Indian Diabetes Prevention Programme[29] had demonstrated the effectiveness that lifestyle modification involving moderate, but consistent, physical activity and diet modification help to prevent diabetes in the Asian Indians, who have a high risk of developing diabetes.

Another study done in Asiad Colony, Tirumangalam of Chennai had provided a model for promoting the construction of public parks near the residential area through the community participation in order to increase the physical activity. In 1998, the eligible people (i.e. people with diabetes and who had shown the impaired glucose tolerance in 1996) recruited in the colony were given awareness and educated on the importance of physical activity. The committee in the colony took an initiative in arranging the fund (₹ 15,00,000) from various organizations and individuals and free space from government for the construction of the public park. After seven years, it was found that there was 58.7 per cent increase in the proportion of people, which was 14.2 per cent at baseline. There was also increase in people who would do some form of physical activity weekly, at least three times, irrespective of their occupation. Followed by this, two other public parks were constructed in other residential areas.[30]

To get an overall picture of pattern of interventions in the form of clinical trials and other community based projects, sources like National Institutes of Health and International Diabetes Federation and World Diabetes Foundation were searched. Out of 316 trials in India, 244 trials were conducted for diabetes. Around 220 of 234 were drug intervention, few interventions with dietary supplements and few with information technology.[31] There were totally 234 projects all over the world funded by World Diabetes Foundation (WDF). Out of 234, 71 projects carried out in South-East Asian region, in which 45 are in India. Project details are given in the Table 2(a) and Table 2(b). The focus was on awareness, screening camps, prevention of gestational diabetes, mass retinopathy treatment, school level education programmes, multimedia campaign, training health care professions in prevention and clinical management of diabetes.[32]

Table 2 (a) *Projects Funded by World Diabetes Foundation*

State	*Year*	*Project No.*	*Project*
AP	2005	WDF04–078	Diabetes Awareness Camps
	2006	WDF 05 137	Health Promotion and Diabetes Prevention
	2007	WDF 07 224	Reduction of Blindness
	2008	WDF 07–279	Diabetic Foot Programme
	2008	WDF 08 330	Capacity Development Project
Karnataka	2005	WDF 05–110	Mobile Diabetic Retinopathy Treatment
	2006	WDF 05 142	Rural Diabetic Foot Care
	2012	WDF 09 456	Comprehensive Diabetes and Eye Care
	2013	WDF 09 469	Improving Foot Care in Urban Areas
	2013	WDF 08 381	Gestational Diabetes among Rural and Tribal People
Kerala	2006	WDF 06– 166	Community based Diabetic Retinopathy Services
	2008	WDF 07–236	Primary Prevention of Diabetes
	2012	WDF 08 353	One step Ahead – A Diabetic Foot Campaign
Tamil Nadu (TN)	2003	WDF 02–39	Diabetic Eye Care – I
	2005	WDF 05–115	Preventing Diabetes and its Complications in Rural Areas
	2006	WDF 04–079	Diabetes Eye Care II
TN, Kerala	2006	WDF 05 148	Diabetic Eye care III
	2006	WDF 06– 163	Diabetic Retinopathy Integrated Programme
	2007	WDF 06–203	Strengthening National Diabetes Care Services
	2008	WDF 11 612	Prevention of Diabetes in Mother and Child
	2008	WDF 08–312	Gestational Diabetes II
	2013	WDF 08 406	Prevention of Diabetes through IT
	2012	WDF 08 385	Diabetes Training for TB Health Personnel

Table 2(b) *Projects Funded by World Diabetes Foundation*

State	*Year*	*Project No.*	*Project*
Assam	2013	WDF 11 654	Comprehensive Type 2 Diabetes Care
Delhi	2008	WDF 07 295	Media Campaign for Prevention of and Care of Diabetes
Gujarat	2008	WDF 07 244	Sam Vedana Eye Care for Diabetes
	2013	WDF 09 477	Diabetes Prevention Programme
Maharashtra	2009	WDF 08–319	Comprehensive Eye Care Model, India
	2012	WDF 08 338	Mumbai Diabetic Retinopathy Study
Manipur	2013	WDF 11 655	Diabetes Prevention Through Community Mobilisation
MP	2007	WDF 06–214	Rural Diabetic Retinopathy Treatment
	2012	WDF 11 592	Jagruti – Awareness Mission for Dibetes
Orissa (Odisha)	2011	WDF 10 540	Institutional Empowerment for Diabetic Foot Care
	2012	WDF 08 338	Reduction of Blindness due to Diabetes
Punjab	2011	WDF 10 551	Gestational Diabetes
	2007	WDF 06 198	Shri Guru Harikrishna Shahib Diabetic Retinopathy project
Rajasthan	2012	WDF 07 275	Prevention of Blindness
UP	2012	WDF 12 678	Gestational Diabetes
	2012	WDF 11 647	Prevention and Control of Diabetes
	2012	WDF 08 390	Eye Care at the Doorsteps of Rural India
	2012	WDF 09 487	Mobile Treatment for Diabetic Retinopathy
West Bengal	2013	WDF 12690	Prevent Diabetic Retinopathy, Protect Sight
TN, Kerala, Karnataka, AP, Gujarat, Orissa (Odisha)	2003	WDF 03–52	National Diabetes Programme
Delhi, Maharashtra, Rajasthan, UP	2006	WDF 05– 120	Preventing Obesity and Diabetes in School Children

Level of Diabetes Care in India

The level of diabetes care depends on the availability, accessibility and affordability towards the health services system. For instance, the people who had been staying in semi-urban or rural areas were diagnosed with the disease 4 years later than their urban counterparts. People with diabetes living in the semi-urban or rural areas had shown higher rates of complications, despite less duration of diabetes than those in urban settings. This was due to the availability of less health care or absence of total health care. Similarly, employed and working people with diabetes had fewer complications compared to those non-working or those in rural areas engaged in agricultural labour. Among people with similar diabetes duration, majority from high socio-economic group were found to have very few complications or were free of complications. It was observed from the same study that 54 per cent of diabetes patients in this group were free of complications and only 8 per cent were presenting with 3 complications. Whereas the people in the low socio-economic group, it was noted that only 23 per cent of the people did not have any complications and 26 per cent of the people were found to have 3 complications.[33, 34, 35]

Meanwhile, the study was conducted during 2004 to 2005 to assess the availability and price of essential drugs in public and private sector in 5 major states. The results of the public sector had shown that availability of glibenclamide (which is given in first line treatment of diabetes) was 100 per cent in Karnataka, 95 per cent in Tamil Nadu, 83.3 per cent in Haryana, whereas in Maharashtra and West Bengal, it was found to be very minimum i.e 15 per cent and 3.8 per cent respectively. Despite 26 facilities were surveyed in West Bengal, only 1 facility had the drug glibenclamide.[36]

The study which was done by Chronic Care Foundation (2010) had shown that the indirect cost was found to be higher among the rural diabetic population than those in urban areas. From this, it was also revealed that the loss of work and loss of wage were also high. Another population based study conducted in Chennai had shown that the annual direct cost was estimated to ₹ 25,391 and the annual indirect cost was ₹ 4,970 towards the diabetes care. The amount spent towards the hospital admission account for the highest i.e 54 per cent (₹ 12,992) followed by the expenditure for drugs and monitoring which was 34 per cent (₹ 8,595). The people with diabetes could meet their treatment expenses through indebtedness and mortgaging property. The patients from low socio-economic status were found to be more into indebtedness which further worsened their living condition.[37, 38, 27]

A study conducted among 112 diabetic patients in Tiruvannamalai district had revealed various reasons for the interruption of the treatment – lack of health facility, lack of transport, lack of drug availability, cost of drug, lack of family cooperation, lack of motivation and awareness about complications. It was found that more emphasis was given to sociologic reasons rather than looking into the disease condition.[39]

Conclusion

To conclude, the prevalence of diabetes in India shows an increasing trend in urban areas. This trend is also observed in rural areas gradually. The response of physicians and patients shows a fragmented approach in the management of diabetes. There have been multiple efforts taken by different national and international actors through scientific meetings to set standard treatment guidelines. An important aspect that this study highlights is the gaps in the translation and adherence of these guidelines by physicians in the treatment of diabetes.

It also vividly demonstrates the socio-economic constraints that impinge on the management of the disease. These findings point to the gaps in the manner in which several projects by World Diabetes Foundation have addressed diabetes control. Our study raises some important dimensions that go beyond detection and treatment in order to address the issue in a more comprehensive manner. On the one hand burden in terms of prevalence of diabetes and its complications is rising, on the other hand it is being dealt with interventions in a piecemeal manner – such as giving only awareness or mass remedies to treat the complications like retinopathy or foot care at different levels. There is no consistency in focusing each aspects of disorder and care as it has multi and complex interactions since its' onset to everyday management. Few projects such as Chunampet Rural Diabetes Prevention Project, Tamil Nadu and Comprehensive Type II Diabetes Project, Assam have focused broadly the community participation and inter-sectoral coordination in providing a comprehensive care to people affected with diabetes.

There are few cross-sectional studies which would show the socio-economic inequalities in terms of diabetes care and quality of life among people affected with diabetes. It is sketchy and it does not address the question as to why such condition existed. Hence, in order to have a comprehensive understanding about this complex interaction between the individual, social condition, disease condition (diabetes) and health services system, it needs a multilevel interdisciplinary inquiry at all levels such as Individual level (Individual's perception and experiences of diabetes, treatment management, social conditions at household level) societal level (social groups, networks and support) and Institutional level (health care resources, professional skills, quality of services, availability, accessibility, affordability and acceptability of the services provided).

Note: The major content of this paper is taken from the review part of my M. Phil Dissertation. The research entitled 'Social Dimensions of Coping with Type 2 Diabetes: An Exploratory study in Chennai' has been submitted for the partial fulfilment of my M. Phil, under the supervision of Professor Rama V. Baru at the Centre of Social Medicine and Community Health, School of Social Sciences, Jawaharlal Nehru University, New Delhi. I would like to thank and acknowledge Professor Rama V. Baru for her inputs and comments towards this research paper.

Notes

1. Summary Report on Causes of Death: 2001–03. Office of Registrar General, Government of India. http://censusindia.gov.in/vital_ statistics/summary_report_death_01_03.pdf
2. International Diabetes Federation. 2011. *IDF Diabetes Atlas*. 5th edition, Brussels, Belgium: International Diabetes Federation.

3. National Health Profile (NHP) of India. 2011. www.cbhidghs.nic.in/index2.asp?slid=1208&suslinkid=944 (accessed online on 21 February 2013).
4. Siegel, K., Venkat Narayan, R.M. and Kinra, S. 2008. Finding a Policy Solution to India's Diabetes Epidemic. *Health Affairs*, 27 (4): 1077–1090.
5. Beaglehole, R., Bonita, R., Alleyne, G. et al., 2011. UN High Level Meeting on Non-Communicable Diseases: Addressing Four Questions. *Lancet*, 378: 449–455.
6. Weaver, L.J. and Narayan, V. 2008. Reconsidering the History of Diabetes in India: Emerging or Re-Emerging Disease? *NMJI*, 21 (6): 288–291.
7. Report of the WHO Expert Committee. 1965. *Diabetes Mellitus*. Technical Report Series No. 310, Geneva: WHO.
8. Mohan, V., Sandeep, S., Deepa, R., Shah, B. and Varghese, C. 2007. Epidemiology of Type 2 Diabetes: Indian Scenario. *Indian J Med Res*, 125: 217–230.
9. Misra, P., Upadhyay, R.P., Misra, A. and Anand, K. 2011. A Review of the Epidemiology of Diabetes in Rural India. *Diabetes Res Clin Prac*, 92: 303–311.
10. Ramachandran, A., Mary, S., Yamuna, A., Murugesan, N. and Snehalatha, C. 2008. High Prevalence of Diabetes and Cardiovascular Risk Factors Associated with Urbanization in India. *Diabetes Care*, 31: 893–898.
11. Anjana, R.M. et al., 2011. The Need for Obtaining Accurate Nationwide Estimates of Diabetes Prevalence in India: Rationale for a National Study on Diabetes. *Indian J Med Res*, 133: 369–380.
12. ICMR-INDIAB Collaborative Study Group. 2011. Prevention of Diabetes and Pre-Diabetes (Impaired Fasting Glucose and/or Impaired Glucose Tolerance) in Urban and Rural India: Phase 1 Results of the Indian Council of Medical Research – India Diabetes (ICMR – INDIAB) Study. *Diabetologia*, 54: 3022–3027.
13. Misra, A., Vikram, N.K., Arya, S. et al., 2004. High Prevalence of Insulin Resistance in Postpubertal Asian Indian Children is Associated with Adverse Truncal Body Fat Patterning, Abdominal Obesity and Excess Body Fat. *Int J Obesity*, 28: 1217–1226.
14. Gupta, R., Misra, A., Vikram, N.K. et al., 2009. Younger Age Escalation of Cardiovascular Risk Factors in Asian Indian Subjects. *BMC Cardiovascular Disorder*, 9 (28): e1–e12.
15. Mohan, V., Mathur, P., Deepa, R. et al., 2008. Urban Rural Differences in Prevalence of Self-Reported Diabetes in India: The WHO-ICMR Indian NCD Risk Factor Surveillance. *Diabetes Res Clin Pract*, 80: 159–168.
16. Raman, R., Aditi, G., Suganeswari, K., Vaitheeswaran, K. and Tarun, S. 2012. Prevalence and Risk Factors for Diabetic Microvascular Complications in Newly Diagnosed Type II Diabetes Mellitus. Sankara Nethralaya Diabetic Retinopathy Epidemiology and Molecular Genetic Study (SN-DREAMS Report 27). *Journal of Diabetes and its Complications* (available online doi:10.1016/j.jdiacomp. 2012.02.001).
17. Pradeepa, R., Rema, M., Vignesh, J., Deepa, M., Deepa, R. and Mohan, V. 2008. Prevalence and Risk Factors for Diabetic Neuropathy in an Urban South Indian Population: The Chennai Urban Rural Epidemiology Study (CURES–55). *Diabetic Medicine*, 25: 407–412.
18. Viswanathan, V., Thomas, N., Tandon, N. et al., 2005. Profile of Diabetic Foot Complications and its Associated Complications: A Multicentric Study from India. *J Assoc Physicians India*, 53: 933–936.
19. Harries, A.D., Murray, B.M., Jeon, C.Y. et al., 2010. Defining the Research Agenda to Reduce the Joint Burden of Disease from Diabetes Mellitus and Tuberculosis. *Tropical Medicine and International Health*, 15 (6): 659–663.

20. Vijay, V., Satyavani, K., Vigneswari, A. et al., 2012. Prevalence of Diabetes and Pre-Diabetes and Associated Risk Factors among Tuberculosis Patients in India. *PLOS One*, 7 (7): e41367.
21. http://nihfw.nic.in/ndc-nihfw/html/programmes/nationaldiabetescontrol.htm
22. Pandve, H.T., Chawla, P.S., Fernandez, K. and Singru, S.K. 2010. Recent Developments in Diabetes Control and Prevention in India. *Int J Diab Dev Ctries*, 30 (3): 171–172.
23. Report of the Working Group on Disease Burden for 12th Five-Year Plan. 2011. New Delhi: MoH&FW.
24. Indian Guidelines for Management of Type 2 Diabetes. 2002. *Assoc Physicians India*, 50: 297–366.
25. Indian Council of Medical Research. 2005. *ICMR Guidelines for Management of Type 2 Diabetes*. New Delhi: Indian Council of Medical Research. http://www.icmr.nic.in/guidelines_diabetes/guide_diabetes. html
26. API-ICP Guidelines on Diabetes. 2007. *J Assoc Physicians India*, 55: 1–50.
27. Shabana, T., Arutselvi, D., Satyavani, K. and Vijay, V. 2010. Socioeconomics of Diabetes Care in India: A Community Based Cost of Illness Study. *Diab Res Clin Prac*, 89 (3): 334–340.
28. Kumar, D., Bajaj, S. and Mehrotra, R. 2006. Knowledge, Attitude and Practice of Complementary and Alternative Medicines for Diabetes. *Public Health*, 120: 705–711.
29. Ramachandran, A., Snehalatha, C., Mary, S., Mukesh, B., Bhaskar, D. and Vijay, V. 2006. The Indian Diabetes Prevention Programme Shows that Lifestyle Modification and Metformin Prevent Type 2 Diabetes in Asian Indian Subjects with Impaired Glucose Tolerance (IDDP – 1). *Diabetologia*, 49: 289–297.
30. Mohan, V., Shanthirani, C.S., Deepa, M., Datta, M., Williams, O.D. and Deepa, R. 2006. Community Empowerment: A Successful Model for Prevention of Non-Communicable Diseases. *JAPI*, 54: 858–862.
31. Clinical trials.gov (accessed online on 12 March 2013).
32. www.worlddiabetesfoundation.org/projects/ (accessed online on 14 March 2013).
33. Kapur, A., Bjork, S., Nair, J., Kelkar, S. and Ramachandran, A. 2004. Socioeconomic Determinants of the Costs of Diabetes in India. *Diabetes Voice*, 49 (3): 1–4.
34. Shobana, R., Christina, A., Vijay, V. and Ramachandran, A. 2005. Improving Psycho-Social Care: The Indian Experience. *Diabetes Voice*, 50 (1): 1–3.
35. Kapur, A. 2007. Economic Analysis of Diabetes Care. *Indian J Med Res*, 125: 473–482.
36. Kotwani, Anita. 2007. Prices and Availability of Common Medicines at Six Sites in India Using a Standard Methodology. *Indian J Med Res*, 125: 645–654.
37. Chronic Care Foundation of India. 2009. *A Report on Non-Communicable Chronic Diseases in India: A Study of the Gaps, Quality and Cost of Care*. New Delhi: Chronic Care Foundation of India.
38. Shabana, T., Arutselvi, D., Burman, H., Mahesh, U. and Vijay, V. 2011. How Far has Translation of Research been Implemented into Clinical Practice in India? Are the Recommended Guidelines Adhered To? *International Journal of Diabetes Mellitus*, Vol. 3, Issue I, 25–30.
39. Srinivas, G., Suresh, E., Jagadeesan, M., Amalraj, E. and Datta, M. 2002. Treatment-Seeking Behavior and Compliance of Diabetic Patients in a Rural Area of South India. *Ann N Y Acad Sci*, 958: 420–424.

10

Public Health Infrastructure in Child Health Care Services

Regional Situational Analyses in Rural Madhya Pradesh

Chander Shekhar, Garima Dutta and Sarang Pedgaonkar

As per sample registration system report 2010,[1] Madhya Pradesh ranks highest in infant mortality in India at the level of 67 per 1,000 live births and highest in neonatal mortality i.e. 44 per 1,000 live births. Further, huge regional variation in infant mortality prevails in rural settings. For example, it stands at 83 infant deaths per thousand births in central region as compared to 45 in south-western region. The situation is much gloomy in rural areas of Madhya Pradesh where infants beyond the first year of their life do not survive out of every 1,000 live births despite several initiatives like Universal Immunization Programme (UIP) to improve child survival by the Government of India. In Madhya Pradesh, the percentage of children who received complete immunization is only 36 per cent[2] aged 12–23 months and there also exists huge regional variation. To reduce infant and child mortality, the Madhya Pradesh government and population policy had set some of the goals like, total immunization of 70 per cent by 2005 and 90 per cent full immunization aged 12–23 months by 2009. But still the state is far behind from the goal. Evaluation study of National Rural Health Mission (NRHM)[3] by government of India reveals that human resource shortage seems to be still serious in the state of Madhya Pradesh. Against 1,080 required specialists the state has only 220 in position. There are 262 PHCs functioning without a doctor. IPHS facility survey has recommended upgradation of 96 CHCs and the physical upgradation work has started only in 27 CHCs.

The health care system in India has expanded considerably over the last few decades; however, the quality of services is not uniform, due to various reasons like non-availability of manpower, problems of access, acceptability and lack of community involvement. Hence, Indian Public Health Standards (IPHS) standards are being introduced in order to improve the quality of public health level.[4] As highlighted by Majumder and Upadhya, India's health care system at present has a three-tier structure to provide health care services to its citizens. The first tier, known as primary tier, has been developed to provide health care services to the vast majority of rural people. The primary tier comprises three types of health care institutions: Sub-Health Centre (SHC), Primary Health Centre (PHC) and Community Health Centre (CHC)[5]. These standards are being applied to SHC (Sub-Health Centre), PHC (Primary Health Centre) and CHC (Community Health Centre). This paper elaborates the situation only at the primary level in the state of Madhya Pradesh by regions.

Review of Literature

The rapidly growing population had been a major concern for health planners and administrators in India since independence. In 1951, India was the first country in the world to launch a family planning programme. Since then, approaches aimed at reducing population growth have taken a variety of forms. Till 1977, the major focus of health activities was family planning, which was changed into family welfare programme with maternal and child health becoming an integral part of family planning programme. In the year 1978, Government of India launched diarrhoeal disease control programme[6] with a main objective to prevent death due to dehydration caused by diarrheal diseases among children under 5 years of age. Thereafter, the national health policy came in the year 1983[7], envisioned significant reduction in infant mortality rate, neonatal mortality and child mortality rate by 2000. As cited by Kulkarni,[8] Universal Immunization Programme (UIP) against six preventable diseases, namely, diphtheria, pertusis, childhood tuberculosis, poliomyelitis, measles and neonatal tetanus was introduced in the country in a phased manner in 1985. UIP became a part of the Child Survival and Safe Motherhood (CSSM) Programme in 1992.[9] The programmes seek to sustain high coverage levels achieved under the Universal Immunization Programme (UIP) in good performance areas and strengthen the immunization services of poor performing areas. Thereafter, following the recommendations of the International Conference on Population and Development (ICPD) in 1994, Government of India came up with national population policy in 2000, to address the unmet needs of contraception, health care infrastructure, health personnel and to provide integrated service delivery for basic reproductive and child health care.[9] In the year 2002, Government of India again formulated the national health policy[10] with main objective of achieving an acceptable standard of good health by decentralizing public health system by upgrading infrastructure and to ensure a more equitable access to health services across the social and geographical expanse of India. National Rural Health Mission[11] came in the year 2005, with a primary goal providing accessible, affordable and quality health care services to rural population with the special focus on 18 states which have week public health indicators and health infrastructure. Madhya Pradesh is one of the states among high focused states. To see the improvement in the quality of health care delivery in the country under the mission, Indian Public Health Standard (IPHS) was set.

It is evident from the many existing studies that a good health infrastructure plays a very significant role in providing good health to its people. A study was done by Lakshmi and Sahoo, on health infrastructure and health indicator in the state of Andhra Pradesh and there they indicated that good health infrastructure has significant and positive bearing on health indicators. They created a health infrastructure index and found that 1 per cent increase in health infrastructure decreases Crude Birth Rate (CBR) by 37.966 per cent, Crude Death Rate (CDR) by 27.816 per cent and Infant Mortality Rate (IMR) by 30.598 per cent respectively.[12] According to Datar et al., larger and better-equipped facilities such as PHCs or hospitals have a bigger effect on vaccine coverage. One notable exception is that having a PHC or hospital within 2 or 5 km significantly increased the likelihood of full-cover for polio vaccine. Rural health infrastructure, especially hospitals and PHCs, played an important role in expanding vaccine coverage and preventable diseases.[13] Leipziger, et al., emphasized the role of infrastructure in achieving three health related Millennium Development Goals. They found that apart from traditional variables (income, assets, education and direct health interventions), better access to basic infrastructure services has an important role to play in improving child health outcomes.[14] Ghei et al., found positive association between child immunization and availability of health infrastructure.[15] Datar et al., showed that the availability of health infrastructure had only a modest effect on immunization coverage. Larger and better-equipped facilities had bigger effects on immunization coverage. Health infrastructure in terms of hospitals, hospital beds, doctors, nurses, pharmacists, etc. has a significant direct and positive contribution to health outcomes of any country.[13] Senavirathne,[16] reported that in countries like Sri Lanka which have registered improvement in maternal mortality rate and infant mortality rate, the availability of health infrastructure care substantially improved in the early part of 20th century.[16] Bitner,[17] found that a poor service environment is not conducive to good interaction between service provider and their clients. As revealed in a report,[18] underutilization of facilities is also caused by the lack of training. In a large project in India, very expensive imported vacuum extractors were provided to First Referral Units (FRUs), but the doctors were not trained in this procedure; and hence, this expensive equipment remained unused.

Objectives

The core objective of the study is to understand health infrastructure situation that can be seen critical in view of child health status in rural areas of different regions of Madhya Pradesh. This paper is prepared to assess the utilization of the child health care services from PHCs and CHCs at regional level and to examine situation of human resource, drug and essential equipments.

Methods and Materials

The data used for this study has been obtained from DLHS (district level household and facility survey) 2007–08, SRS (sample registration survey) 2010. DLHS is designed to provide district level estimates on maternal and child health, family planning and other reproductive health services and other important interventions of National Rural Health Mission (NRHM). DLHS–3 also collected information regarding facilities available at the sub-health centre, Primary Health Centre (PHC), Community Health Centre (CHC) and district hospital. The health facility questionnaires contained information on human resources, infrastructure and services. For the first time, population-linked facility survey was conducted in DLHS–3. At the district level, all community health centres (CHC) and district hospital were covered. Further, all sub-health centres (SHC) and primary health centres (PHC) which were expected to serve the population of the selected primary sampling unit (PSU) were also covered. In this study, unit level facility data for SHC, PHC and CHC have been analysed.

There are total 50 districts in Madhya Pradesh; we clubbed all district into different regions according to the NSSO (national sample survey organization) classification namely Vidhyanchal, Central, South-central, Malwa, South-western and Northern region. The study requires regional level analyses for utilization of child health care services. Therefore, regional weights need to be generated to provide regional level estimates. The working mechanism to develop regional weight is given below:

Regional weight= $W^{w*} [(Ni^{R}/N_{c})/(ni^{R}/n_{s}^{R})]$

Ni^{R} – Number of household in census in a region

N_{c} – Total number of household in census of the whole state

ni^{R} – Number of household sampled in a region.

n_{s}^{R} – Number of household sampled in a state

In this paper we mostly have used percentages to understand the situation of the utilization of various services availability of drugs, equipments, human resources at CHC, PHC and SHC level.

It is always cited that workload on any level of health facility is directly linked with quality of service provided. Table 1 shows large regional variations in the catchment population of each type of facility. In case of PHC, it ranges from 29,698 on the South-central region to 56,042 in the Malwa region. As per the IPHS norms, a PHC should cater primary health care needs of around 30,000 people. Looking into average size of population served by CHC shows that on average workload is one and half times higher than (1,49,413 per CHC) the prescribed norms (1,00,000 population per CHC) under IPHS. It also presents huge regional variations starting from 1, 23,058 per CHC in the South-central region to 1,86,462 in the northern region. IPHS also suggests the size of population to be catered at SHC level is 5,000 people. In contrast, a SHC served up to 5,912 persons on average in whole of Madhya Pradesh. Regional band is spread between 5,210 persons in South-central region to 6,830 persons in Vindhyanchal region.

Level of Full Immunization in Regions of Madhya Pradesh

The complete immunization of children helps greatly in reducing child mortality as shown by studies in the past and it is an important for programme managers. The immunization of children against six potentially deadly, but preventable

Table 1 *Average Population Covered by CHC, PHC and SHC in Different Regions of Madhya Pradesh*

Region	*No. of PHCs*	*Population*	*Average population*	*No. of CHCs*	*Population*	*Average population*	*No. of SHCs*	*Population*	*Average population*
Vindhyanchal	99	42,02,195	42,446	49	89,68,138	1,83,023	264	18,03,212	6,830
Central	47	19,86,084	42,257	34	47,50,417	1,39,718	176	11,01,332	6,257
Malwa	104	58,28,442	56,042	51	71,41,809	1,40,035	291	15,91,913	5,470
South-central	109	32,37,090	29,698	55	67,68,212	1,23,058	259	13,49,464	5,210
South-western	58	22,49,790	38,789	33	41,70,350	1,26,374	169	9,16,775	5,424
Northern	59	31,50,058	53,390	37	68,99,102	1,86,462	203	12,89,076	6,350
Madhya Pradesh	476	2,06,53,659	43,390	259	3,86,98,028	1,49,413	1,362	80,51,772	5,911

Figure 1 *Different Regions of Madhya Pradesh*

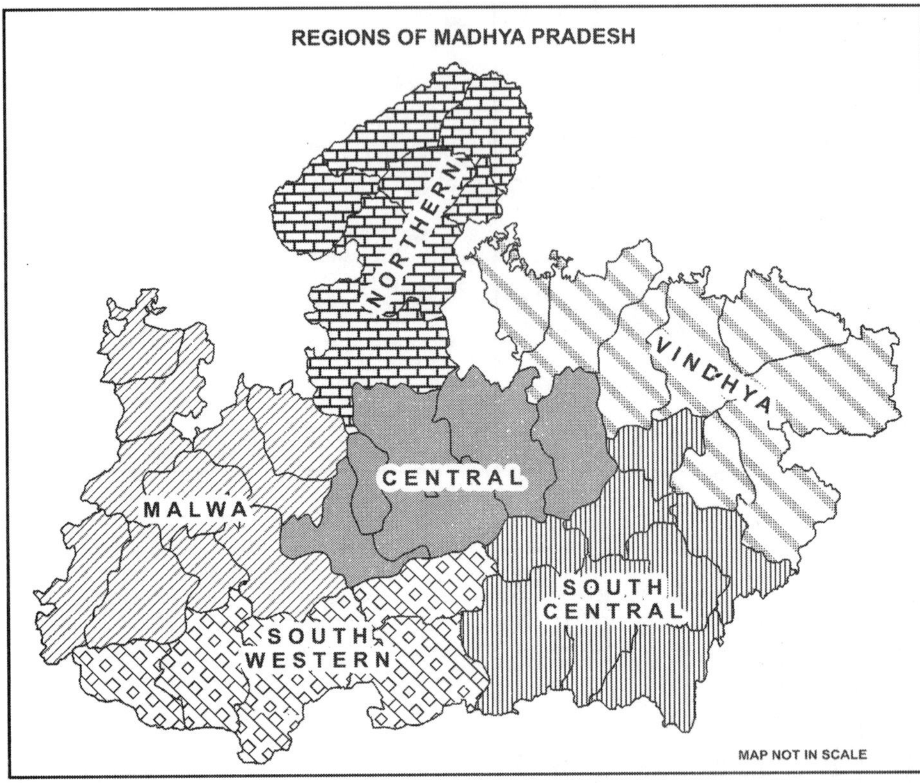

Graph 1 *Percentage of IMR and Level of Full Immunization in Rural Madhya Pradesh*

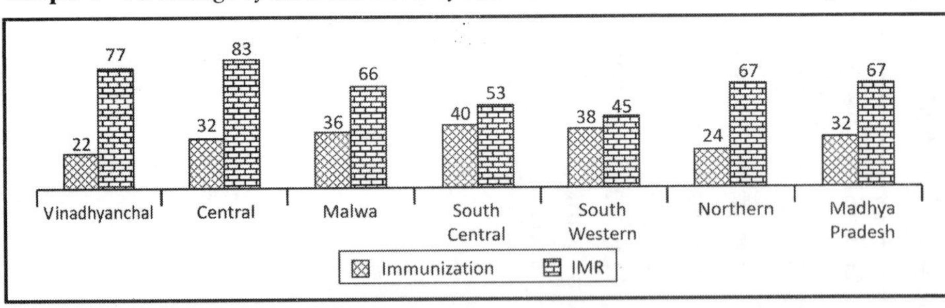

diseases – tuberculosis, diphtheria, pertussis, tetanus, polio and measles – has been an important cornerstone of the child-health-care system. Graph 1 gives an idea how infant mortality rate and level of child immunization are linked in different regions of Madhya Pradesh. The level of IMR is 67 per cent against 36 per cent children aged 12–23 months who are fully immunized. As it is clearly seen that inverse relationship exists between infant mortality rate and level of complete immunization. However, the Central and Malwa regions do not show strong relationship between the two indicators. It may be because only preventive reasons may not be solely responsible for child mortality in these two regions.

To explain the level of full immunization in rural area, one needs to analyse the sources of immunization. Table 2 suggests that majority of children received immunization from Integrated Child Development Services (ICDS) centres. It implied that we need to improve the functioning of these centres and integration between health and family welfare and women and child departments. As it is known that ICDS workers only facilitates or organize activities on immunization day where Auxiliary Nurse Midwife (ANM) or local workers from health department actually provide vaccination. It is good to see that 85 per cent children receive immunization from public health system. Regional variation in these figures is not so high. Role of sub-health centres is found to be relatively higher in South-western region than others.

Table 2 *Place of Vaccination Received (12–23 Months) in Rural Areas in Different Regions of Madhya Pradesh, 2007–08*

Regions	*Place of Receiving Immunization*				
	CHC	*PHC*	*SC*	*ICDS Centres*	*NGO/PVT*
Vindhyanchal	8.0	4.5	4.7	61.8	15.8
Central	5.2	4.6	3.9	57.3	19.4
Malwa	5.0	8.0	5.0	62.8	16.3
South-central	2.7	3.9	3.9	82.3	7.9
South-western	6.2	8.7	9.4	67.3	12.9
Northern	4.0	6.3	6.8	57.4	18.0
Madhya Pradesh	5.2	6.0	5.6	65.4	14.7

Utilization of Selected Services from SHCs, PHCs and CHCs

Diarrhoeal diseases are another fatal disease among children under age of five years. Therefore, one needs to understand what kind of treatment seeking prevails in different regions. This section is looking into the utilization of selected services for treatment seeking from government, private/NGOs. Table 3 show the treatment seeking behaviour for diarrhoea and fever from different sources across regions of Madhya Pradesh. It is clearly evident that most of the children were receiving treatment from the private facilities which is completely opposite in comparison with the immunization. In Madhya Pradesh, 37 per cent children were taking treatment for diarrhoea from government facilities. South-central region (46%) is showing the highest percentage among all the regions for taking treatment from government facilities. Among all the regions, northern region (71%) had highest percentage for taking treatment from the private facility. For the treatment of fever also, the picture is very much similar to diarrhoeal diseases. Most of the children have taken treatment from the private facilities. Although in the South-central region the contribution of both private and government was nearly equal, but in most of the regions, private facilities are having higher percentage. Northern region (73%) had highest percentage among all the regions for taking treatment from the private facilities followed by Malwa and central regions.

Table 3 *Percentage of Children Received Treatment for Diarrhoea and Fever in Rural Areas from Different Sources in Regions of Madhya Pradesh, 2007–08*

Regions	*Government*	*NGO/Private*	*Government*	*NGO/Private*	*CHC*		*PHC*		*SHC*	
	Diarrhoea		*Fever*		*Diarrhoea*	*Fever*	*Diarrhoea*	*Fever*	*Diarrhoea*	*Fever*
Vindhyanchal	36.6	63.4	33.4	66.6	11	11	10	10	3	3
Central	36.2	63.8	31.7	68.3	9	6	7	8	5	5
Malwa	36.2	63.8	31.1	68.9	11	9	8	8	6	5
South-central	46.0	54.1	48.8	51.2	11	9	13	13	5	3
South-western	42.3	57.7	33.1	66.9	14	11	16	11	5	4
Northern	28.9	71.1	27.5	72.5	12	11	5	6	3	3
Madhya Pradesh	37.1	62.9	34.0	66.0	11.1	9.7	8.9	9.5	4.5	3.8

Table 3 also shows percentage of those children who received treatment for diarrhoea and fever from different levels of government health facilities like CHCs, PHCs and SHCs. Among all the three type of facilities, CHCs are playing a major role in providing treatment for both diarrhoea and fever. The south-western region (14%) shows the highest percentage for receiving treatment for diarrhoea from CHCs and PHCs as well. For the treatment of fever, Vidhyanchal, south-western and northern regions are showing relatively high utilization of CHCs (11%) than the other regions. The utilization of PHCs (13%) in south-central region is found to be above all the regions in seeking treatment for fever among children. The utilization of sub-health centres is quite low for both the diseases.

Availability of Human Resources for Child Health Care Services

In order to provide good health facilities and round the clinical services, there is need to have a complete bunch of human infrastructure at each level of facility. To provide quality of care at CHCs, PHCs and SHCs, Indian Public Health Standards (IPHS) are being prescribed to provide optimal expert care to the community and achieve and maintain an acceptable standard of quality of care. This section is dealing with the availability of human resource at CHCs, PHCs and SHC level. As it is given in the IPHS guidelines in regard to manpower, there should be two specialists at CHC level.

Graph 2 showing the availability of at least one paediatrician at CHC in regions of Madhya Pradesh. In Madhya Pradesh 17 per cent of CHCs are having at least one paediatrician. Northern region is showing good picture in regards with the availability of man power. The region has the highest percentage (35%) of paediatrician among all the regions. And the south-central region is showing the poorest picture among all the regions, where only less than one in 10 CHC (9%) had at least one paediatrician.

Graph 2 *Percentage of at Least 1 Paediatrician at CHC in Regions of Madhya Pradesh*

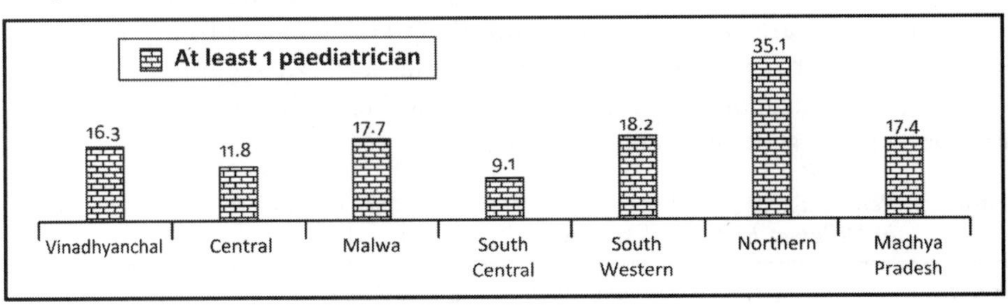

Training of Health Personnel for Child Health Care Services

Table 4 is showing the availability of human resource i.e. medical officers, staff nurses, pharmacists and ANM at different facilities government facilities. In Madhya Pradesh, 66 per cent of PHCs are having at least one medical officer. The south-western region is showing highest percentage (71%) and south-central region is showing lowest percentage (55%) of medical officers (MO) available at PHC level. But if we look into the availability of staff nurses the picture is really gloomy. Madhya Pradesh is having availability of only 19 per cent of staff nurses at PHC level. With regard to the availability of ANM/female health workers, both PHC and SHC are showing an impressive picture but availability of additional staff nurse/ANM at PHC level is very poor (33%). The variations in case of additional staff nurse ranges between 28 per cent for central region and 41 per cent for northern region.

Table 4 *Percentage of Availability of Human Resource at PHC and SHC in Different Regions of Madhya Pradesh, 2007–08*

Regions	*Medical Officer (PHC)*	*Staff Nurse (PHC)*	*Pharmacist (PHC)*	*ANM/Female Health Worker*		*Additional Staff Nurse/ANM*	
				PHC	*SHC*	*PHC*	*SHC*
Vindhyanchal	64.7	15.2	42.4	74.8	88.3	35.4	8.7
Central	68.1	23.4	34.0	76.6	88.9	27.7	5.1
Malwa	67.3	23.1	30.8	80.8	87.6	35.6	5.0
South-central	55.1	18.4	30.3	80.7	94.2	29.4	8.9
South-western	70.7	10.3	17.2	77.6	91.7	31.0	7.1
Northern	79.7	22.0	33.9	88.1	92.6	40.7	14.3
Madhya Pradesh	66.0	18.7	32.1	79.6	90.2	33.4	8.2

Availability of human resource play a very crucial role in proving health services to people, but if health personnel are well trained, then they will be more effective in delivering the services. Table 5 is showing the percentage of medical officers who received child health care training in last five years. In the state of Madhya Pradesh only 21 per cent medical officers received immunization training and Integrated Management of Neonatal and Childhood Illness (IMNCI) training in last five years at PHC level. In IMNCI training, central region is showing the highest percentage (38%) and Vindhyanchal shows the lowest percentage of MOs who received IMNCI training in Madhya Pradesh. The variation in case of receiving immunization training ranges from 31 per cent for south central region to 56 per cent for the northern region. The level of receiving immunization training is comparatively better than IMNCI training at PHC level in the state of Madhya Pradesh.

Table 5 *Percentage of Training Received by Medical Officers in Last 5 Years At PHCs in Different Regions of Madhya Pradesh, 2007–08*

Regions	*Immunization*	*IMNCI*	*Both Trainings*
Vindhyanchal	37.4	17.2	14.1
Central	53.2	38.3	21.3
Malwa	40.4	36.5	24.0
South-central	31.2	26.6	16.6
South-western	39.7	20.7	15.5
Northern	55.9	57.6	37.2
Madhya Pradesh	40.8	31.1	20.6

Availability of Equipments for Child Health Care

Neonatal care is concerned with the health condition of the newborn during first four weeks of life. Neonatal survival is highly sensitive indicator of population growth and socio-economic development. Low birth weight, therefore, is a key factor of adverse outcome in early life. It is seen commonly that unavailability of newborn care equipments and management of low birth weight babies services can be directly linked with a proportion of infant deaths.For example, babies suffering with breathlessness, hypertension and low birth associated complications need emergencies support of equipments meant for revival of normally in-health conditions. The most important of them are neonatal resuscitation; baby warmer and a separate corner for complete set of low birth weight babies management services. In Madhya Pradesh, the availability of newborn care and neonatal resuscitation is around 33 per cent (Table 6). And it is highest in Malwa region (46%) followed by south-central region (34%). In case of availability of baby warmers the situation is really poor, only 20 per cent surveyed PHCs possess baby warmers at the state level. And among the six regions, only 34 per cent PHCs in Northern region had baby warmer which is highest in the state. On the other hand, only 10 per cent PHCs had these critical equipments in the south-western region.

Table 6 *Percentage of Availability and Functionality of Baby Care Equipments at PHC and CHC Level in Different Regions of Madhya Pradesh, 2007–08*

Regions	*Equipment for new born care and neonatal resuscitation (PHC)*		*Baby warmer (PHC)*		*Low birth weight babies managed services at CHC*
	Available	*Functional*	*Available*	*Functional*	
Vindhyanchal	28.3	86.2	14.1	85.7	36.7
Central	27.7	92.3	14.9	57.1	44.1
Malwa	46.2	93.8	32.7	94.1	58.8
South-central	33.9	83.8	11.9	92.3	34.6
South-western	24.1	92.9	10.3	100.0	63.6
Northern	30.5	94.4	33.9	85.0	75.7
Madhya Pradesh	33.2	89.9	19.8	88.3	50.6

These levels show merely the availability of these equipments. However, considering the state of functionality it can further bring down these percentages to fairly low level at least in the central and northern region. Nearly half of the CHCs have capacity to managed low birth babies. The levels of such facility differ greatly by regions. Slightly above one-third (35%) of CHCs has the capacity to manage low birth babies.

Cold chain equipments are very important for heat-sensitive vaccines and it is essential for safe transportation of vaccines from the place of manufacturing to the place of field storage and final carriage to the place of immunization. Cold chain equipments include ice lined refrigerators (ILR), deep freezers, cold box and vaccine carrier. Table 7 is showing the percentage of cold chain equipments at the PHC level in regions of Madhya Pradesh. The availability of ILR in

Madhya Pradesh is 57 per cent. Malwa region is showing highest percentage regarding availability of ILR i.e. 76 per cent and Vindhyanchal shows lowest availability of 38 per cent. Availability of vaccine carrier is comparatively better across the regions. It may be noted that south-central (49%) and Vindhyanchal (44%) are lagging behind in percentage of PHCs having cold box.

Table 7 *Percentage of Availability of Cold Chain Equipment at PHC in Different Regions of Madhya Pradesh, 2007–08*

Regions	*ILR*	*Deep Freezer*	*Cold Box*	*Vaccine Carrier*
Vindhyanchal	38.3	39.9	44.4	75.8
Central	61.7	68.1	70.2	95.7
Malwa	75.9	75.9	76.9	92.3
South-central	47.8	47.7	48.6	89.0
South-western	65.5	72.4	70.7	93.1
Northern	59.3	54.2	74.6	91.5
Madhya Pradesh	56.9	57.9	62.0	88.5

Drugs Availability for Child Health Care

The Table 8 is showing the percentage of availability of drugs at CHC and PHC level in regions of Madhya Pradesh. In anti-allergic drugs at PHC and CHC level, south-central region is showing highest percentages with 91 per cent and 96 per cent of their availability respectively. Anthelmintic are drugs that are used to treat infections with parasitic worms. Availability of these drugs at CHC level (83%) was better than PHC level in the state. Northern region suffers heavy shortage of these drugs at PHC level (61% showing availability of stock) as compared to low level of shortage in south-western (88% showing availability of stock). The variation at the CHCs level was lower than PHCs across the region.

Table 8 *Percentage of Essential Drugs Available at CHC and PHC in Different Regions of Madhya Pradesh, 2007–08*

Regions	*Anti-allergics*		*Anthelminthic*		*Electrolyte*	
	PHC	*CHC*	*PHC*	*CHC*	*PHC*	*CHC*
Vindhyanchal	85.9	95.9	76.8	89.8	62.6	73.5
Central	83.0	76.5	80.9	73.5	70.2	64.7
Malwa	83.7	88.2	76.0	82.4	72.1	82.4
South-central	90.8	96.4	78.0	83.6	68.8	85.5
South-western	87.9	84.9	87.9	84.9	79.3	78.8
Northern	83.1	89.2	61.0	78.4	71.2	91.9
Madhya Pradesh	86.1	89.6	76.7	82.6	70.0	79.9

Electrolyte is basically used during dehydration, the shortage of which sometimes can also be fatal especially in case of children. Only 70 per cent surveyed PHCs reported the availability of their stock at the state level. Once again, situation is relatively better at the CHCs level. The south-western region indicates relatively higher percentage of PHCs possessing electrolytes, whereas northern region leads with 92 per cent of availability of the drugs at CHCs level.

Discussion

In Madhya Pradesh, regions like Central and Vindhyanchal in rural areas show higher infant mortality rate of 83 and 77 infant deaths per thousand live births. It means under-five mortality rate must have been much higher in these regions as its overall level is 96 per thousand live births in rural Madhya Pradesh. In this situation, low level of immunization is a cause of concern in rural area of all the regions. Most of the children received the vaccinations from ICDS centres. It brings a point of policy discussion that there is a need of high level of integration between health and women and child development departments. It is indicting that primary health centres and community health centres must focus and closely monitor outreach services. On the contrary, majority of children (67%) who suffer from diarrhoeal diseases and fever receive treatment from private sector providers. In south-western and south-central regions, utilization of public health facilities, especially PHCs and CHCs are relative high in case of treatment seeking among those children who suffer from diarrhoea and fever.

According to Indian Public Health Standards, one medical officer at PHC level and six medical officers (including specialists) at CHC level must be appointed. One cannot imagine regular functioning of any health facility without a medical officer. However, most of the regions in the state indicate shortage of medical officers with at least one-third of PHCs and CHCs. The situation further deteriorates in the northern and south-central regions (almost half of the facilities without MOs). Similarly pharmacist is one of the key personnel at these facilities. Nearly one-third of PHCs (32%) had pharmacists in position in the state as a whole. The shortage of these personnel is acute (83%) in case of the south-western region. In the absence of such key staffs like MOs and pharmacists, one cannot expect increase in utilization of public health facilities. Therefore, state needs to make immediate provisions to hire more medical personnel in these categories. It is well understood that merely availability of staff may not yield the desired results. The staff should possess the updated skills through departmental trainings and specialized guidelines to be adopted. Merely less than one-third of medical officers (31%) appointed at PHCs were trained in the important training of the integrated management of neonatal and childhood illnesses. Vidhanchal region depicts much gloomy picture of having only 17 per cent MOs trained in this area. Therefore, there is an urgent need of placing well trained health personnel to treat neonates and children for life threatening diseases and infections. A relatively high proportion of CHCs (51%) have reported low birth weight baby managed services over there. On the contrary, only 17 per cent of CHCs had a paediatrician. It is really beyond the imagination that such facilities can handle low birth weight babies and its complications with such a shortage of paediatricians, e.g. only nine per cent of CHCs in central region have these specialist. The task becomes more difficult when only 33 per cent PHCs in the state have critical facilities like newborn care and neonatal resuscitation equipments. The equipments for storing vaccines are also not showing very encouraging though majority of PHCs reported that they had vaccine carrier (89%). It means once a PHC does not have capacity to store vaccines in required environment it may lose its effectiveness or turn to be life threatening rather than life saving. Carrier has its own capacity and time to preserve the vaccines but actually good ILR or deep freezer with 24x7 hours power must be available at least at CHCs level.

In terms of drug supply and availability, all regions show a much better picture than human resource and equipment. But it is question to ponder that in absence of pharmacist and medical personnel who can prescribe these medicines to patients and how the drug resistance and other contraindication of them are managed.

Conclusion

This paper clearly illustrates the immediate need of strengthen the outreach services to reduce mortality due to preventable diseases. In this regard, Central and Vindhyanchal regions require special attention to improve the childhood mortality. Scarcity of human resources, in particular trained and specialist, has direct impact on service utilization in. Therefore, not only their independent effects but also compounded with unavailability of equipments and drugs might have marred the utilization of essential services and their health impacts in almost all regions. Therefore, a comprehensive plan to improve the public health infrastructure in the line of Indian Public Health Standards is the need of the hour to meet the NRHM goals in Madhya Pradesh.

Notes

1. Registrar General of India. 2012. *Sample Registration System Statistical Report 2010*. New Delhi: Office of the Registrar General.
2. International Institute for Population Sciences (IIPS). 2010. *District Level Household Survey (DLHS–3) Report 2007–08*. Mumbai: International Institute for Population Sciences.
3. Planning Evaluation Organization and Planning Commission. 2011. *Evaluation of National Rural Health Mission in 7 States of India*. New Delhi: Planning Commission, February.
4. Directorate General of Health Services, Ministry of Health and Family Welfare. 2006. *Indian Public Health Standards (IPHS) for Primary Health Centres Guidelines*. New Delhi: Ministry of Health and Family Welfare, March.
5. Majumder, A. and Upadhyay, V. 2004. An Analysis of the Primary Health Care System in India with Focus on Reproductive Health Care Services. *Artha Beekshan*, 12 (4): 29–38.
6. Ministry of Health and Family Welfare. 1982–83. *Diarrhoeal Diseases Control Programme: Plan of Operation*. New Delhi: Ministry of Health and Family Welfare.
7. Ministry of Health and Family Welfare. 1983. *National Health Policy*. New Delhi: Ministry of Health and Family Welfare.

8. Kulkarni, Manu N. 1992. Universal Immunization Programme in India: Issues of Sustainability. *Economic and Political Weekly,* July, 4: 1431–1437.
9. Bhende, A. and Kanitkar, T. 2006. *Principle of Population Studies*. 18th Revised Edition, Mumbai: Himalayan Publication Press.
10. Ministry of Health and Family Welfare. 2002. *National Health Policy*. New Delhi: Ministry of Health and Family Welfare.
11. Ministry of Health and Family Welfare. 2005. *National Rural Health Mission*. New Delhi: Ministry of Health and Family Welfare.
12. Lakshmi, T. and Sahoo, D. 2013. Health Infrastructure and Health Indicators: The Case of Andhra Pradesh, India. *Journal of Humanities and Social Sciences*, January–February, 6 (6): 22–29.
13. Datar, A., Mukherji, A. and Sood, N. 2007. Health Infrastructure and Immunization Coverage in Rural India. *Indian J Med Res*, 125: 31–42.
14. Leipziger, D., Fay, M., Wodon, Q. and Yepes, T. 2003. Achieving the Millennium Development Goals: The Role of Infrastructure. World Bank Working Paper No. 3163, November.
15. Ghei, K., Agarwal, S., Subramanyam, M.A. and Subramanian, S.V. 2010. Association between Child Immunization and Availability of Health Infrastructure in Slums in India. *Arch Pediatr Adolesc Med*, 164 (3): 243–249.
16. Senavirante, H.R. and Rajapaksa, L.C. 2000. Safe Motherhood in Sri Lanka: A 100-Year March. *International Journal of Gynaecology and Obstetrics*, 7: 113–124.
17. Bitner, M.J. 1992. The Impact of Physical Surroundings on Customers and Employees. *Journal of Marketing*, 56: 57–71.
18. Mothercare. 1999. *Child Survival and Safe Motherhood Programme Review and Assessment: Lessons Learned and Recommendations*. An Evaluation Report Prepared for the Ministry of Health and Family Welfare of India by Mothercare, 30 September 29 October, Section 8, p. 65.

11

Benefit Incidence of Public Expenditure in Health

A Study of Karnataka

Varun Sharma, Jyotsna Jha and Divya Krishnaswamy

The prime objective of a health care system is to meet the health care needs of people in the most efficient and effective manner. Aligned with the objectives of the National Rural Health Mission (NRHM), Karnataka has implemented various programmes to attain the goals of the National Population Policy (NPP) and the Millennium Development Goals (MDGs). Karnataka has also recognized the immeasurable value of enhancing the health and well-being of its people. As a result of the state's focus on these issues, the health infrastructure in Karnataka is better placed than that of other states in the country. The health indicators in the state are much better positioned when compared with the corresponding national averages: Total Fertility Rate (TFR) in Karnataka is 2.0 which is less than the national average of 2.6 (Registrar General of India, 2012); the Infant Mortality Rate (IMR), Maternal Mortality Rate (MMR) and Sex Ratio (SR) in the state are 35/1000, 178 and 968 per '000' males respectively and are better than the corresponding national averages at 44, 212 and 940 (Registrar General of India, 2012; Registrar General and Census Commissioner, n.d.).

Health care financing plays a significant role in sustaining the improvement in health outcomes. Considering the rising cost of medical care and high Out of Pocket (OOP) health spending, greater attention needs to be paid to equitable health financing. It is essential that the government plays a multifaceted role as the financing source, a financing agent and the service provider. Health insurance schemes, prepayment schemes, selection of cost-effective strategies such as use of generic drugs, central purchasing and better management of infrastructure, equipments and transport enhance both the quality and coverage of health care (Government of Karnataka, 2004). Such measures help the poorest strata of society in accessing health care services at affordable prices. This paper attempts to investigate the distributional incidence of public spending on health for different groups of interest.

Public spending can take the form of public transfers, taxes, subsidies or policy change in terms of prices of services provided by public institutional bodies. In the health sector, it has been noticed that public health care facilities which cater to people from the lower economic strata are highly subsidized – National Sample Survey Organisation (NSSO).

Addressing the needs of poor people in terms of their access to health care is the critical objective of most governments. Measuring benefits of government expenditures across income, race and other characteristics of individuals is an extensive empirical exercise. The poor often have limited access to services because of their compromised economic status. Hence, the government is expected to target the provision of these services to the poor. But how does one ascertain the extent to which either existing allocation or the increased allocation is reaching the poor (Tiongson, Davoodi and Asawanuchit, 2003)? Benefit incidence analysis (BIA) is a tool that addresses this question.

BIA brings together the elements of the supply of and the demand for public services and can provide valuable information on inefficiencies and inequities in government allocation of resources for social services and on the utilization of these services. Benefit incidence tells us who benefits from the services, transfers, subsidies or policy changes while estimating the size of benefits received by people. Benefit incidence helps to estimate the distributional benefit of public spending on health among different economic strata in Karnataka state.

Review of Literature

The literature on benefit incidence previously had three distinct periods. Prior to 1975, benefits were allocated to households either on a per capita basis or in proportion to the income of the household. Both allocation mechanisms yielded obvious conclusions about benefit incidence. There was also a preoccupation in early literature about allocating the entire budget including the benefits of so-called pure public goods such as defence. Aaron and McGuire (1970) attempted to reduce the inherent arbitrariness of the allocation of pure public goods benefits to households by deriving benefit measures based on a specific utility function. The parameters of their utility function suggest a strong pro-rich distribution of benefits, at least in developed countries (Selden and Wasylenko, 1992).

The approach adopted by social scientists since 1975 has great potential for informing policy choices on the transfer of resources within programmes to target the poor more accurately. Nonetheless, researchers studying the benefits derived from public spending in developing countries may need to pay extra attention to (i) expenditures made through off-budget programmes such as public enterprises, (ii) benefit shifting especially for agricultural programmes, (iii) differential public service quality, especially between urban and rural areas, (iv) the effects of benefits on inter- and intra-family transfers and (v) the effects of benefits on urban-rural migration.

Gertler and Paul (1990) and Gertler, Luis and Warren (1987), had estimated demand curves for various social services in an extended analysis of benefit incidence. Changes in welfare-based measures (or compensating variation) of social services benefits can be estimated by using demand curves for particular population subgroups. Studies using welfare-based measures of benefits for a wide range of public functions can yield valuable information to policymakers and help target limited resources towards those public services that provide maximum benefit to the poor. However, these studies do not, till date, offer benefit measures on the broad range of government services that more traditional benefit incidence studies have to offer (Selden and Wasylenko, 1992).

Households incur OOP expenses to obtain in-kind subsidies embodied in health care services and these should be incorporated in benefit incidence analysis. Some can be considered as transaction costs (such as transport expenses) while others add to the benefits that are obtained from the service (such as user-charges). Benefit incidence refers only to the distribution of public subsidy; it is often useful to incorporate an analysis of the household spending for the service to obtain a full account of the service involved.

The rest of the paper is organized as follows: Section III describes the process of benefit incidence analysis; Section IV details the data sources; Sections V, VI and VII provide the methodology, estimation of distributional incidence, and assumptions and limitations of study respectively; and Section VIII describes the findings and provides a discussion about the findings.

How is Benefit Incidence Analysis Conducted?

The following information is essential for estimation of the incidence of public spending on various services:

- Government spending from the budget reports released by the Department of Finance.
- An understanding of the quantum of public utilization of resources.
- The socio-economic characteristics of the population using the service.

All this data is typically reported on an aggregate basis.

In order to conduct benefit incidence analysis, the first step is to obtain the average unit cost of providing a public service by dividing the government spending by the total number of users of the service. Figures from the state budget for the health sector may be used to obtain total public spending on health services; this includes both recurrent and capital expenditure. The total number of beneficiaries of the service is estimated from household surveys.

Data on the following parameters is required to conduct such an analysis:

- public expenditure to estimate the value of benefits;
- individual or household level data from household surveys on the usage of service; and
- socio-economic characteristics of users of service.

Data Sources

Information on public expenditure: This was obtained from budget documents of the government to estimate value of benefits. The present analysis uses data from the health sector, Programme Budget Analysis (PBA) report (Centre for

Budget and Policy Studies, 2012) to estimate total public spending on health care.

Number of beneficiaries: These have been estimated from the District Level Household and Health Facility Survey-III[1] (or DLHS-III) (International Institute for Population Sciences, 2010) data for Karnataka state and extrapolated for the population figures as per Census 2001.

Quintile-wise distribution of the population accessing health care in public health facilities have also been estimated from DLHS-III. A Wealth Index was constructed based on the methodology proposed by Filmer and Pritchett[2] as a proxy for income/consumption quintile. The Wealth Index was constructed based on the information on nature of housing, access to basic amenities and possession of durable goods. Based on the Principle Component Analysis (PCA), factor loading to amenities, assets and durables was derived and used for the computation of the Wealth Index. The Wealth Index score was categorized into five categories ranging from the poorest to the richest at the state level. This categorization was used as a proxy for income/ consumption quintile to ascertain the benefit incidence across income/wealth classes of public spending/expenditure on health care.

Methodology

The four basic steps in BIA are as follows:

- All individuals are ranked from the poorest to the richest as per the chosen measure of welfare (in the current analysis this measure is the Wealth Index). Groups are typically ordered from lowest to highest with respect to the classifying variable.
- Identify which individual used each type of publically provided service (net of cost recovery in terms of user fees or charges).
- Calculate the average unit cost of providing the service.
- Multiply the utilization figure with the government's unit cost of provisioning of services to estimate the total amount of public spending per group of interest.

Estimation

Xj = Ó Eij (Si/Ei)

Where, j = 1, 2, 3, 4, 5, i =1, 2

Xj is the benefit analysis in local currency accrued to wealth group *j* from (net) government spending denoted as *S*, also measured in local currency;

Eij represents the number of total beneficiaries in level i from group *j* where each group is a quintile; and

Si/Ei is the unit cost of providing *health care at level i*.

Assumptions and Limitations

- Only primary, secondary and tertiary (development and recurring expenditure) expenditures were considered while estimating total public health spending; expenditure on administration and other overheads was not included.

— Public spending on health care was estimated using the budget documents of Karnataka for the financial year 2007–08

- Total number of beneficiaries was estimated based on the population figures as per Census 2001.
- DLHS-III provides household level data about access to health care when any household member falls sick[3]; this was used to analyse health seeking behaviour. However, information on access to secondary/tertiary health care in DLHS-III was ambiguous; as a result, data on access to secondary and tertiary health care was clubbed together.
- Estimation of costs:
  — Unit cost was assumed to be uniform for a particular level of health care.
  — Cost recovery in terms of user charges collected constitutes a very small proportion and hence was not considered while estimating unit cost.
  — No distinction was made regarding the rural-urban divide.

Findings and Discussion

The present paper provides two estimates for the average cost of providing service – one based on total health spending (development and recurrent) and one based on recurrent spending only. Recent practices confine analysis to recurrent spending only, thereby avoiding the difficulties encountered in estimating the flow of services/benefits from capital expenditures. However, when capital budgets are large, they have a profound effect on the benefit incidence of public spending. Average cost has been estimated by dividing total public expenditure on health care by the total number of beneficiaries.

The total number of beneficiaries was estimated from the Census 2001 population figures: Karnataka population as per Census 2001 was 52.85 million; the total number of households was 10.36 million; and the average household size was 5.1. Considering that 42.9 per cent of households in DLHS-III responded affirmative to seeking treatment at public health facilities; this translates into 22.67 million (4.44 million households) when the figures are extrapolated for the entire state.

Based on the estimated figure of total beneficiaries, the average unit cost of providing public health care services was estimated for both primary health care and secondary/tertiary health care.

Table 1 shows the distribution of sample by wealth categories and source of treatment. It was noticed that in Karnataka, 42.9 per cent of households seek treatment in a public health facility when any member of their household falls sick. A few observations that emerge from the Table 1 are: (1) fifty-two per cent of the poorest access health care in public health facilities, (2) from the poorest to the richest wealth class, the percentage of households accessing health care at public health facilities declines, and (3) even amongst the richest wealth quintile,

23.8 per cent households seek treatment in public health facilities. Though at a glance this 23.8 per cent seems high as the assumption is that rich people do not access public health facilities; however, this figure is in line with real scenarios as is shown from findings of various studies (National Sample Survey Organisation, 2006).

Table 1 *Wealth Class and Source of Treatment*

Characteristics	*Households as per DLHS-III*	*Accessing health care at public health facility*	*Not accessing health care at public health facility*	*Percentage accessing health care in public health facilities*	*Distribution of those accessing health care in public health facility by wealth classes*
Poorest	5,598	2,913	2,685	52.0	23.3
Poor	6,027	2,995	3,032	49.7	24
Medium	5,813	2,783	3,030	47.9	22.3
Rich	5,811	2,396	3,415	41.2	19.2
Richest	5,813	1,383	4,430	23.8	11.1
Total	29,062	12,470	16,592	42.9	100.0

Source: District level Household and Facility Survey (DLHS-III) 2007–08.

Table 2 shows the distribution of households by wealth quintile and the level of health care facilities they access; it also provides the socio-economic classification of users of public health services. Here public health facilities include government hospitals, PHC, CHS, SC, UHC, AYUSH hospitals, Anganwadi/ICDC centre, government mobile clinic and other public health facilities. It is seen that in general, a majority of those who seek treatment in public health facilities primarily belong to the poorest, the poor and the medium socio-economic sections. From Table 2 it is seen that of the 12,470 households that access health care at public health facilities, 71.7 per cent have availed primary health care while the rest have availed secondary or tertiary health care services. When we look at which wealth classes access primary health care services from public health facilities, we see that the percentage of those accessing such services declines as we move from the poorest to the richest wealth classes; a mere 8.4 per cent from the richest wealth quintile have availed primary health care in public health facilities.

Table 2 *Wealth Quintile-wise Distribution of Level of Health Care*

Level of health care	*Wealth quintile*					*Total*
	Poorest	*Poor*	*Medium*	*Rich*	*Richest*	
Primary	2,267 (25.4)	2,246 (25.1)	2,017 (22.6)	1,660 (18.6)	752 (8.4)	8,942
Secondary and tertiary*	646 (18.3)	749 (21.2)	766 (21.7)	736 (20.9)	631 (17.9)	3,528
Total	2,913 (23.4)	2,995 (24.0)	2,783 (22.3)	2,396 (19.2)	1,383 (11.1)	12,470

Source: DLHS-III 2007–08

Note: *Secondary and tertiary health care level is clubbed, figures in bracket shows the percentage distribution.

Table 3 shows the estimated number of beneficiaries of public health spending in Karnataka as against the Census 2001 population figures. Extrapolating the findings from DLHS-III the total number of beneficiaries of public health services is estimated to be 22.67 million.

Table 3 *Estimation of Beneficiaries of Public Health Spending*

Characteristics	*Number*	*Per cent*
Total population (Census 2001)	5,28,50,562	100.0
Estimated number of total beneficiaries (based on DLHS-III)	2,26,72,891	42.9
Estimated number of total beneficiaries of primary health care (based on DLHS-III)	1,62,56,463	71.7
Estimated number of total beneficiaries of secondary and tertiary health care (DLSH-III)	64,16,428	28.3

Source: Census 2001, DLHS-III 2007–08

Table 4 shows the distribution of estimated beneficiaries assessing health care by level of health care and wealth quintile. More poor people access primary health care in public health facilities than the rich as was seen in Table 2. However, not much difference was observed when we look at data on access to secondary and tertiary health care.

Table 4 *Estimated Beneficiaries* Accessing Health Care in Public Health Facilities by Wealth Quintile and Level of Facility*

Level	*Primary health care*	*Secondary and tertiary health care*	*Total*
Q1 (Poorest)	41,21,382	11,74,890	52,96,273
Q2 (poor)	40,83,205	13,62,218	54,45,423
Q3 (Medium)	36,66,885	13,93,136	50,60,021
Q4 (Rich)	30,17,863	13,38,575	43,56,437
Q5 (Richest)	13,67,128	11,47,609	25,14,738
Total	1,62,56,463	64,16,428	2,26,72,891

Note: * To estimated number of beneficiaries in respective wealth class by level of health care refer to Table 2

The Tables above provide the data related to utilization of public health facilities and socio-economic characteristics of beneficiaries of public health facilities required to conduct benefit incidence analysis.

Health expenditure includes expenditure incurred for medical care, drug and supplies, institutional build-up, medical education, training and research, public health and family welfare. The total budgeted health expenditure for the three sectors (primary, secondary and tertiary) in 2007–08 was found to be ₹ 73,277 lakh (primary health care ₹ 39,523 lakh and secondary and tertiary care ₹ 33,754 lakh). These figures include development expenditure in the respective health care sector. Based on this information, we estimated ₹ 323.2 to be the average cost of providing public health services. Table 5 shows the per capita public expenditure on health in Karnataka in different sectors based on total expenditure in all three sectors and recurrent expenditure.

Table 5 *Per capita Public Expenditure* on Health in Karnataka*

(In Rupees)

Health sector	*Per capita expenditure (development and recurrent)*	*Per capita expenditure (recurrent)*
Primary health sector	243.1	224.9
Secondary and tertiary health sector	526.1	302.1
Total	323.2	246.8

Note: * Per capita expenditure figures are arrived at by dividing total expenditure in respective sector by estimated number of total beneficiaries in respective sector (refer to Table 3)

Table 5 shows that in Karnataka ₹ 323.2 (absolute figures) per capita is spent on health care (development and recurrent expenditure). The per capita health expenditure on primary health care is ₹ 243.1; together, the secondary and tertiary care sectors account for ₹ 526.1 per capita health expenditure. However, considering recurrent expenditure, per capita expenditure in Karnataka in the different sectors is ₹ 224.9 (primary sector) and ₹ 302.1 (secondary and tertiary sector).

Multiplying the utilization figures (Table 2 or Table 4) with the government's unit cost of provision (Table 5) gives the amount of public spending on services going to each group.

Table 6 shows the benefit incidence of health spending to different wealth groups. It is observed that public health spending in Karnataka in the primary health sector is more pro-poor when compared to secondary or tertiary health sectors. Table 6 also shows the incidence of the entire expenditure across all the quintile classes; aggregate expenditure on health in a particular quintile is taken into consideration.

Table 6 *Benefit Incidence of Spending Accrued to the Wealth Group*

(In Rupees)

Level	*Total expenditure (development and recurrent)*			*Recurrent expenditure*		
	Primary health care	*Secondary and tertiary health care*	*Total (per capita)**	*Primary Health care*	*Secondary and tertiary health care*	*Total (per capita)**
Q1 (Poorest)	10,020# (61.6)	6,181 (96.3)	17,117 (75.5)	9,270 (57.0)	3,550 (55.3)	13,069 (57.6)
Q2 (poor)	9,927 (61.1)	7,166 (111.7)	17,599 (77.6)	9,184 (56.5)	4,115 (64.1)	13,437 (59.3)
Q3 (Medium)	8,915 (54.8)	7,329 (114.2)	16,354 (72.1)	8,248 (50.7)	4,209 (65.6)	12,486 (55.1)
Q4 (Rich)	7,337 (45.1)	7,042 (109.7)	14,080 (62.1)	6,788 (41.8)	4,044 (63.0)	10,750 (47.4)
Q5 (Richest)	3,324 (20.4)	6,037 (94.1)	8,127 (35.8)	3,075 (18.9)	3,467 (54.0)	6,206 (27.4)
Total	39,523 (243.1)	33,754 (526.1)	73,277 (323.2)	36,564 (224.9)	19,385 (302.1)	55,949 (246.8)

Note: # figures are in lakhs * figures in brackets show per capita distribution of benefit of public spending in rupees.

Figure 1 *Concentration Curve Showing the Incidence of Public Spending on Health in Karnataka*

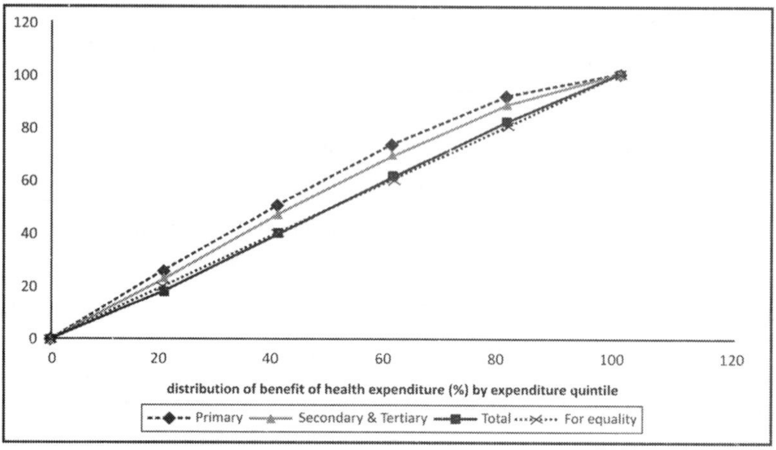

To summarize the expenditure pattern further, the benefit incidence of public spending on health can also be illustrated by a concentration curve graph. A concentration curve of government spending plots the cumulative proportions of households, ranked from the poorest to the richest, on the horizontal axis, against the cumulative proportion of benefits received by the household, plotted on the vertical axis. Figure 1 shows this cumulative distribution – it shows three concentration curves (one each for the primary and secondary/tertiary sectors, and one for total health care) and the 45 degree line (purple coloured line) called the line of equality across all sectors. The graph is an illustration of the structure of benefit derived from government spending.

Benefits from public spending are said to be pro-poor if the concentration curve lies above line of equality; this type of concentration curve is concave and implies that authorities follow policies that target the poorer section of society. From Figure 1 it is quite evident that the concentration curve for primary health care is more concave than that of secondary/tertiary health care or of total health care; hence, it is safe to say that Government of Karnataka follows policies which target the poorer sections of society.

Discussion

The analysis of distribution of public spending on health care shows that public spending on health care in Karnataka is more pro-poor at the primary care level; this highlights the commitment of the government to provide affordable health care services to needy people particularly for preventive health care. However, at the secondary/tertiary level as the concentration curve almost runs along the line of equality, the distribution of public spending on health care is almost equally distributed across economic categories.

On an overall level, benefits of public health spending are pro-poor in Karnataka showing the government's commitment to provide policies and to increase its outlay on health so as to benefit people that are disadvantaged either socially or economically.

Considering that most of the people belonging to poor economic strata access health care in public health facilities, it is essential on the part of financing and implementing authorities to invest even more on public health facilities so that benefits flow to the economically weaker sections of society.

Notes

1. DLHS-III collected the data from 29,062 households in Karnataka state in 2007–08 regarding their demographic, socio-economic, health-seeking behaviour and reproductive and child health-related issues. The survey included 27,864 ever-married women and 6,452 unmarried women in Karnataka. Information was collected at various levels and for different dimensions.
2. Filmer, D. and Pritchett, L.H. 2001. Estimating Wealth Effect without Expenditure Data – or Tears: An Application to Educational Enrollments in States of India. *Demography*, 38: 115–132.
3. The question in DLHS-III was 'When members of your household get sick, where they mainly go for treatment?' It is assumed that as per DLHS-III those who had responded affirmative to accessing health care from a particular type of health facility would eventually access services from that type of health facility when need arose.

References

Aaron, H.J. and McGuire, M.C. 1970. Public Goods and Income Distribution. *Econometrica*, 38 (2): 907–920.

Centre for Budget and Policy Studies. 2012. *Program Budget Analysis: A Review of Health Expenditure in Karnataka*. Bangalore: CBPS.

Gertler, P. and Paul, G. 1990. The Willingness to Pay for Education in Developing Countries. *Journal of Public Economics*, 42: 251–275.

Gertler, P., Luís, L. and Warren, S. 1987. Are User Fees Regressive? The Welfare Implications of Health Care Financing Proposals in Peru. *Journal of Econometrics*, 33: 67–88.

Government of Karnataka. 2004. *The Karnataka State Integrated Health Policy*. Proceedings of the State Cabinet, Bangalore: GoK.

International Institute for Population Sciences. 2010. *District Level Household and Facility Survey (DLHS–3): Karnataka (2007–08)*. Mumbai: IIPS.

National Sample Survey Organisation. 2006. *Morbidity, Healthcare and the Conditions of the Aged: NSS 60th Round*. New Delhi: MoSPI and GoI.

Registrar General and Census Commissioner. n.d. Retrieved from www.censusindia.gov.in: http://www.censusindia.gov.in/census_data_ 2001/census_data_online/

Registrar General of India. October 2012. Retrieved from www.censusindia.gov.in: http://http://www.censusindia.gov.in/vital_ statistics/srs_bulletins/srs_bulletin-october_2012.pdf

Selden, T.M. and Wasylenko, M.J. 1992. *Benefit Incidence Analysis in Developing Countries*. Washington, D.C.: World Bank.

Tiongson, E., Davoodi, H.R. and Asawanuchit, S.S. 2003. *How Useful are Benefit Incidence Analyses of Public Education and Health Spending*. Washington, D.C.: IMF.

12

Access to In-Patient Health Care in West Bengal

A Benefit Incidence Analysis

Montu Bose

In the post-globalization era, the transition towards the market economy garnered a structural modification on the role of the state. Increasingly, higher shares of population across the globe started depending on for-profit and not-for-profit private organizations for their health care needs. However, along with this, most of the developing countries are also turning back towards the policy of Universal Health Care, where the poorest and the most vulnerable section of the population is expected to be covered by essential primary care. Therefore, subsidization of health care from public purse appears to be a common and desired goal for most of the developing countries. The public intervention in finance and provision of health care is an attempt to promote efficiency through correcting various market failures, and also to uphold equity by improving the distribution of economic welfare. More specifically, pro-poor subsidy spending from public is endorsed for its instrumental value in improving the health of the population and so the productivity of the labour force and consequently, economic growth. India and its states are not an exception in this regard. With Universal Health Coverage (UHC) on the policy anvil across the globe, India, representing a kaleidoscopic mosaic of people from different groups, caste, religion, language, has started to focus on UHC. It is defined as 'ensuring equitable access for all Indian citizens, resident in any part of the country, regardless of income level, social status, gender, caste or religion, to affordable, accountable, appropriate health services of assured quality (promotive, preventive, curative and rehabilitative) as well as public health services addressing the wider determinants of health delivered to individuals and populations, with the government being the guarantor and enabler of health and related services'. Thus, it becomes extremely important for a government to target the subsidies well, to cover the poor population with needed timely health interventions.

In this backdrop the performance of health system can be judged from two distinct angles: the efficiency perspective and the equity perspective; while the former talks about getting the maximum out of given resources, the latter talks about the distribution of this benefit across different socio-economic classes. A few recent studies undertaken on the public-run hospitals in West Bengal have already shown the presence of deficiency in provisioning of health care services. This insufficient provision, if not distributed properly would challenge the desirability of the system even more. The system is subsidized and the crucial question is 'who is reaping benefit of this subsidy?' To get a holistic view of the situation, one needs to look simultaneously at the access and benefit incidence (BI) of government run facilities across different economic classes.

West Bengal, a middle-income state in the eastern region of India is a medium performer in terms of health (with fourth lowest Infant Mortality and full vaccination coverage above the national average). However, significantly high rural-urban gap in almost all health indicators and lack of access to specialty services bring West Bengal to the public debate of 'almost non-performance of government-run hospital services' in all forms of media. It has the oldest and probably the largest public health and hospital-based health care delivery infrastructure and network among the states of India. In West Bengal, according to NSSO 60th Round, over 27 per cent of the population still lived below the poverty line and about 75 per cent of the hospitalized seek treatment in government-run hospitals (against the national average of 40%). This signifies the importance of public health system in West Bengal in general and also the seriousness of impact of this malfunctioning on the common people of the state at large. This paper intends to examine whether in West Bengal, economically the most vulnerable section of the society is able to access the public health care services and enjoy government subsidies or not. More specifically the objectives are:

- To analyse the access pattern of hospitalization in public-run hospitals across monthly per capita consumption expenditure (MPCE) classes in the state.
- To identify the actual beneficiaries of this public subsidies.

The paper attempts to find out the access and benefits derived across different services provided to the in-patients of different socio-income groups.

The rest of the paper is organized as follows: a brief review of literature is presented in section 2 and sections 3 and 4 contain the detailed description of methodology to be adopted and data sources of the study. Results are presented in section 5 followed by an overall assessment in the concluding section.

Literature Survey

Access to health care is a multidimensional and complex notion. Various barriers exist which limit equitable access to and utilization of health care services by different socio-economic domain. Studies from India portrays the widening gap between the 'urban and rural' and the 'haves and have-nots'. Literatures also focus on social group and gender related disparities in access to health care. A recent study by Palmer (2008) presents a vast literature on utilization by socio-economic status or other equity-related subgroups.

Measuring the benefits of publicly provided goods to individuals is a matter of longstanding concern in the economics literature. For market based goods and services, the prices consumers pay can be taken as reflecting underlying values and can be used to yield measures of welfare that can be compared across individuals. But when governments subsidize the provision of goods and services like health, education etc. supply is usually rationed and the price paid (if any) does not necessary reflect the shadow price to an individual consumer. To measure the value to the beneficiaries of government-subsidized goods and services, one can use Benefit Incidence Analysis (BIA) which has been broadly applied in many studies.

A recent paper by McIntyre and Ataguba (2011) provides detail method of the BIA analysis with a critical review of its limitations. Using data from the VHLSS[1] Wagstaff (2010) examined the basic methodology of BIA and its assumptions. Another study by O'Donnell et al. (2008) shows that the distribution of public health care is pro-rich in most developing countries and pro-poor incidence is easier to realize for higher national incomes. Many other studies have conducted the BIA to find out the distribution of social spending in health and education.

A number of studies have also used this method to calculate the distribution of public subsidies in India. Using the NSS data Mahal et al. (2001) found that in terms of curative care and tertiary level hospital services, richer section of the society are enjoying more benefits than their poorer counterparts. In a recent paper by Chakraborty, Singh and Jacob (2011) use the access and utilization of health care services related NSSO data of 60th Round (2004–05) for BIA calculation and compared the inter-temporal changes using NSSO data on health care of 52nd Round (1995–96). Relying on the same data sources, Acharya et al. (2011) tries to find out answers to health care related public policies for two Indian states – Tamil Nadu and Orissa (Odisha). There has been no study, however, on benefit incidence for separate services categories, which are largely used for hospitalized care. This paper attempts to bridge this gap.

Methodology

To estimate benefit incidence information is needed on the share of group *j* in the utilization of service *i* (α_{ij}/α_i) and government's net expenditure on service i (ρ_i). Mathematically, Benefit Incidence is estimated by the formula:

Where,

η_j = Benefit of public subsidy enjoyed by group j,
α_{ij} = utilization of service i by group j,
α_i = utilization of service i by all groups together,
ρ_i = government's net expenditure on service i and
θ_{ij} = group j's share of utilization of service i.

We have taken i = bed, test, medicine, doctor and
j = poor, lower middle, upper middle and rich section of the society.

Data

National Sample Survey (NSS)[2] provides household level information on monthly per capita consumption expenditure (MPCE), which can be taken as a proxy for economic status. Following NSSO we have clubbed all individuals into four broad categories – Poorest (P), Lower Middle (LM), Upper Middle (UM) and Richest (R), separately for rural and urban areas.[3]

Information on ten different services accessed by individuals during hospitalization at the public hospitals and dispensaries are recorded in NSSO unit level data. We have clubbed these services into four broad categories – Doctor or surgeon's fee (DOC), medicines (MED), diagnostic tests (TEST) and bed and related services (BED)[4].

Access is assessed on the basis of Yes/No responses and to calculate benefit incidence the following steps have been followed for each sector separately.

1. First we have calculated the number of in-patients who have utilized the services of government hospitals across different MPCE classes (α_{ij}). The share of a MPCE class in utilization of a service gives us the utilization share for the MPCE class (θ_{ij}).
2. To calculate public subsidy (or expenditure) on in-patient and out-patient across rural and urban areas no specific information was available in a readily usable form. National Health Accounts (NHA, 2004–05) provides data [13] on total public health care expenditure for each state including West Bengal which has two components: current expenditure and capital expenditure. However, for BIA calculation one needs to have information on only current expenditure. This decomposition of *total* between *current* and *capital* heads is available only at the All-India level. Hence, in the absence of any better proxy we have used the All-India share to cull out the current public health expenditure from the state-level total. A further decomposition of this total current expenditure is needed between out-patient and in-patient for both rural and urban sectors. Population share of in-patient (IP) and out-patient (OP) for both rural and urban regions available from NSSO data has been used for this purpose, which yields information on OP-Rural, IP-Rural and OP-Urban, IP-Urban.
3. For service-wise break-up of in-patient care (IP-Rural and IP-Urban), *incremental apportionment rule* (IAR) has been devised and implemented. For each beneficiary we have information on types of services accessed and total out-of-pocket expenditure borne as in-patient. So, we can calculate the relative access of different services in both Rural and Urban sector where the sequence may not be identical.[5] Since, by definition all in-patients have to access bed hence, those who have accessed only bed their average out-of-pocket expenditure has been taken as the cost of BED. Next the subgroup of patients who have accessed both BED and TEST have been taken (as TEST is the next most demanded service in both rural and urban areas) and their average expenditure on these two services taken together has been calculated. Now, the cost of BED has been deducted from this to get the cost of TEST as an incremental cost. At the subsequent

stages the third and then fourth most important item has been incorporated and the incremental cost of this inclusion has been isolated as cost of that service. For all the four services in both Rural and Urban areas the unit cost is thus obtained and the *share* of each item in the total cost has also been estimated. Multiplying the government expenditure by these *shares* we got the region specific as well as service specific government expenditure like IPD_R_BED, IPD_R_MED, IPD_U_TEST, etc.

4. To get per capita government expenditure for a service (say IPD_R_BED_PCGE), we have divided the government expenditure by the number of patients who have used the service of the sector.
5. To calculate out of pocket (OOP) expenditure, NSS information has been used.
   - (a) Total expenditure incurred by an individual during hospitalization gives us the amount of OOP payment of the individual for a specific service. Where individuals were unable to report the actual amount of expenditure which they have made ('Y' in NSSO data), the average expenditure for the MPCE class for the service has been used as proxy.
   - (b) Since the patients belonging to different expenditure classes have different purchasing power, hence to normalize that difference an OOP-weight has been used. The share of government expenditure in total expenditure (government plus OOP) has been taken as the weight.
   - (c) This adjusted OOP expenditure has been used as the representation of actual OOP payment.
6. To calculate the net-subsidy (ρ_i), actual OOP expenditure has been deducted from the per capita government expenditure (PCGE).

Multiplying the net subsidy amount with the initially calculated utilization ratio we can have the measure of benefit incidence (BI) for the service (η_j).

Results and Discussion

Access and Utilization: According to NSSO data in 2004–05, 18.08 per cent of rural and 22.84 per cent of urban population in West Bengal reported morbidity, and out of them, 49.74 per cent in rural and 44.57 per cent in urban were admitted to hospitals as in-patients. The majority of them availed public facilities (76.60 per cent in rural and 65.36 per cent in urban). In cases of hospital bed and medicine, the access in both rural and urban areas are pretty close. Access pattern is showing an increasing association with the extent of deservingness where the poorest group has the maximum access and the richest group has the minimum, the range varies between 90.91 per cent for BED for poorest (P) to 51.98 per cent for DOC for richest (R) in rural sector and 89.00 per cent for BED for P to 41.97 per cent for DOC for R in urban sector (Table 1). In general the access is marginally better for the rural area where both the availability and affordability of private health care institution is less. Among the services, BED is the mostly accessed one as without BED one cannot be identified as in-patient.

Next to BED the highest access is revealed by medicine (MED), next comes TEST and DOC is the last one. The pattern is uniform across sectors; however, the magnitudes in rural are always higher than those of urban for all types of services confirming a stronger presence of private infrastructure and manpower in urban centres.

Table 1 *Access to Public Health Services Across Economic Classes and Regions (%)*

MPCE	*Rural*						*Urban*					
	Morbid	*IPD*	*BED*	*MED*	*TEST*	*DOC*	*Morbid*	*IPD*	*BED*	*MED*	*TEST*	*DOC*
P	12.95	55.69	90.61	89.52	91.35	88.00	17.40	48.78	89.00	88.24	82.54	80.00
LM	16.01	51.81	84.11	83.40	77.42	71.62	20.10	42.70	80.40	83.33	75.71	76.34
UM	19.77	46.88	74.84	75.66	68.58	66.91	21.61	46.95	68.42	68.78	64.71	64.29
R	23.93	48.39	60.00	56.37	54.72	51.98	29.34	42.60	45.34	44.33	41.97	37.65
All	18.08	49.74	76.60	75.17	69.77	65.52	22.84	44.57	65.36	64.96	59.60	57.65

Source: Computed from NSS 60th Round Data and NHA.

Note: P-Poorest, LM-Lower Middle, UM-Upper Middle, R-Richest; IPD – in-patient department.

Benefit Incidence: In general, the average per capita benefit enjoyed in the rural sector (₹ 1,416.80) is marginally greater than that by the urban area (₹ 1,374.10). In both sectors wide variation of benefit incidence is observed across income-classes. In rural West Bengal the range varies between ₹ 663.40 to ₹ 1,753.10, whereas in urban area the range is between ₹ 561.40 and ₹ 1,890.20, indicating a wider variation for the latter. It is interesting to note that in both sectors the lowest per capita benefit goes to the poorest class (P) and the maximum is reaped by the upper middle class (UM). The richest class (R) is getting lesser benefit than the middles classes (both LM and UM) but much higher than the poorest ones (Table 2). Since the mean values of average benefit enjoyed by each economic class in each location are pretty close to their median, hence, no intra-class disparity is suspected. When a service-specific analysis is carried out this middle-class bias becomes most prominent for DOC, which has lowest access, (in both rural and urban) and very negligible for BED in urban. For other two services like MED and TEST, the middle band is getting the maximum, followed by the rich, keeping the poor at the most deprived state. Though this pattern is uniformly prevailing in both rural and urban areas, the MED-subsidy in rural is higher than that in urban, whereas the opposite holds for TEST-subsidy. So, the benefit incidence is suggesting a very different picture than the previously discussed access pattern.

Subsidy Distribution across Services: At this juncture it would be interesting to explore the pattern of subsidy distribution across services. This pattern would throw some light on the socially inequitable pattern of benefit distribution observed so far. A closer look at the services provided during hospitalization suggests each service has some uniqueness in its nature. For BED, recurring cost to provide the service is very low. This is reflected in the subsidy-distribution for the service also – here for all economic classes, the benefit derived is very low for both rural and urban areas. For MED, government just reimburses the cost of medicines used for the treatment. Here, due to better utilization and access to better quality products by the upper income classes, subsidy amount varies across income categories and the middle class gets bigger reimbursement than the poorest one. After all, the amount of reimbursement is directly related to the ability to spend. So, the reimbursement policy itself would create some affordability-bias. For TEST, recurring cost depends on the maintenance cost and cost of hiring technicians to run the service. Here, we can see better benefit for the urban sector where due to availability of better services these costs are higher compared to the rural areas. Recurring cost is the highest for the DOC service. Here, both the sectors experience maximum level of benefit compared to the other services along with high level of inequality in subsidy distribution across income classes.

Table 2 *Per Capita Benefit-Subsidy Across Types of Service, Economic Class and Region (₹)*

Area	*MPCE*	*BED*		*MED*		*TEST*		*DOC*		*All*	
		Q_2	$\overline{X}$	Q_2	$\overline{X}$	Q_2	$\overline{X}$	Q_2	$\overline{X}$	Q_2	$\overline{X}$
Rural	P	50.5	40.2	120.4	119.5	78.2	73.5	434.6	429.5	669.7	663.4
	LM	148.7	121.3	293.7	291.1	183.3	174.7	1080	1077.0	1690.0	1664.3
	UM	102.3	89.3	284.2	292.7	178.3	166.9	1211	1204.0	1778.0	1753.1
	R	13.5	31.5	140.8	136.4	86.0	88.0	638.3	654.0	940.2	910.2
	All	77.2	83.8	286.7	239.9	165.2	142.4	1080	950.7	1639.0	1416.8
Urban	P	35.6	31.5	88.7	87.3	132.8	124.2	325.6	318.5	581.1	561.4
	LM	25.0	35.1	178.2	177.3	253.7	227.8	904.2	904.1	1353.0	1344.3
	UM	0.0	26.3	252.6	253.8	320.3	316.6	1290	1294	1892.0	1890.2
	R	0.0	24.8	169.5	168.0	243.2	189.5	841.1	825	1241.0	1207.3
	All	4.6	29.1	170.5	186.9	272.5	232.4	903.8	925.8	1366.0	1374.1

Source: Computed from NSS 60th Round Data and NHA.

Note: P-Poorest, LM-Lower Middle, UM-Upper Middle, R-Richest, Q_2-Median, $\overline{X}$-Mean.

Social Equity: Then the question arises about the intra-sectoral distribution of subsidy benefit. Median benefit from bed-related services is highest for the lower middle class (about ₹ 150) followed by the upper middle income category in the rural sector. Here, richest class people are enjoying least benefit from the service followed by the poorest one. For other three services, least amount of the subsidy benefit is enjoyed by the poorest, understandably, the most deserving income class in the rural and urban West Bengal. This analysis highlights the existence of both inter-region and inter-class disparities in distribution of the benefits of the public subsidy. Maximum subsidy benefit can be observed in doctor's services; where, middle class patients have a benefit of more than ₹ 1,000 and ₹ 900 respectively for rural and urban areas. Two, middle-income groups mostly benefited by the public spending over different subsidies. The richest section in almost all service categories, in both areas receives lower subsidy benefit per capita compared to the middle class, because even when they take access, they actually buy additional services from private market to ensure quality care.

In quite a few cases poor economic class has fared even worse than the richest one in terms of benefit-absorption of public subsidy in 'in-patient care'. Therefore, it is clear from the discussion that public subsidies on different services are unevenly distributed among different income class. Here, disparity is mostly across classes and not so much within class.

Conclusion

The study reveals succinctly that access to public in-patient health care facilities in West Bengal is quite impressive and the average is greater than 76 per cent in rural and 65 per cent in urban areas. However, the benefit distribution of this access is highly biased towards the middle income classes, and the poorest class is fared even worse than the richest class. This inequitable skewness in benefit distribution can be explained in terms of the reimbursement policy followed by the government. To be reimbursed one has to make the required expenditure first, and those who are financially more deficient and less connected face higher economic costs in availing these opportunities. Crowding-in by the middle income group into the public health care system drives out the economically weaker section in the state. Those poor, who manage to get an access to public health care facilities, actually fail to receive other services and/or the subsidies associated with the services like medicines, tests and doctor.

This essentially portrays a targeting problem. The poorest and understandably the most vulnerable section of the population gets the least benefit out of this highly elaborate and deep structured public health care system. Access to hospitalization and benefit of public subsidies also varies across sectors. Rural sector enjoys more public subsidy benefit compared to the urban counterpart but inter-class inequality and pro-rich distribution of this subsidy dampens the welfare implication of the prevailing situation.

Notes

1. Vietnam Household Living Standards Survey, 2006.
2. 60th Round Unit Level Dataset, 2004.
3. Due to difference in cost-of-living the MPCE classes in Rural and Urban areas do not always correspond. However, in each region the total sample is spread over 12 MPCE classes. So, we have clubbed three consecutive classes in each economic sub-stratum.
4. DOC – hospital staff and physiotherapy; MED – medicines received from hospitals; TEST – diagnostic tests and BED – bed, attendant charges, food, other services, blood and expenditure not reported elsewhere.
5. In fact, the sequence is BED-TEST-MED-DOC in Rural and BED-TEST-DOC-MED in Urban.

References

Acharya, D., Vaidyanathan, G., Muraleedharan, V.R., Dheenadayalan, D.S. and Dash, U. 2011. *Do the Poor Benefit from Public Spending on Healthcare in India? Results from Benefit (Utilization) Incidence Analysis in Tamil Nadu and Orissa*. Chennai: CREHS.

Chakraborty, L., Singh, Y. and Jacob, J.F. 2011. Public Expenditure Benefit Incidence on Health: Selective Evidence from India. Working Paper No. 2012–111, New Delhi: National Institute of Public Finance and Policy.

Dilip, T.R. 2005. *Extent of Inequality in Access to Health Care Services in India*. Mumbai: Centre for Enquiry into Health and Allied Themes (CEHAT), pp. 247–268.

Dutta, A., Bandyopadhyay, S. and Ghose, A. 2011. *Efficiency in Secondary Hospitals in West Bengal*. Department of Health and Family Welfare, GoWB.

Lingam, L. 2007. *Gender and Health: Emergent Issues beyond Equitable Access*. Forum 11, Beijing: People's Republic of China.

Mahal, A., Yazbeck, A.S., Peters, D.H. and Ramana, G.N.V. 2001. The Poor and Health Service Use in India. Health, Nutrition and Population (HNP) Discussion Paper.

McIntyre, D. and Ataguba, J.E. 2011. How to Do (or Not to Do) … . A Benefit Incidence Analysis. *Health Policy and Planning*, 26: 174–182.

National Health Accounts India 2004–05. *National Health Accounts Cell*. Ministry of Health and Family Welfare, Government of India.

O'Donnell, O., Doorslaer, E.V., Wagstaff, A. and Lindelow, M. 2008. Who Benefits from Health Sector Subsidies? Benefit Incidence Analysis. In *Analyzing Health Equity Using Household Survey Data: A Guide to Techniques and Their Implementation*, Washington, D.C.: The World Bank, pp. 165–175.

Palmer, N. 2008. Access and Equity: Evidence on the Extent to Which Health Services Address the Needs of the Poor. In S. Bennett, L. Gilson and A. Mills (eds), *Health, Economic Development and Household Poverty*, London: Routledge, pp. 61–74.

Planning Commission Report. Government of India, 2012. Available from http://planningcommission.nic.in/reports/genrep/index.php?repts=b_repgen.htm. Searched on 20 February 2013 at 1.35 p.m.

Sen, G. and Iyer, A. 2012. Who Gains, Who Loses and How: Leveraging Gender and Class Interactions to Secure Health Entitlements. *Social Science and Medicine*, 74: 1802–1811.

Wagstaff, A. 2010. *Benefit Incidence Analysis: Are Government Health Expenditures More Pro-Rich Than We Think?* World Bank: Development Research Group and Human Development and Public Services Team.

Section III

Maternal Health Care

13

Maternal Complications and Utilization of Maternal Health Care Services with Special Reference to West Bengal

Dipika Subba

Globally, maternal mortality is the leading cause of death among women in the reproductive age. It is the consequences of pregnancy and childbirth or the consequences of utilization of health care services during pregnancy and childbirth. Utilization of maternal health care services is a proximate determinant of maternal morbidities and mortalities (McCarthy and Maine, 1992; Bhatia and Cleland, 1995). It is of paramount importance as it affects the well-being of the mother as well as her children. Several studies have shown that the majority of maternal deaths can be prevented through early and timely access to and utilization of quality maternal health care services (Bhatia and Cleland, 1993; Babalola and Fatusi, 2009 as cited by Hauwa 2011). But implementing and assuring utilization of effective maternity care for women in the developing world is not an easy task United Nations Population Fund (UNFPA, 2005). Since, late 80s improvement on maternal health and reducing maternal mortality became an area of concern for several international summits and conferences. Government of India has also initiated many programmes and policies to curb the maternal mortality and improve the health condition of women. The goal to improve the maternal health received further momentum from the UN Summit on Millennium Development Goals (MDGs) in 2000. In India, the maternal mortality ratio (MMR) dropped from 600 deaths per 100,000 live births in 1990 to 390 in 2000 and to 200 in 2010 (Office of registrar general, GOI, 2011 as cited by Saxena et.al, 2013). Though the maternal mortality ratio has improved over the period of time but to meet the UN Millennium Development Goal (MDG), India needs to achieve the MMR of 109 by 2015. Another programme i.e. Reproductive and Child Health Programme emphasizes the need for mothers to deliver babies in hygienic conditions under the supervision of skilled health professionals, but most women in India deliver their babies at home without professional help. DLHS III, 2007–08 estimates that out of total birth 52 per cent were delivered at home and out of which only 5 per cent were assisted by a skilled person.

In the present study, the eastern region of India is taken into consideration. This region consists the states of Bihar, Jharkhand, West Bengal and Odisha. The maternal complications is very high in this region. They alone accounted 25 per cent of total maternal complications. Bihar has a highest maternal complications in India followed by Jharkhand and West Bengal. The three states i.e. Bihar, Jharkhand and Odisha fall under Empowered Action Group States and has already been an area of concern in many studies. So, for further micro study, only West Bengal has been considered. It shows a unique picture. It has the dubious distinction of achieving low fertility and mortality along with high maternal complications. The level of infant mortality, maternal mortality and fertility are well below the respective national average. West Bengal has already achieved the replacement level of fertility with an average of 1.9 children in her lifetime Sample Registration Survey (SRS) 2008. It is also worth noting that the state of West Bengal has reached close to the target set by Millennium Development Goals (MDG) of the United Nations of achieving Maternal Mortality Ratio of 109 per lakh live births by 2015. Age at marriage, educational level, use of antenatal care services have also increased over the period of time. But despite all these improved indicators, the maternal complications in West Bengal are very high and rank third in India, just after Bihar and Jharkhand.

Objectives

The present study aims to examine the level of prevalence of maternal complications in eastern states. Further, it looks at the utilization of health care services and examines the influence of socio-economic factors on it by currently married women in the selected state of West Bengal.

Data and Methodology

The study is based on District Level Household Survey III (2007–08). For the selected state West Bengal, a total of 21,878 ever-married women aged 15–49 years were interviewed. Out of these ever-married women, 20,542 currently married women were selected for the present study. The method used in the study is logistic regression. For logistic regression, the dependent variables i.e. full antenatal care (ANC), safe delivery, institutional delivery and postnatal care have been categorized into 0 and 1. The '0' category represents those women who did not seek any health care services and '1' represents those women who sought health care services.

Results

Maternal Complications in Eastern States

In all the eastern states, maternal complications are above the national average of 80.2 per cent (Table 1). In India, at an average, around 58 per cent of women experience at least one pregnancy complication, 61 per cent any of the delivery complications and 36 per cent any post-delivery complications. The highest maternal complications were observed in Bihar (93.3%) followed by Jharkhand (92.2%) and West Bengal (91%). In case of pregnancy and post-delivery complications, Bihar has the highest complications with 75 per cent and 57 per cent respectively. Similarly, in case of delivery complications, Jharkhand experienced highest complications with 83 per cent.

Table 1 *Percentage of Currently Married Women (15–49) Who Had Complications During Pregnancy, Delivery and Post-Delivery, Eastern States, 2007–08*

Complications	*Bihar*	*West Bengal*	*Jharkhand*	*Odisha*	*India*
		Pregnancy Complications			
Swelling of hands, feet and face	28.3	25	29.4	27.2	24
Paleness/giddiness/weakness	56.7	51.6	44.8	35.7	35
Visual disturbances	23.6	15	24.3	15.5	13.6
Excessive fatigue	31.6	27.2	36.3	22.7	24.4
Convulsion not from fever	7.8	3.1	11.4	8.1	6.5
Weak or no movement of foetus	11	3.7	21	9.2	7.7
Abnormal position of foetus	2.4	1.9	4.3	2.7	2.8
Excessive vomiting	27.8	27.9	19.2	26.5	23.3
Excessive bleeding	1.4	1.7	1.8	1.8	1.7
Virginal discharge	3.3	5.2	2.4	1.8	3.2
Others	2.8	5.8	1	0.9	1.8
Any complication	75.4	70.8	66.1	58.5	57.8
		Delivery Complications			
Premature labour	35.3	31.6	51.5	40.6	29.7
Excessive bleeding	8.5	11.8	16.5	14.2	9.1
Prolonged labour	30.1	28.4	30.2	26	20.8
Obstructed labour	65.7	53.5	65.7	43.8	42
Breech presentation	4.6	4.1	7.7	4.2	5
Convulsion	5.8	3.9	12	4.3	4.8
Other	1	2.3	0.6	0.3	0.9
Any complication	81.3	73.1	83.5	68.8	61.1
		Post-delivery Complications			
High fever	35	19.7	25.3	18.8	20.2
Lower abdominal pain	36.3	28.7	29.3	16.2	20.8
Foul smelling vaginal discharge	14.1	11.1	13.6	3.3	6.9
Excessive bleeding	11.3	13.5	11.1	8.1	8.1
Convulsion	7.6	1.8	8.3	6.3	4.3
Severe headache	27.8	20.9	23	13.9	16.7
Other	2.7	4.3	1.5	1.4	1.6
Any complications	57.4	45.9	46.7	33	36.8
Any complications during maternity	93.3	91	92.2	82.8	80.2

Source: Unpublished dissertation by Subba D. (2012), based on DLHS 3, 2007–08.

In all the eastern states, a large percentage of women had reported paleness/giddiness/weakness as pregnancy complications. The reporting of excessive fatigue, excessive vomiting and swelling of hand, feet and face were also high. Excessive bleeding and vaginal discharge are the less reported complications in all the eastern states. In case of delivery complications, obstructed complication had emerged out as very high reported complication by the women in all the eastern states with 65 per cent highest in Bihar and Jharkhand. But, breech presentation and convulsion remained poorly reported complications by the women in all the eastern states. Because the breech presentations can be identified only through sonography and the percentage of sonography conducted in the eastern states is 16.8 per cent against 35.6 per cent of the national average. In case of post-delivery complications, all the eastern states except Odisha have complications above national average. Lower abdominal pain, high fever and severe headache are frequently reported complications among women. Lower abdominal pain was the highest complication reported in all the eastern states with 36.3 per cent highest in Bihar, whereas convulsion and foul discharge are two complications which remained poorly reported.

The analysis of Table 1 clearly indicates that the three eastern states i.e. Bihar, Jharkhand and West Bengal have complications above national average. Further, in all the eastern states, similar reporting of complications was observed. The highest reporting was found on those complications which was easy to identify and can be mentioned without any hesitation or awkwardness. Contrastingly, the health problems that carry a sense of shyness and strict medical examination were poorly reported.

Further in order to provide better interpretation of findings, background characteristics of currently married women has also been discussed (Table 2). It was observed that the age of consummation of marriage and age of motherhood in all the eastern states, except Odisha, is very low. Around 39 per cent of women in Bihar and 18 per cent in West Bengal get married before 15 years of age. And around 60 per cent women in West Bengal, 57 per cent in Bihar and 52 per cent in Jharkhand give birth to their first child at 15–19 years of age. In case of birth order, West Bengal and Odisha are comparatively better. Here, almost 40 per cent of currently married women have single birth. But in the states of Bihar and Jharkhand large percentage of women i.e. 39.7 per cent and 31.3 per cent have above 4 births. In all the eastern states, Hinduism is the dominant religion. In case of caste groups, a large percentage of currently married women in Bihar, Jharkhand and Odisha are OBC, whereas Jharkhand and Odisha have a considerable percentage of tribal women. But in case of West Bengal, large percentage of currently married women are of general caste followed by schedule caste. Coming towards the educational level of women, West Bengal is far better than other eastern states. Large percentages of women, around 60 per cent in West Bengal are literates. The distribution of currently married women by wealth quintiles also reveals that West Bengal is fairly better compared to other eastern states. More than 30 per cent of current married women fall in high wealth index, as against 15 per cent in Bihar and Jharkhand. Similarly, large percentages of women (18.8%) in West Bengal reside in urban areas.

Table 2 *Percentage Distribution of Currently Married Women at Age 15–49 Years by Selected Background Characteristics, Eastern States, 2007–08*

Background characteristics	*Bihar*	*Jharkhand*	*West Bengal*	*Odisha*
	Percentage	*Percentage*	*Percentage*	*Percentage*
AGE AT MARRIAGE (below 15)	38.8	16.1	18	6
15–17	37.6	39.5	41.4	36.4
18+	23.6	44.5	40.7	57.6
AGE OF WOMEN AT BIRTH (below 15)	1.4	1.7	3.3	0.8
15–19	56.9	52.4	60.2	45.4
20–24	37	38.5	30.3	43.8
25+	4.7	7.4	6.2	10
BIRTH ORDER (1)	21.7	26	38.7	40
2	20.5	23.6	31	26.9
3	18.1	19.1	15.3	14.5
4+	39.7	31.3	15	18.6
RELIGION (Hindu)	86.7	69.1	74.2	96
Muslim	13.1	10.2	24.1	1
Others	0.2	20.7	1.6	2.9
CASTE (SC)	20.5	14	34.7	20
ST	2.1	32.5	8.7	27.5
OBC	59.3	42.6	11.7	29.2
Others	18.2	10.9	45	23.3
MOTHER'S YEARS OF SCHOOLING (illiterate)	65.9	63.1	39	46.1
1–5	11.8	11.3	24.4	19.9
6–10	18	20.5	29.7	27.1
Above 10	4.2	5	6.8	6.9
HUSBAND YEARS OF SCHOOLING (illiterate)	35.6	34.3	29.1	28
1–5	14.7	15.5	25.8	24.2
6–10	34	36.7	32.5	34
Above 10	15.8	13.5	12.6	13.7
WEALTH INDEX (lowest)	29.7	40.1	25.6	42.8
Second	36.1	28.1	21.8	17.9
Middle	17.9	13.5	20.3	15.3
Fourth	10.9	9.5	19.1	13.4
Highest	5.4	8.8	13.3	10.6
PLACE OF RESIDENCE (Rural)	91.3	86	81.1	87.5
Urban	8.7	14	18.9	12.5

Source: Unpublished dissertation by Subba D. (2012), based on DLHS 3, 2007–08.

The background characteristics of currently married women in eastern states clearly indicate that the state of West Bengal is comparatively better than the other Eastern states. The state fairs in terms of the proportion literate (61%), proportion living in urban areas (19%), proportion in high wealth quintile (33%) and women with single births (40%).

Utilization of Maternal Health Care Services in West Bengal

In West Bengal out of the total currently married women only one-fifth (Figure 1) received full ante-natal care. Similarly, in case of routine antenatal check-up it is observed that the check-up was never near completion. However, blood pressure, weight measure, haemoglobin test and abdomen checks were among the highest (Figure 2). Antenatal advice was even poorer. Most of the women (more than 50%) received information regarding nutrition, breast feeding, institutional delivery and cleanliness (Figure 3). Place of delivery (Figure 4) shows that about half of the deliveries were conducted at home and the rest in different hospitals. Though the proportion of institutional deliveries (49%) in West Bengal is much above the national average but the home delivery (50%) is higher than institutional delivery. Out of total institutional delivery 38.3 per cent was conducted at public sector and only 10.8 per cent at private sector. Around 85 per cent of deliveries (Figure 5) were normal which is more common and only half of the delivery (Figure 6) were safe which include institutional delivery or home delivery assisted by a skilled person (i.e. Doctors, ANM, nurses and other health personnel).

Logistic Regression

To examine the impact of the set of all variables, multi variant technique has been applied. Table 3 presents odd ratio of multivariate logistic regression for the four indicators of utilisation of maternal health care services i.e. full antenatal care, safe delivery, place of delivery and post-natal care. The table depicts that the age at marriage do not hold a significant relation with full antenatal care, safe delivery and place of delivery but has a significant relation with post-natal care. But, birth order holds a significant relation with all the four indicators of health care services. Compared to first birth order, women with 2–3 births and above 4 are less likely to utilise health care services. Social groups also show a significant relation with maternal health care services. Muslim women are 39 per cent, 66 per cent, 67 per cent and 25 per cent less likely to have full ANC, safe delivery, institutional delivery and post-natal care than Hindu women. In case of caste group, compared to General caste women, Schedule Caste and Schedule Tribe women have low chances of utilising health care services. Both mother's as well as husband's years of schooling have a significant influence on the utilisation of maternal health care services. Women who had completed above 10 years of schooling are twice more likely to utilize health care services than women who are illiterate. Similarly women whose husband have completed above 10 years of schooling are 57 per cent, 68 per cent and 43 per cent more likely to go for full ANC, safe delivery, and institutional delivery. Wealth index, pregnancy wastage and place of residence also hold a significant relation with maternal health care services. The women in the higher wealth index are seven times more likely to have a safe delivery and institutional delivery, four times more for post-natal care and twice more for full ANC. Similarly, women with pregnancy wastage have higher probability to use maternal health care services. Urban women are also twice more likely to seek health care services than rural women.

Figure 1 *Full ANC, West Bengal 2007–08*

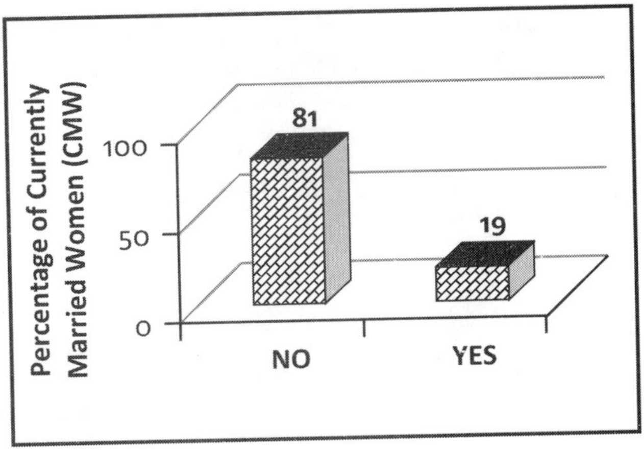

Figure 2 *Routine Antenatal Check-up, West Bengal, 2007–08*

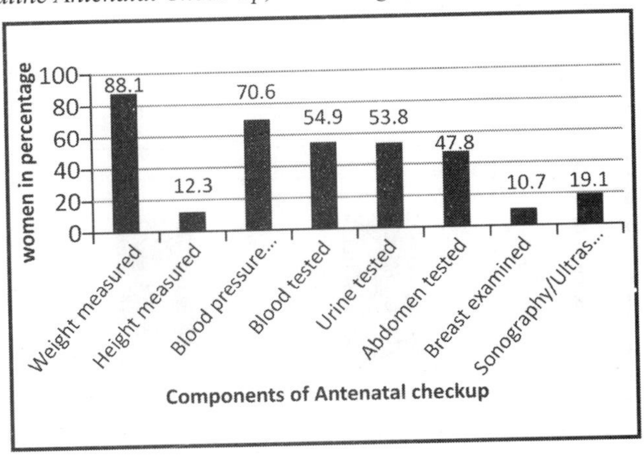

Figure 3 *Advice Received on Different Component During ANC, West Bengal, 2007–08*

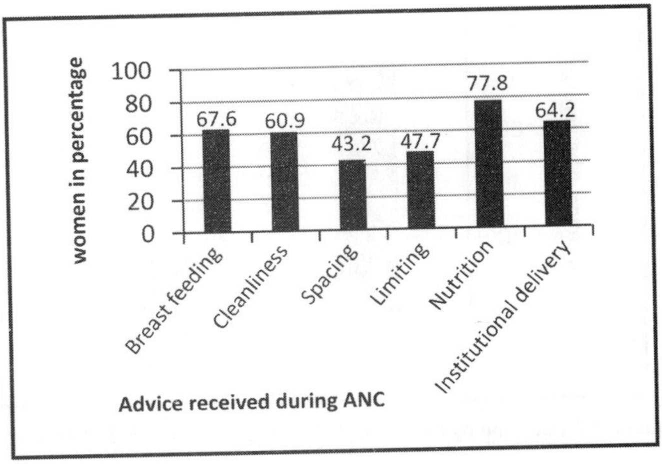

Figure 4 *Place of Delivery West Bengal, 2007–08*

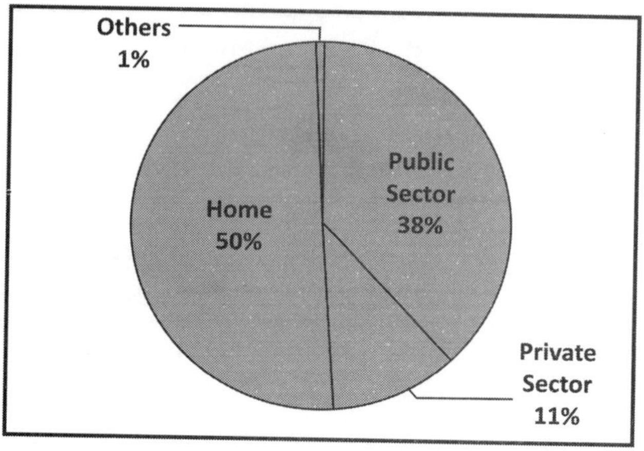

Figure 5 *Type of Delivery West Bengal, 2007–08*

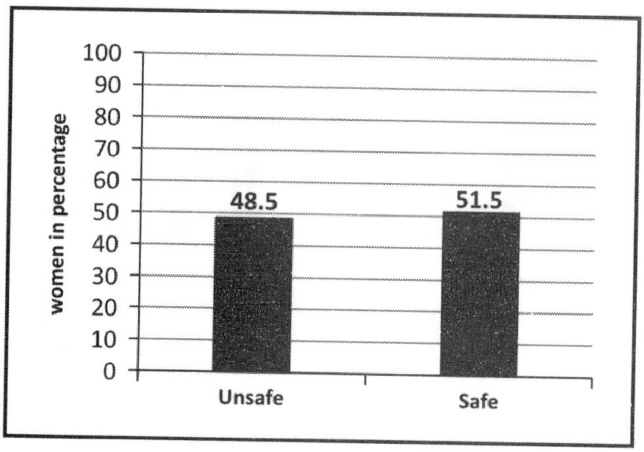

Figure 6 *Safe Delivery West Bengal, 2007–08*

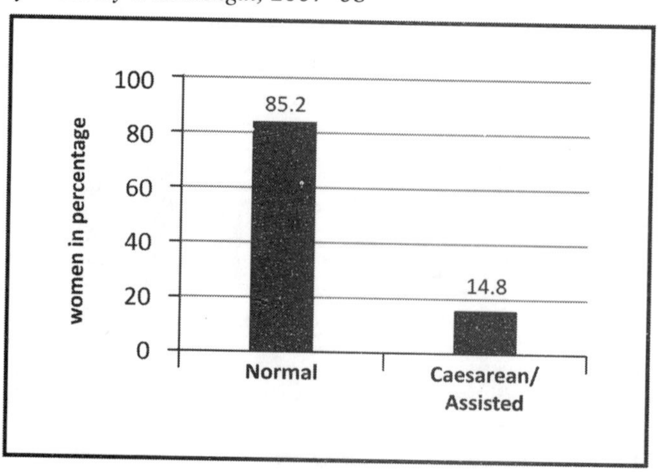

Source: Unpublished dissertation by Subba D. (2012), based on DLHS 3, 2007–08.

Table 3 *Odd Ratio of Logistic Regression for the Indicators of Utilisation of Maternal Health Care Services*

Variables	*Full ANC*	*Safe Delivery*	*Place of Delivery*	*Post Natal Care*
	Exp(B)	*Exp(B)*	*Exp(B)*	*Exp(B)*
AGE AT MARRIAGE (below 15)				
15–19	0.90	1.04	1.11	1.26**
20–24	0.86	1.14	1.21	1.29*
25+	1.04	0.97	0.85	0.90
AGE OF WOMEN AT BIRTH (below 15)				
15–19	1.11	0.71	0.67	0.79
20–24	1.38	0.75	0.74	0.80
25+	1.34	1.10	1.13	0.95
BIRTH ORDER (below 2)				
2–3	0.77***	0.37***	0.38***	0.59***
4+	0.54***	0.22***	0.21***	0.44***
RELIGION (Hindu)				
Muslim	0.61***	0.44***	0.43***	0.75***
Others	0.96	0.44**	0.41***	0.35***
CASTE (General)				
SC	0.83*	0.73***	0.78**	0.89
ST	0.93	0.46***	0.49***	0.53***
OBC	0.90	1.10	1.00	0.83
MOTHER'S YEAR OF SCHOOL (illiterate)				
Primary	1.26	1.24**	1.24**	0.98
Middle and Secondary	1.52***	1.56***	1.61***	1.10
Above Secondary	2.08***	2.76***	2.89***	1.60**
HUSBAND YEARS OF SCHOOLING (illiterate)				
Primary	1.24*	1.00	0.98	1.05
Middle and Secondary	1.10	1.14	1.08	1.14
Above Secondary	1.57***	1.68***	1.43**	1.31
WEALTH INDEX (lowest)				
Second	1.12	1.26**	1.30***	1.30***
Middle	1.41***	1.43***	1.48***	1.60***
Fourth	1.58***	3.30***	3.19***	2.20***
Highest	2.08***	7.58***	7.64***	4.91***
PREGNANCY WASTAGE (No)				
Yes	0.92	1.47***	1.50***	1.45***
PLACE OF RESIDENCE (Rural)				
Urban	0.96	2.80***	2.72***	1.69***

Source: Unpublished dissertation by Subba D. (2012), based on DLHS 3, 2007–08.

Discussion

The present study provides a better understanding to the level of prevalence of maternal complications in the Eastern States of India. It was observed that the complications which were easy to identify and can be mentioned without any hesitation or awkwardness are the ones which were frequently reported, but in contrast to this the complications which carries a sense of shyness and strict medical examination were poorly reported. The background characteristic of currently married women in Eastern states clearly shows that the state of West Bengal is comparatively better than other Eastern states. However, the maternal complications are very high. Routine antenatal care has been never near completion. Antenatal advice was even poorer. Full utilization of ANC which is essential for safe motherhood is just above national average. Large number of deliveries still take place out of the institution. Out of total institutional deliveries, large number of deliveries were conducted in public sector. Because the mean cost of delivery at public sector (₹ 2,366) is much lower than (₹ 9,625) private sector (DLHS 3, 2007–08). Since last 2 decades, the Government of India has taken major steps to curb the maternal mortality and improve the health condition of women. One of the major schemes was NRHM under which Janani Suraksha Yojana (JSY) has been implemented with an objective of full institutional deliveries by providing financial incentive for the mothers who choose institutional delivery. Though JSY is playing its role in providing cash assistance for institutional delivery but the cash assistance given to pregnant women during delivery is not enough to cover all expenses for institutional deliveries (CORT, 2007). Around 51 per cent of deliveries have taken place out of the institution attended mostly by dais. Out of these non-institutional deliveries only 5 per cent was safe. While stating the reason behind not availing the institution for delivery, it appeared that 40 per cent did not find it necessary and 31 per cent did not get time to go (DLHS 3, 2007–08).

The findings of the multi-variant logistic regression in the study suggest that age at marriage and age at motherhood do not hold any significant relation with full ANC, safe delivery and institutional delivery. But, age at motherhood has a significant influence on post-natal care which is similar to the finding of Fielder, 1981 and Elo, 1992. Because mother's age sometimes serves as a proxy for the women's accumulated knowledge of health care services which may have a positive influence on the use of health services (Chakraborty et.al, 2003). Another demographic variable i.e. birth order shows that women with higher birth order have low utilisation of health care services which is similar to the finding of Bhatia and Cleland 1995, Chakraborty et.al 2003, Elo 1992. This is mainly due to the fact that women give greater attention to their first pregnancy, as they are inexperienced with pregnancy and therefore less likely to utilise health care services with the increase in birth order. Socioeconomic variables such as caste, religion, women year of schooling, husband's years of schooling and wealth index also reveals a significant relation with maternal health service use. SC/ST women are less likely to utilise health care services than general women which is similar to the studies done by Navaneetham et.al, 2002, Sontakke et.al, 2009 and Appasamy et.al, 1995 as cited by Navaneetham et.al, 2002. This may be due to the fact that these SC/ST women are less educated and economically backward leading to least aware of the availability of health care services and benefits in using them. Muslim women also use less health care services compared to Hindu women because Muslim women have low education, low autonomy and rigid social custom (Salam and Siddiqui, 2006, and Maana et.al, 2011). It was also observed that women and her husband's years of schooling have a positive impact on utilisation of maternal health care services. Similar finding was observed by Becker et.al, 1993, Elo, 1992 and Chakraborty, 2003 because better educated women are more aware of existing health care services and use them more effectively to maintain or achieve good health status. Further, education also empowers women and provides greater confidence and capacity to make the decision to use modern health care services (Caldwell et al. 1983, Mosley and Chen 1984). Wealth index which is used as a proxy indicator for standard of living indicates that with the increase in wealth index the likelihood of utilising health care services also increases. Similarly women with pregnancy wastage utilise more health care services which is similar to the findings of Bhatia and Cleland 1995. Likelihood of utilizing maternal health care service is low among rural women because rural women are least aware of modern health service and have strong traditional beliefs. It has also been mentioned in several studies that even if women are interested in checkups there are cost of transport and related services where a poor section of rural population cannot afford to pay.

Conclusion

The finding of the study suggests that in order to improve the utilization of maternal health care services in West Bengal effort is to be made to create awareness especially among women of rural area about the benefits of using health services. The analysis also highlighted the fact that social position (caste) plays an important role in utilisation of maternal health care services. The need for a target approach especially for schedule caste and tribe for improving the utilisation of maternal health services is realised. Further comprehensive efforts are also needed to target women of lower economic status with basic health care services. Thus, in order to achieve targets and goals set out by MDG's, effective policies should be implemented by focusing mainly on these disadvantaged groups.

References

Becker, S., Peters, D.H., Gray, R.H., Gultiano, C. and Blake, R.E. 1993. The Determinants of Use of Maternal and Child Health Service in Metro Cebu, the Phillippines. *Health Transition Review*, 3: 77–89.

Bhatia, J.C. and Cleland, J. 1993. Levels and Causes of Maternal Mortality in South India. *Studies in Family Planning*, 24: 301–318.

——. 1995. Determinants of Maternal Care in a Region of South India. *Health Transition Review*, 5: 127–142.

Caldwell, J., Reddy, P.H. and Caldwell, P. 1983. The Social Component of Mortality Decline: An Investigation in South India Employing Alternative Methodologies. *Population Studies*. 37: 185–205.

Chakraborty, N., Islam, M.A., Chowdhury, R.I., Bari, W. and Akhtar, H. 2003. Determinants of the Use of Maternal Health Services in Rural Bangladesh. *Health Promotion International*, 18: 327–337.

CORT. 2007. Assessment of Janani Suraksha Yojana in West Bengal. http://www.cortindia.in/rp%5crp–2007–0503.pdf

Elo, T.I. 1992. Utilisation of Maternal Health Care Services in Peru, the Role of Women's Education. *Health Transition Review*, 2: 49–69.

Fiedler, J.L. 1981. A Review of the Literature on Access and Utilisation of Medical Care with Special Emphasis on Rural Primary Care. *Social Science and Medicine*, 15: 129–142.

Hauwa, S.A. 2011. Utilization of Maternal Health Care Services in Nigeria: An Analysis of Regional Differences in the Patterns and Determinants of Maternal Health Care Use. Dissertation, University of Liverpool.

Manna, P.K., De, D. and Ghosh, D. 2011. Knowledge, Attitude and Practices for Antenatal Care and Delivery of the Mothers of Tea Garden in Jalpaiguri and Darjeeling Districts, West Bengal. *National Journal of Community Medicine*, 2: 4–8.

McCarthy, J. and Maine, D.A. 1992. Framework for Analyzing Determinants of Maternal Mortality. *Studies in Family Planning*, 23: 23–33.

Mosley, W.H. and Chen, L.C. 1994. An Analytical Framework for the Study of Child Survival in Developing Countries. *Population and Development Review*, 10: 25–45.

Navaneetham, K. and Dharmalingam, A. 2002. Utilisation of Maternal Health Care Services in Southern India. *Social Science and Medicine*, 55: 1849–1869.

Office of the Registrar General, Ministry of Home Affairs, Government of India. 2011. *Special Bulletin on Maternal Mortality in India 2007–09*. New Delhi, India: Government of India, p. 4.

Salam, A. and Siddiqui, S.A. 2006. Socioeconomic Inequalities in Use of Delivery Care Services in India. *Journal of Obstetric Gynecology India*, 56: 123–127.

Saxena, D., Vangani, R., Mavalankar, D.V. and Thomsen, S. 2013. Inequity in Maternal Health Care Service Utilization in Gujarat: Analysis of District Level Health Survey Data. *Global Health Action*, 6: 1–9.

Sontakke, P., Reshmi, R.S. and Sebastian, D. 2009. Obstetric Morbidity among Currently Married Women in Selected States in India. *Journal of Family Welfare*, 55: 17–26.

Subba, D. 2012. Determinants of Maternal Complications in Eastern States with Special Reference to West Bengal, India. Dissertation, New Delhi, India: Jawaharlal Nehru University.

Wong, E.L., Popkin, B.M., Cullkey, D.K. and Akin, J.S. 1987. Accessibility, Quality of Care and Prenatal Care Use in the Philippines. *Social Science and Medicine*, 24: 927–944.

14

Involvement of Men in Maternal and Newborn Care

A Study Among Farmers in Mahnar Block of Vaishali District, Bihar

Gunjan Gaurav and Suhas Kadam

Introduction and Review of Literature

Maternal and child health in India: India has high infant and under-5 mortality and was reported 50 and 64 respectively in Sample Registration Survey (SRS) 2007–09. The target of Infant Mortality Rate (IMR) and Under-five Mortality Rate (U5MR) under Millennium Development Goals (MDG) is 28 and 42 respectively. National Family Health Survey (NFHS-3) has found a great difference in infant mortality in rural and urban area. Early age of marriage, low level of education and poverty was found to be associated with infant mortality in India. There is great regional disparity in India in terms of health outcome. In the slow progress of maternal and child health achievement one of the constraints in India is how to involve men who acts as gatekeepers to the access and utilization of services to women and children.

Involvement of men – an international consensus: The International Conference on Population and Development (ICPD) held in 1994 in Cairo was a landmark in the history of population and development, as it advocated a shift from achieving demographic target to meeting the individual needs of men and women. The conference presented a programme of action which had pledges to achieve the goal of universal access to reproductive health services for everyone in all countries till 2015.

Policy discourse of male involvement in India: ICPD conference was the landmark when India started giving a look on the male involvement in policy of family welfare. Two major policies related to male involvement in reproductive and child health were National Population Policy, 2000 and Reproductive and Child Health (RCH-II), 2005.

National Population Policy in its action plan stressed on involving men in promoting small family norms by emphasizing on raising awareness about benefits of few children, spacing, health, nutrition and education. The report particularly emphasized on popularizing the vasectomy, in particular, non-scalpel vasectomy among client and health care professionals.[1]

It has been now been widely recognized that involvement of men has not moved beyond the family planning measures in India which is reflected in the policies. However, NFHS-3 for the first time tried to capture the data related to men. The findings of NFHS-3 clearly reflects that even after fifteen years of ICPD, male's participation in maternal health has not reached its desirable level. The strong patriarchal society where women's work is still limited to cooking, taking care of family and rearing child, where women's decision-making power is marginalized and man is like a gatekeeper to the family for the outside world, it is challenging to involve men in maternal and child health care.

Male assistance in ANC and pregnancy: Antenatal Care (ANC) service is an important component of maternal and child health care. With the increase in proportion of mothers taking care in health facilities during pregnancy and child-birth, health risks to mothers and their children get reduced.[2] ANC is the first point of linking the woman and her family with the health system and increases the chances of using a skilled attendant at birth. Barriers to male involvement in ANC are not only limited to male attitude and preferences but the societal allocation of roles to men and power structure in the society. A study done by Britta et al., in 2004 in Nepal revealed that husbands accompanied only 40 per cent of their women attending ANC and that greater decision-making power for women was associated with lower accompaniment to ANC by husband and lower overall male involvement.[3] In the same study it was found that men prefer to accompany women who is younger and has no child compared to women who is older and has previously given birth to a child, and reason of not accompanying was mostly job constraints and not the childcare responsibilities.[3]

In India only half of the males (50%) reported that they were present during ANC.[4] NFHS–3 also found that male presence in rural Ahmednagar district was found 81 per cent during ANC which was considerably high.[6] Another study in urban slums of Agra showed only 18 per cent of male accompanied wife for ANC.[5] Presence during ANC is higher in urban areas and increases with education of male.

Male involvement in delivery of child: One of the underlying issues of maternal mortality is delivery not attended by the skilled birth attendant and it is partly attributed to the low male partner involvement in delivery care and low involvement in making wife access to the delivery by skilled birth attendants.

In a study in slums of Agra it was found that only 18.33 per cent husbands were present during antenatal check-ups but in case of delivery 87.5 per cent were present during delivery.[5] However, India has two different populations – rural and urban. The gap between their practices and health outcome is also different. There is a great divide between urban and rural India. In a study in rural Ahmednagar district of Maharashtra, Singh found that only 52 per cent of husbands were present during delivery. The major reason of not being present was as quoted 'wife at parent's house' (85%).[6] The decision to choose place of birth is mainly determined by the husband and sometimes elders in family like it to be with the mother-in-law.

Male involvement in new-born care: Parents usually have a high emotional attachment with the newly-born child as early as the first day after delivery and fathers have an equally emotional attachment as the mothers.[7] Father involvement in infant care refers to the tasks father develops on a daily basis and which can be identified by any person. Fathers who attend their infant births and receive hospital contact during postpartum period were more involved in infant caretaking responsibilities.[8]

Gender attitude and male involvement: Barker defined gender equitable men as 'young men who are respectful in their relationship with women and seek relationships based on equality with their partners and intimacy rather than sexual conquest'.[9] Male role is derived from patriarchy and in most society's dominance of men is felt, and men control the actions and interactions of their families in all spheres of social relationship.[10] There is male supremacy embedded in the society. Male involvement in safe motherhood is limited due to social system and culture in India. Male dominance in terms of physical, social and sexual relationship can be a risk to women in terms of sexual behaviour, pregnancy and overall health, and in more egalitarian gender relations it is easier to achieve better sexual and reproductive health for both men and women.[11] The present study has focussed on all the aspect of pregnancy and new-born care. It has tried to understand the knowledge, support in maternal care and new-born care for wider understanding of linkages between these aspects, apart from the socio-economic and cultural determinants. In a nutshell, the present study was taken in Bihar among farmers with a focus on knowledge, gender attitude, support in pregnancy care and new-born care. As no study has been done in Bihar and in farmer's community with an aim to capture all these aspects comprehensively, the study will be an important contribution in the literature available in the area of men's involvement in maternal and child health.

Objectives

Objectives of the study were: (1) To determine the male assistance in maternal care in terms to visit to ANC, access to delivery care and household support. (2) To determine the male involvement in new-born care in terms of immunization, sickness and day-to-day care. (3) To identify factors associated with the men's knowledge, awareness and their involvement in providing assistance in pregnancy, delivery and new-born care.

Methods and Materials

The study was carried out in Vaishali district which is located in the state of Bihar. There are three sub-divisions and sixteen blocks in the district. One, block Mahnar was purposively selected out of sixteen blocks for the study. *Study Design*: The study was a cross-sectional community-based household survey. The study employed quantitative techniques of data collection with few open-ended questions. *Sample Selection:* Sample size for present study is one hundred twenty (120). The criteria for selection of sample were males who are involved in farming and related activities for at least three months and whose wives had given birth to a child in the past six months. *Sampling Procedure:* The list of all villages was made in the Mahnar block as per the list of land and revenue office. The ten villages were selected by simple random method. The process involved were writing the names of all villages which was 50 in number on the separate pieces of paper, folding the papers, putting them in one container and vigorously shaking the container, after which one paper was picked without replacement until ten villages got selected. The list of all the families where child has born in past six months was made with the help of subcentre for that village. The list was further cross-checked with the data available at various Anganwadi centres. From the selected villages, we found 870 eligible respondents. So as to get sample size of 120, by systematic random sampling we selected every 7th respondent for study. *Data Collection Tools:* The structured questionnaire was prepared with few open-ended questions. The questionnaire was divided into five parts, such as (i) Socio-economic and Demographic Features, (ii) Knowledge of Pregnancy and its Complications, (iii) Assistance in Maternal Health, (iv) Involvement in Newborn Care, and (v) Gender Equitable Men Scale to measure attitude towards gender equitable norms. *Data Analysis:* Data analysed by using SPSS (Version 20) with statistical tests such as univariate analysis, Chi-square test and cross tabulations. *Limitations of the Study:* Due to small sample size the present study cannot be generalized for the area and further research is required in the given area.

Results

Socio-Demographic Background: There were respondents of all age groups. About 42.5 per cent was found to be from the age group of below 25 years and 57.5 per cent were from the age of more than 25 years. Nearly 30 per cent had no formal education and were mostly illiterate (Table 1).

Male Involvement in Newborn Care

(i) *Husband's knowledge about newborn care:* Men were found knowledgeable about the aspect of newborn care. Around 68.3 per cent of the men had knowledge of more than two aspects of newborn care while only 4.2 per cent had no knowledge of any of the aspects of newborn care (Table 2).

(ii) *Source of information for newborn care:* Most of the respondent reported public health professionals (44%) and friends and relatives (37%) were main source of information on newborn care. Media has played very little role in enhancing knowledge on newborn care and has been reported as a source of information by 14 per cent only.

(iii) *Knowledge about amount of water to be given in diarrhoea:* Diarrhoea is one of the major killer diseases for the infants in developing countries. Almost 72 per cent of the men said correctly that in case of diarrhoea more than usual amount of water should be given to the children (Table 3).

(iv) *Knowledge about immunization:* Around 81 per cent men had the knowledge that immunization has a schedule and child needs to get immunization as per the schedule. However, men were found least involved in accompanying child for the immunization and only 15.8 per cent of men were found to accompany the child for immunization. Wife plays an active role in accompanying child for immunization and 71.7 per cent of the times she accompanied the child for immunization.

(v) *Accompany the child for immunization:* In case of accompanying the child for immunization, most of the times around 72 per cent the mother of the child accompanied her child for immunization. The percentage of husband and relatives is more or less the same (Table 4).

(vi) *Knowledge about breastfeeding:* Around 58.3 per cent of men responded correctly that child should be breastfed within the first two hours of the delivery (Table 5).

(vii) *Behaviour towards feeding of child:* The study shows 43.3 per cent of men motivate their wife for breastfeeding but also 31.7 per cent of men motivate wife for giving food other than milk in the first six months which is made for exclusive breastfeeding (Table 6).

(viii) *Decision of treatment of child:* In terms of treatment of child, men are cooperative and 74.4 per cent had taken decision themselves for the place of treatment of their child. Further 79.0 per cent (34/43) men accompanied their child for the treatment. Reason given for not accompanying was mainly due to involvement in work and presence of other members in the house (Table 7).

(ix) *Men accompanying child for treatment:* Out of forty-five children who had fallen ill men accompanied in thirty-four cases (75.55%). Reasons cited for not accompanying was being not present and presence of relatives to accompany the child.

(x) *Factors affecting male involvement in child care:* As contrary to the domain of pregnancy and maternal care, age was not found significant in case of child care. Education was found significant for knowledge of newborn care and among above primary educated men, 79.4 per cent were found to have knowledge of more than two aspects of newborn care compared to those up to primary educated(56.1%). Caste was found significant for accompanying child for immunization and knowledge about newborn care. Larger proportion of men in nuclear family (91.7%) motivated wife for giving food other than miik compared to joint family (62.5 %). Higher proportion of men from joint family had knowledge of more than two dimensions of newborn care (74.0%) compared to men from nuclear family (45.8%) (Table 8 and 9).

Table 1 *Socio-demographic Background*

Characteristics	*Frequency N=120*	*Percentage*
Age		
Less than 25 years	51	42.5
26–30 years	58	48.3
More than 30 years	11	9.2
Education		
No formal Education	36	30.0
Primary Education	21	17.5

Cont'd...

...Cont'd

Secondary education	31	25.8
Matriculate and above	32	26.7
Religion		
Hindu	112	93.3
Muslim	08	6.7
Caste		
Schedule castes	55	45.8
OBCs	41	34.2
General	24	20.0
Wife Education		
No formal education	55	45.8
Primary education	46	38.3
Above primary education	19	15.8
No. of Children		
0–2 children	65	54.2
More than two children	55	45.8

Table 2 *Knowledge About Newborn Care*

Knowledge	*Frequency*	*Frequency per cent*
No knowledge of newborn care	5	4.2
Knowledge of one aspect of newborn care	15	12.5
Knowledge of two aspects of newborn care	18	15.0
Knowledge of more than two aspects of newborn care	82	68.3
Total	120	100

Table 3 *Knowledge About Amount of Water to be Given in Diarrhoea*

Amount of water	*Frequency*	*Frequency percentage*
More than usual	87	72.5
About the same	12	10.0
Less than usual	03	2.5
Don't know	18	15.0
Total	120	100.0

Table 4 *Accompanying Child for Immunization*

Accompany	*Frequency*	*Per cent*
Husband himself	19	15.8
Wife	86	71.7
Relatives	15	12.5
Total	120	100

Table 5 *Knowledge of Ideal Time to Start Breastfeeding*

Breastfeeding	*Frequency*	*Frequency percentage*
Immediate within two hours	70	58.3
Same day after two hours	43	35.8
1–3 days	06	5.0
Don't know	01	0.8

Table 6 *Behaviour Towards Feeding of Child*

Behaviour	*Frequency*	*Frequency percentage*
Motivate wife to breastfeed	52	43.3
Motivate wife for giving other food	38	31.7
Ensures proper diet to child	110	91.7

Table 7 *Decision of Treatment of Child*

Person who had taken decision	*Frequency N = 43*	*Frequency percentage*
Husband himself	32	74.4
Wife	02	4.7
Jointly by husband and wife	07	16.3
Relatives	02	4.7
Total	120	100

Table 8 *Men's Profile on Accompanying Child for Immunization, Motivating for Food Other than Breastfeed and Knowledge of more than Two Aspects of Newborn Care*

Characteristics	*Accompany child for immunization (%)*	*Don't motivate for other food than breastfeed (%)*	*Knowledge of more than two aspects of newborn care (%)*
Age			
Up-to 25 years	13.7	70.6	58.8
More than 25 years	17.4	66.7	75.4
Education of male partner			
Up-to primary	17.5	73.7	56.1
Above Primary	14.3	63.5	79.4
Caste	*		
SC	7.3	76.4	56.4
OBC and General	23.1	61.5	78.5
Type of Household		**	*
Joint	17.7	62.5	74.0
Nuclear	8.3	91.7	45.8
Standard of living			
Low	13.0	73.9	62.3

Cont'd…

...Cont'd

Medium and high	19.6	60.8	76.5
Media Exposure			
Low	15.1	72.1	62.8
High	17.6	58.8	82.4
Farm Ownership			
Own or family land	21.3	65.3	73.3
Rented or other's land	6.7	73.3	60.0
Gender attitude			***
Traditional	10.5	69.7	53.9
Egalitarian	25.0	65.9	93.2
Total no. of children			
0–2 children	13.8	80.0	66.2
More than 2 children	18.2	54.5	70.9
Education of Wife			
Up to primary	17.8	71.3	66.3
Above Primary	5.3	52.6	78.9

(***p<0.001, **p<0.1, *p<0.05)

Table 9 *Adjusted or [With 95% Cumulative Incidence (CI)] of Indicators of Male Involvement in Newborn Care Using Binary Logistic Regression*

Characteristics	*Accompany child for immunization (%)*	*Don't motivate for other food than breastfeed (%)*	*Knowledge of more than two aspects of new- born care (%)*
Age			
Up to 25 years®	1.00	1.00	1.00
More than 25 years	1.05	0.22*	0.52
Education of male partner			
Up to primary®	1.00	1.00	1.00
Above Primary	1.94	0.99	0.49
Caste			
SC®	1.00	1.00	1.00
OBC and General	0.27	0.98	0.45
Type of family			
Joint®	1.00	1.00	1.00
Nuclear	1.16	0.15	1.84
Standard of living			
Low®	1.00	1.00	1.00
Medium and high	0.79	1.95	1.74
Media exposure			
Low®	1.00	1.00	1.00
High	1.85	0.76	0.62

Cont'd...

...*Cont'd*

Farm ownership			
Own or family land®	1.00	1.00	1.00
Rented or other's land	1.98	1.15	0.63
Gender attitude			
Traditional®	1.00	1.00	1.00
Egalitarian	0.35	0.99	0.12**
Total no. of Children			
0–2 children®	1.00	1.00	1.00
More than 2 children	0.75	10.67**	1.54
Education of wife			
Upto primary®	1.00	1.00	1.00
Above Primary	5.32	3.76	1.10

(***p<0.001, **p<0.1, *p<0.05) ®=*Reference category*

On doing logistic regression (Table 8) age and total number of children was found significantly associated with not motivating for food other than milk. Gender attitude was found significantly associated with knowledge of newborn care. Male more than 25 years are more likely to motivate their wives for giving food other than breast milk compared to less than 25 years in period made for exclusive breast-feeding. Male having more than two children were also found to motivate for food other than breast milk compared to those who had up to two children.

Discussion and Conclusion: Male assistance in antenatal and delivery care: The present study finds nearly 80 per cent of wives visited the health facility for ANC. Nearly half of the men do not accompany wives for ANC. Among those who accompanied, majority of them did not accompany their wives for every visit. The study is in accordance to similar study done in Nepal and NFHS-3 but in contrast to study in Ahmednagar district. In a study in Nepal, Britta found nearly 40 per cent men accompany wife for ANC.[3] Similarly, Bhatta in Nepal also found only 40 per cent accompanied wife for ANC.[12] NFHS-3 also shows 50 per cent of men accompanied wife for ANC. However, study of Singh in rural parts of Ahmednagar district revealed 84 per cent men accompanied wife for ANC. The reason for this may be that Bihar is underdeveloped and has fairly bad indicators on maternal and child health, compared to Maharashtra which is developed and has good maternal and child health indicators. One-fifth of the males cited that they do not accompany as Action for Securing Health for All (ASHA) is there to accompany. It seems that ASHA just tries to meet the target of ANC visits. However, the positive benefits are that ASHA is contributing towards the goals of ANC visits by pregnant ladies. The grassroots workers need to orient towards importance of involving men in ANC. 74 per cent men reported their child has been delivered in institution. It is highly in contrast to the report of IIPS (2007-08)[15], which reported 27.7 per cent of institutional delivery. The reason may be the high focus of NRHM and lot of NGOs working in the maternal and child health in given areas. More than half of the men (60%) were present during delivery. Most of them (67%) had reported wife to be at mother in-law's home for not being present during delivery. The study was in lines of finding in Ahmednagar district where 52% of men were found to accompany wife during ANC and 85 per cent reported the reason for not being present as wife was at her parent's home.

Only one-tenth reported they made joint decision with wife for place of delivery and in most cases, husband himself or elders in family made the decision for the place of delivery. It shows lack of women autonomy and interaction between couple for deciding place of delivery. Further, when mother of husband takes decision for place of delivery it is more likely to be in the home. The findings are in line with the study done in rural Maharashtra where mother-in-law was found to have an attitude that pregnancy is a natural phenomenon and did not require much care.[13] Males reported themselves as supportive to their partners in day-to-day pregnancy care and majority of them had given support on two or more than two features. Similar study in Ludhiana also found that majority of husbands gave good emotional (84%), social (73.3%), economical (57.3%) and informational (41.3%) support during pregnancy.[14]

Male assistance in newborn care: More than three-fourth of men had knowledge of two or more than two aspects of newborn care. Men have better knowledge of newborn compared to maternal care which was reflected by their low knowledge on complications of pregnancy compared to newborn care. It was further reflected when 79 per cent of men accompanied child for treatment. However, men do not support their child in immunization and only 15.8 per cent accompanied child for immunization. It was similar to the finding in Nepal where only 10.3 per cent men accompanied their child for immunization.[12] About 40 per cent of men do not know ideal time for breast-feeding and 30 per cent of men motivated wife for giving food other than milk in the first six months which is exclusive for breast-feeding. The study showed that there is need to increase awareness among the men about breast-feeding practices as it will lead the father to be more supportive and involved in breast-feeding. As studies have shown role of support of husband in decision of mother to initiate and continue breast-feeding so it is important to involve men in breast-feeding for future policies. Men were found to accompany their child for treatment and most of them accompanied child for treatment. Men possibly perceive that their involvement is needed only in case of emergency, so although they do not help in immunization and day-to-day care but they try to make health care available in case of serious illness.

Notes

1. National Population Policy. 2000.
2. Mwaniki, P., Kabiru, E. and Mbugua, G. 2002. Utilisation of Antenatal and Maternity Services by Mothers Seeking Child Welfare Services in Mbeere District, Eastern Province, Kenya. *East African Medical Journal*, April, 79 (4): 184–187

(cited 29 June 2013). Available from: http://www.ncbi.nlm.nih.gov/pubmed/12625672

3. Mullany, B., Hindin, M. and Becker, S. 2004. Women's Autonomy and Male Involvement in Antenatal Care: Associations and Tensions. 25th International Union for the Scientific Study of Population Conference, 1–18 (cited 29 June 2013). Available from: http://onlinelibrary.wiley. com/doi/10.1002/cbdv.200490137/abstract
4. NFHS–3 India. 2006.
5. Awasthi, S., Nandan, D., Mehrotra, A.K. and Shankar, R. 2008. Male Participation in Maternal Care in Urban Slums of District Agra. *Indian J Prev Soc Med*, 39 (3): 4–6.
6. Singh, A. and Ram, F. 2009. Men's Involvement During Pregnancy and Childbirth: Evidence from Rural Ahmadnagar, India. *Population Review*, 48 (1) (cited 29 June 2013). Available from: http://muse.jhu.edu/ content/crossref/journals/population_review/v048/48.1.singh.html.
7. Figueiredo, B., Costa, R., Pacheco, A. and Pais, A. 2007. Mother-to-Infant and Father-to-Infant Initial Emotional Involvement. *Early Child Development and Care*, July, 177 (5): 521–532 (cited 29 June 2013). Available from: http://www.tandfonline.com/doi/abs/10.1080/ 03004430600577562
8. Keller, W., Hildebrandt, K. and Richards, M. 1985. Effects of Extended Father-Infant Contact During the Newborn Period. *Infant Behavior and Development*, 8 (3): 337–350 (cited 29 June 2013). Available from: http://onlinelibrary.wiley.com/doi/10.1002/cbdv.200490137/abstract
9. Barker, G. 2000. Gender Equitable Boys in a Gender Inequitable World: Reflections from Qualitative Research and Program Development with Young Men in Rio de Janeiro, Brazil. *Sexual and Relationship Therapy*, 15 (3): 263–282.
10. Nwokocha, E. 2007. Maternal Crises and the Role of African Men: The Case of a Nigerian Community. *African Population Studies*, 22 (1): 35–56.
11. Saraswati, R. 2001. Negotiating with Patriarchy: Addressing Men in Reproductive and Child Health. *Economic and Political Weekly*, 36 (49): 4589–4592.
12. Bhatta, D.N. 2013. Involvement of Males in Antenatal Care, Birth Preparedness, Exclusive Breastfeeding and Immunizations for Children in Kathmandu, Nepal. *BMC Pregnancy and Childbirth*, January, 13 (1): 14 (cited 27 May 2013). Available from: http://www.pubmedcentral.nih.gov/articlerender.fcgi?artid=3558464&tool=pmcentrez&rendertype=abstract
13. Foundation for Research in Health Systems. 1996.
14. Haobijam, J., Sharma, U. and David, S. 2010. Study to Assess the Family Support and its Effect on Outcome of Pregnancy in Terms of Maternal and Neonatal Health in a Selected Hospital, Ludhiana, Punjab. *Nursing and Midwifery Research*, 6 (4): 137–145 (29 June 2013). Available from: http://medind.nic.in/nad/t10/i4/nadt10i4p137.pdf
15. IIPS. 2007–08. *District Level Household and Facility Survey*. Mumbai: IIPS.

15

Maternal Health Care Service Utilization in Nepal

Role of Women's Education

Komal Prasad Dulal

Various studies showed that maternal mortality ratio in Nepal before 1990s was very high as there was effect of various factors associated on it. It was the break-through year in this area in 1994 which resulted in various changes, especially change in national policy and programme all over the world. Government of Nepal also made some changes in her policy and programme. Establishment of new birthing centre, improvement in quality of services, training to the manpower, free maternity services etc. are the major ones. Utilization of maternal health care services (ANC, delivery care and postnatal care) is most essential to save maternal health as well as to increase the tendency to give birth to child under health personnel supervision.

Maternal Health in developing countries is still a matter of great concern as each country is facing the problem of persistent poor maternal health care due to ignorance of the issue for a long period of time. It is due to high fertility in the past which has contributed to degrade the overall reproductive health of women. Nepal no more remains exceptional to this aspect. The importance of maternal health care services in reducing maternal and infant morbidity and mortality has received increasing recognition since the International Conference on Population and Development (ICPD), Cairo in 1994. According to the ICPD programme of action, maternal health services should include education on safe motherhood, effective and focused prenatal care, maternal nutrition programmes, adequate delivery assistance that avoids excessive recourse to caesarian sections and provides for obstetric emergency, referral services for pregnancy, childbirth and abortion complications, postnatal care and family planning.[1] Several studies are concentrated to know the hindrances for safe motherhood. Some of the studies are covered here in order to support the studies of Nepal's maternal health care service utilization. Most of the studies incorporated here are concentrated separately on three components of maternal health care. Those studies are covered here in expecting that the covariate for one component is also the reason for the other.

Several studies have shown that there exists an association between the use of antenatal care and positive maternal outcome. Study from Vietnam and Zaire also indicated to have improved maternity.[2] Unlike the use of antenatal care, the place of delivery, if adequate facilities are provided effectively, has consistently been found to be associated to reduce maternal mortality.[3]

The maternal characteristic such as education of women has been found to have the strongest association with the use of maternal health care services.[4] Maternal education exerts a significant influence on the use of maternal health care services.[5] Similarly, women's exposure to information through the radio, television and newspaper significantly increases the utilization rates for all services in India.[6] Utilization of family planning/maternal and child health (FP/MCH) is associated with woman's status and such improved status results in the tangible change of services utilization.[7] Studies based on Bangladesh also showed that there is significant relationship with socio-economic and demographic factors with maternal health care services.[8]

Since older and younger women have different experience and influence, their behaviour on seeking health care also vary. Women over the age 35 are less likely to utilize prenatal care but more likely to utilize delivery and postnatal care.[9] However, a study in Bangladesh indicated that type of assistance utilized at delivery does not differ significantly with the age of the mother and place of delivery.[10] A study in Morocco also indicated that urban women are two or three times more likely to use health services.[11] The importance of place of residence in determining women's use of maternal health care can be explained through the availability of health facilities and the educated women of urban area. Similarly, women who delivered their first child were found to be significantly more likely to use prenatal care and trained assistance during the birth delivery than women in the higher order.[12]

When family planning is strategically targeted to women below 20 and above 40 years as well as to the higher parity women, the noticeable amount of changes were found in fertility which ultimately reduces the maternal health complications. This further justifies the relationship of contraception, fertility and maternal health.[13] Behavioural scientists strongly believe that the adoption and use of contraceptives may facilitate the more rapid adoption of the use of health care services or vice versa.[14]

Increasing investments in programmes that are effective in improving the use of MCH services can also be a viable strategy to improve use of modern family planning techniques.[15] Similarly, the maternal health care utilization has significant relationship with wanted and unwanted pregnancy.[16] An approach to increase MCH depends on improvement of availability of services, physical infrastructure to reach institution and poverty of the people.[17] Similarly, in another study, high survival rate of son excludes the use of maternal services.[18] Some socio-cultural factors may also play such role to restrict a woman not to have health services.

Role of Government of Nepal to reduce gender differences in education through female literacy programme and some programmes designed and implemented to save lives of women during maternity has, to some extent, resulted improved situation of ANC, delivery care and postnatal care as can be observed through NDHS–2011.[19] Similarly, other different variables in addition to education such as religion, mass media exposure, place of residence, birth order etc. may influence Full Maternal Health Care Services Utilization(FMHCSU) and are also associated with women's education.

Objective

The main objective of this work is to analyse the role of women's education in full utilization of maternal health care services. Other specific goals include:

- Identify the association of background variables to full utilization of maternal health care services.
- Analyse the Gross and Net effects of women's education to full utilization of Maternal Health Care Services.

Analytic Framework

My model, constructed based on the various literature surveys that are also included in the introduction part of maternal health care utilization, is the main gateway for women to remain safe due to maternity. There are many propositions that determine the maternal health care utilization:

- Age, sex, household composition, structure and size, head of the household, region, etc.
- Characteristics of illness cost and benefits of health care, wealth quintile, distance to reach health institution, place of residence, employment status, etc.
- Quality of health care system, beliefs and values.

Among the many variables, education variable is taken as an important variable that influences maternal health care utilization. Currently, Government of Nepal has also focused its literacy programme for female to change their status totally from household chores to classrooms of school/college. Women's education is likely to be associated with many other variables too. An educated woman has fewer births than uneducated women and the use of contraception, both modern and traditional are also seemed to be used more consciously. Increased level of female education has multiphasic effects too. For example, educated women have improved economic status of household which further helps to be conscious to seek better health. Educated women would like to live in well facilitated areas. In Nepal, currently Government of Nepal has targeted for female education, women employment. A lot of changes have occurred in mass media and information technology. Schools/colleges are being expanded to rural areas as well as there are improvement in transportation facilities. Sub Health Post are being upgraded to provide maximum level of basic health care including ANC. Training manual and components are being changed annually to provide skilled birth training to the health manpower. Modern contraceptive methods like condom, pills and injectables are available free of cost in almost all lowest level of health services. All these factors are more likely to confound the association between women's education and maternal health care utilization.

There are other different variables, in addition to education such as religion, mass media exposure, place of residence, birth order etc. that may influence FMHCSU and are associated with women's education. Therefore, a strategy employed here in this study is to estimate the relationship of education for one model of analysis and the second model with other explanatory variables to see further influence in FMHCSU, expecting that these other variables are acquired at different stages of women's reproductive life.

The schematic diagram showing the role of women's education in FMHCSU:

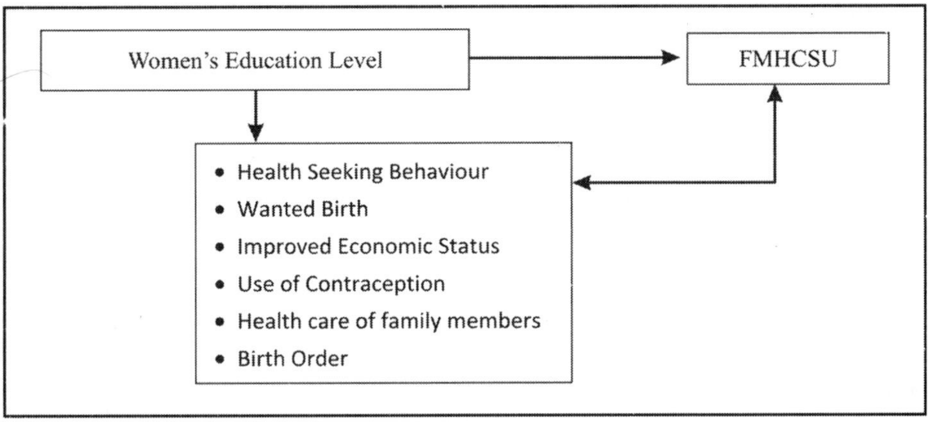

Source: Drawn by Author.

Data and the Method

This study has utilized Nepal Demographic Health Survey 2011 women's data file. This survey interviewed 12,674 currently married women of reproductive age (15–49 years).Out of them 4,148 (weighted cases) women had given birth to child in the five years preceding the survey time. For the maternal health care utilization, the information was collected only from the last birth in details about ANC, delivery and postnatal care. The three responses such as number of ANC visit, delivery at health institute or not and the postnatal check-up from birth to 42 days of delivery are taken for analysis purpose, supposing that these are most common for all pregnant women to be utilized in order to give healthy babies and also for safety of her own health.

The dependent variable is created by using the antenatal care, delivery care and postnatal care. In antenatal care, the response of questions on how many times did you visit health institutions is further grouped into two categories – No visit and at least one and above visit. Delivery care is also divided into two groups as birth given in health institution of any kind (government, public, private or NGO) and home or elsewhere (not in health institution). Similarly, the postnatal care from birth to 42 days of delivery is categorized as 'Yes' for receiving such service within the time frame and those having no such visit within the time-frame are considered as 'No'. In this way, from these three components and six categories are computed to make one variable. The complete use of three components is considered here as 'Fully utilized' (coded as 1) and the women who failed to receive any one of the services are taken as 'Not fully utilized' (coded as 0). Binary logistic regression is used here for analysis purpose. Two models are constructed to see the role of women's education in FMHCSU. The first model is the role of women's education in FMHCSU and the second model is based on some socio-economic and demographic variables with FMHCSU.

Results

Table 1 shows that there are about 15 per cent of women, among women who had given birth to child in five years preceding the survey, did not visit any of the health institution for pregnancy check-up, whereas majority of them had visited at least one time. There could still be problem seen with these 15 per cent women if this proportion remained same in future. Delivery care at health institution is the best solution to save lives of pregnant women. A well-facilitated institution is required for this. There are still about 62 per cent women who had given birth to a child in the last five-year period outside the health institution despite the free maternity and some allowances provision supported by the government. Comparing antenatal care (ANC) visit and delivery care, there is about 45 per cent reduction in delivery at health institution. However, the analysis does not cover the exact percentage of women who had ANC visit utilize delivery services by the same proportion of women. Similarly, prenatal care (PNC) is most essential to save from worse maternity situation after delivery. But, only about 43 per cent of women had institutional check-up within the time frame. Comparing these three outcomes, there is no such resemblance and consistency with utilization of maternity care in Nepal. Therefore, the problem always lies in those women who missed the services.

Table 1 *Distribution of Respondents of Age 15–49 by Different Components of Maternal Child Health Care Utilization*

Components of Maternal Health Care					
Antenatal Care (%)		*Delivery At (%)*		*Check up After Delivery (%)*	
No Visit	15.2	Not at Health facility	61.5	Yes	43.2
At least One Visit	84.8	Health Institute	38.5	No	56.8
Total			100%		
Total Number			4,148		

It can be seen from the Table 2 that only about 33 per cent of women who had given birth to a child in the last five-year period have gone for FMHCSU. This Table 2 further indicates that two-thirds of the women in Nepal are still at very high risk during childbirth process due to giving birth without full utilization of maternity services. Data on maternal mortality rate (MMR) indicates that MMR is reducing rapidly since 1990. On the other hand, a high percentage of women do not have FMHCSU, and it raises many questions to the researcher to investigate further in this area.

Table 2 *Distribution of Respondents Full Maternal Health Care Service Utilization Index*

Covariates	*Number*	*Percentage*
Not Fully Utilized	2,762	66.6
Fully Utilized	1,386	33.4
Total	4,148	100

Source: Calculated by author.

FMHCSU, without reservation, varies with many other socio-economic and demographic variables. While cross-classified with some selected variables, it can be seen from Table 3 that about 66 per cent of the women living in urban area have FMHCSU, whereas only 30 per cent of the women in rural area have FMHCSU, less than fifty per cent than urban women. This association is highly significant too. Nepal is declared as a secular country currently, but the large share of people is still Hindu and rest are of other religions such as Buddhists, Jain and Muslim etc. On the whole religious people are divided into two groups as Hindu and Non-Hindu for the purpose of studying whether there is any association of it with maternal health care utilization. About 35 per cent of the Hindu women have FMHCSU, whereas only about 27 per cent of Non-Hindu has FMHCSU and the association is also highly significant.

Table 3 *Distribution of Women Age 15–49 who have Given Birth to Child in the Last Five-Year Period and have Utilized Maternal Health Care by Selected Background Variables*

Covariates	*Categories*	*Maternal Health Care Service Utilization (%)*		*Total Number of Women*	X^2
		Not Fully Utilized	*Fully Utilized*		
Place of Residence	Urban	34.1	65.9	418	220.54***
	Rural	70.2	29.8	3,730	
Religion	Hindu	65.3	34.7	3,444	14.33***
	Non-Hindu	72.7	27.3	704	
Wealth Index	Poorest	90.3	9.7	980	846.35***
	Poorer	78.9	21.1	899	
	Middle	69.5	30.5	872	
	Richer	51.9	48.1	748	
	Richest	26.8	73.2	649	
Mass Media Exposure	Not exposed	83.6	16.4	1,165	473.86***
	Partially exposed	66.2	33.8	2478	
	Fully exposed	28.9	71.1	505	
Education Level	No schooling	82.8	17.2	1,869	591.065***
	Class 1–9	61.7	38.3	1,654	
	SLC and above	31.2	68.8	626	

Cont'd...

...Cont'd

Development Region	EDR	64.3	35.7	999	16.35**
	CDR	66.1	33.9	1,293	
	WDR	63.9	36.1	818	
	MWDR	71.7	28.3	598	
	FWDR	71.1	28.9	440	
Contraception Use	Any method	65.3	34.7	1,635	1.83
	Not using any method	67.4	32.6	2,513	
Birth Order	First order	46.6	54.2	1,302	413.54***
	2–3	70.3	29.7	1,894	
	4 and above	86.4	13.6	952	
Current Age	Less than 20	55.1	44.9	334	77.15***
	20–29	63.8	36.2	2,638	
	30 and above	76.0	24.0	1,176	
Region	Mountain	81.6	18.4	305	57.46***
	Hill	69.7	30.3	1,668	
	Terai	62.1	37.9	2,175	
Total		66.6% (2762)	33.4% (1386)	100% (4148)	

Note: EDR=Eastern Development Region, CDR=Central Development Region, WDR= Western Development Region, MWDR= Mid-western Development Region, FWDR= Far Western Development Region.

Source: Calculated by Author.
***=significant at <.001,**=<.01 and *=<.05
SLC – School Leaving Certificate

NDHS 2011 has divided the total people of Nepal into five groups according the wealth they owned. Same variables and the categories are taken for this analysis. While analysing wealth quintile's relation with FMHCSU, about three-fourths of the women in richest wealth quintile has FMHCSU and the lowest percentages are in poorest wealth quintile. Free maternity service has not played a vital role here as can be inferred from this relationship. The association is also highly significant.

Mass media such as radio, TV and newspaper also play a vital role in such a technological society which has reached to most of the village development committee even in remote areas of Nepal in these days. Government of Nepal enacted the use all media to disseminate health-related information. Expansion of FM radio frequency to rural areas and also producing health information in native languages are the major contributing factors to keep people informed. From these three variables, one new variable has been created. It is found from Table 3 that more than two-thirds of the women who are exposed to mass media fully have fully utilized maternal health care whereas those women who are not exposed to any media have only 16 per cent fully utilized. It indicated that media has played vital role in receiving maternal health care fully, which is highly significant too. Similarly, education has also the same relationship with

FMHCSU as in the mass media exposure. As level of education increases, FMHCSU also increases. This is also justified by significant result of chi-square value.

Nepal is divided into five development regions for administrative purpose. While considering the availability of health institutions distributed equally in all development regions, no pattern has been seen in FMHCSU, but the largest percentage of women of Western Development Region have fully utilized it followed by Central Development Region. The association is also significant.

There is no vast difference between contraception users and non-users in utilizing fully the maternal health care service. Birth order is an important indicator to see the relationship with maternal health care utilization. It can be seen from the Table 3 that about 53 per cent of first order women have fully utilized it and it decreases as the order of birth increases. The association is highly significant. Younger women are more likely to utilize maternal health care than older women. It can be seen that the highest percentage of younger women (less than 20 years) having fully utilized maternal health care than other age groups which is in decreasing trend. This is highly associated as chi-square value shows it. Similarly, Terai which is also known as a highly developed region except Kathmandu valley, of hilly region, has utilized services more among three ecological regions of Nepal. The association is highly significant.

Table 4 *Odds Ratio of FMHCSU with Women's Educational Level and Different Background Characteristics of Respondents, Results of Logistic Regression*

Variables	*Categories*	*Model 1 Exp(B)*	*Model 2 Exp(B)*
Education Level	No Education®		
	Class 1–9	2.98***	1.306**
	SLC and above	10.617***	2.093***
Media Exposure	Not Exposed®		
	Partially Exposed		1.092
	Fully Exposed		1.817***
Religion	Hindu®		
	Non Hindu		0.883
Wealth Quintile	Poorest®		
	Poorer		2.270***
	Middle		3.094***
	Richer		5.175***
	Richest		11.435***
Development Region	EDR®		
	CDR		0.961
	WDR		0.974
	MWDR		1.399*
	FWDR		1.382*
Region	Mountain®		

Cont'd...

...Cont'd

	Hill		1.112
	Terai		1.182
Place of Residence	Urban®		
	Rural		0.516***
Contraceptive Use	Using Contraception®		
	Not Using Any Method		1.139
Birth Order	First Order®		
	2–3		0.447***
	4 and above		0.307***
Current Age	Less than 20®		
	20–29		0.795
	30+		0.849
Constant		0.208	0.314
–2 Loglikelihood		4694.72	4083.59

Note: EDR=Eastern Development Region, CDR=Central Development Region, WDR= Western Development Region, MWDR= Mid-western Development Region, FWDR= Far Western Development Region.

®=*Reference category, ***=significant at <.001, **=<.01 and *=<.05, Calculated by Author*

Though the chi-square shows the significant relationship between education and FMHCSU and also with some selected variables, this is further analysed with logistic regression to analyse net and gross effects. Model 1 of Table 4 shows the gross effects of women's level of education to FMHCSU. The chance of FMHCSU by women of education level 1–9 is 2.98 times higher than those having no education. Similarly, as the level of education increases to School Leaving Certificate (SLC) and above, the chances of FMHCSU is highly increased by 10.6 times than the women having no education (illiterate). While analysing the net effect of women's education level with other background characteristics of education such as place of residence, geographical region, current use of contraception, birth order, current age, religion, etc. the net effect has declined sharply than gross effect. According to model 2 the chance of FMHCSU by women of education level 1–9 is only 1.3 times higher than women having no education controlling other variables which has declined by about 50 per cent which is considered as the effects of others covariates. Similarly, in case of education level SLC and above the chances of FMHCU has sharply declined than in model 1 to only 2.09times more. Hence, it can be said that FMHCSU not only depends on education but by the combined effects of different covariates.

The role of media in FMHCSU is seen to be very strong as it has increased by 1.8 times than the women who have not been exposed to any media after controlling other variables. The partially exposed women to media does not play a vital role as it is not significant. The chance of FMHCSU by non-Hindu as compared to Hindu has no significant effect. The chance of FMHCSU by poorer women is 2.27 times higher than women of poorest wealth quintile. The chances of FMHCSU have been increased as the level of wealth quintile increases. It is found 11.4 times higher chances of FMHCSU by women in the richest wealth quintile than women in poorest quintile controlling other variables. This result further indicates that utilization of maternity service depends on the economic condition of women, despite the free maternity service in Nepal. Though there are many places of MWDR and FWDR which are not so much developed as compared to other development regions of Nepal but these two regions have significant effects on FMHCSU. The chance of FMHCSU in MWDR has 1.4 times higher chances than EDR and 1.38 times higher in FWDR controlling other variables. Other two development regions have no effects as compared to EDR. Such results might be the effects of special programme of nutrition as well as other types of integrated programme launched in these two regions. Similarly, ecological regions have not had any effect though the value increased. The place of residence of Nepal is also considered as an affecting factor for FMHCSU. The rural area has 48 per cent less chance of having FMHCSU as compared to urban area by controlling other variables. It might be due to minimum level of service availability and lack of manpower which could assist women during motherhood. Women using contraception has no significant effects to FMHCSU. This result further indicates that the behaviour change has not been observed due to increased accessibility in Nepal. Birth order of women also decides whether to have FMHCSU. Women of birth order 2–3, which is also considered as average level of birth as TFR of Nepal according to DHS is 2.6, has 55 per cent less chance of FMHCSU and this chance further decreases to 70 per cent for higher order birth. The result also shows that chances of FMHCSU by women of age 20+ have no significant effects on FMHCSU as compared to women of age less than 20.

Discussion

The effect of women's education in achieving FMHCSU is analysed along with some background characteristics. Women's education is an important indicator for social change and also sanctions inherent power to bring change in many other sectors. Government of Nepal (GON) has emphasized female education as it has remained with a wide gap between male and female literacy rate in the past. Similarly, GON has started free maternity services since 2008, as stated earlier, to save women and children's life. Along with government efforts, some private hospitals and teaching hospitals are being included as a part of free of cost for maternity services. Travel allowance had been started some few years earlier than free maternity services which are continuing so far. Despite these works from the government side, the access of women for service utilization is very low compared to what it should be. Though there are about 85 per cent of women who go for ANC, percentage of delivery care and postnatal check-up in health institution has reduced more than 50 per cent. It can be said that ANC statistics in Nepal is satisfactory but the other two major part of maternal health has no such acceptable results. Establishment of maternal health care centre is meant for its full utilization. FMHCSU can only reduce the unwanted death of mothers due to pregnancy related cases. Though there is tremendous reduction of MMR observed in Nepal but if one will sees the FMHCSU it is found to be very low (Table 2). Therefore, we have tried to see the net and gross effects of women's education with FMHCSU. It cannot be underestimate the role of female education in FMHCSU but the possible reason for decline in net effect of education as stated in model 2 is the place of residence where the availability of all three types of health services is scarce and always there is a problem of availability of trained health personnel in the rural areas of Nepal. Similarly, some special programmes and targets in some development regions poverty alleviation programme along with some infrastructural development programme might have played a crucial role in achieving FMHCSU. Likewise, expansion of media coverage in most of the rural areas and less awareness to have second birth in health institution, etc. have played the major role in reduction. Rapid increment in the percentage of female higher level education in future may result in better utilization in the country. This increment of service utilization not only improves maternal health but also helps to reduce unwanted maternal morbidity and mortality. Some earlier studies are found to be viewed differently from ANC, delivery care and PNC. But, in the case of free of cost services in the government institution, I hope this could be a new idea for further analysis in developing countries which are trying their best to provide all kinds of maternity services. Further studies can also be done with the same concept in three different surveys of Nepal to see the effects of female education in achieving FMHCSU which ultimately contribute to reduce maternal and child mortality in Nepal.

Conclusion

The emphasis of the government to bring changes in female education only cannot lead to increase FMHCSU, but equally important is considering and laying emphasis on different covariates such as order of birth, place of residence, current age, wealth quintile, religion, development region, media exposure, etc. which may play a significant role in achieving sound utilization of maternity health care services from the very beginning of identification of pregnancy to 42 days after delivery which further leads to save womens' reproductive lives. But, this does not mean to say that female education has no role in FMHCSU.

Notes

1. UNFPA. 1999. *Reproductive Health Situation of Nepal: Nepal Country Report*. Kathmandu, Nepal: United Nations Population Fund.
2. McDonagh, M.I. 1996. Antenatal Care Effective in Reducing Maternal Morbidity and Mortality? *Health Policy and Planning*, 11: 1–15.
3. Thaddeus, S. and Maine, D. 1994. Too Far to Walk: Maternal Mortality in Context. *Social Science and Medicine*, 38: 1091–1110.
4. Elo, I.T. 1992. Utilization of Maternal Health Care Services in Peru: The Role of Women's Education. *Health Transition Review*, 2: 49–68.
5. Raghupathy, S. 1996. Education and the Use of Maternal Health Care in Thailand. *Social Science Medicine*, 43: 459–471.

6. Shariff, A. and Singh, G. 2002. Determinants of Maternal Health Care Utilization in India: Evidence from a Recent Household Survey. Working Paper No. 38, New Delhi: National Centre for Applied Economic Research.
7. Weintraub, H. 1997. Status of Women, Maternal Child Health and Family Planning in Kenya. *International Journal of Public Administration*, 20: 1513–1568.
8. Mostafa Kamal, S.M. 2009. Factors Affecting Utilization of Skilled Maternity Care Services among Married Adolescents in Bangladesh. *Asian Population Studies*, 5: 153–170.
9. Sharma, S.K., Sawangdee, Y. and Sirirassamee, B. 2007. Access to Health: Women's Status and Utilization of Maternal Health Services in Nepal. *Journal of Biosocial Science*, 39: 671–692.
10. Paul, B.K. and Rumsey, D.J. 2002. Utilization of Health Facilities and Trained Birth Attendants for Childbirth in Rural Bangladesh: An Empirical Study. *Social Science and Medicine*, 54: 1755–1765.
11. Obermeyer, C.M. 1993. Culture, Maternal Health Care and Women's Status: A Comparison of Morocco and Tunisia. *Studies in Family Planning*, 24: 354–365.
12. Celik, Y. and Hotchkiss, D.R. 2000. The Socioeconomic Determinants of Maternal Health Care in Turkey. *Social Science and Medicine*, 50: 1797–1806.
13. Winikoff, B. and Sullivan, M. 1987. Assessing the Role of Family Planning Reducing Maternal Mortality. *Studies in Family Planning*, 18 (3): 128–143.
14. McGuire, W.J. 1981. *The Theoretical Foundations of Campaigns*. Beverly Hills, CA: Sage.
15. Hotkiss, D.R., Rous, J.J., Seiber, E.E. and Berruti, A.A. 2005. Is Maternal and Child Health Services Use a Casual Gateway to Subsequent Contraceptive Use? A Multi-Country Study. *Population Research and Policy Review*, 24 (6): 543–571.
16. Raghupathy, S. 1997. Unwanted Pregnancies and Preventive Health Care Use in Thailand. *Population Research and Policy Review*, 16: 579–595.
17. Gage, A.J. and Calixte, M.G. 2006. Effects of the Physical Accessibility of Maternal Health Services on Their Use in Rural Haiti. *Population Studies*, 60: 271–288.
18. Hetson, P. 2001–02. Use of Maternal Health Care among African Women in South Africa. *South African Journal of Demography*, 8: 61–72.
19. Ministry of Health and Population, New ERA and ICF International Inc. 2012. *Nepal Demographic and Health Survey 2011*. Kathmandu, Nepal: Ministry of Health and Population, New ERA and Calverton, Maryland: ICF International Inc.

16

Women's Education and Fertility Regulation in Nepal

Is the Relationship Anomalous?

Ramesh Babu Kafle

'Education enables women to have requisite information on a variety of aspects, increase her power to interact with others, strengthen her capability to take appropriate decisions, improve her autonomy, instill in her a sense of prestige, and, overall, lead to ensuring better status of women in the family as well as in the society'.[1] Female education empowers women mainly through their involvement in family decision-making, autonomy and control over household resources, knowledge and awareness of the modern world and inter-spousal communication.[2] Education enhances women's status within and outside their immediate family and increases their exposure to the information and ideas which brings changes in their general behaviour involving breastfeeding, use of contraception and hence fertility.[3] As a result, more educated women are more aware about contraception in terms of knowledge, acceptability, accessibility and use. They are more capable to make rational choice for the number of children they would have and more likely to behave accordingly. Consequently, they are more likely to use effective means of contraception to regulate fertility. Generally, there is positive relationship between women's education and the use of contraception, thus supporting the negative relationship between women's education and fertility.

Women's education is not a single variable affecting fertility regulation, but it is one of the most influencing factors among all the socio-economic variables. Saleem and Bobak highlighted women's education as one of the most important predictor of contraceptive use, whose effect is not even mediated by autonomy. To have negative impact on fertility, women's education should have positive relationship with the use of contraceptives.[4] Gardon et al., stated that all socio-demographic factors affect women's education, which in turn has effect on knowledge/access to family planning and other attitudinal factors and finally affect the use status of modern contraception.[5] Bongaarts demonstrated negative association of education levels with fertility according to which, better-educated women marry later and less often, use contraception more effectively, have more knowledge about and access to it and more motivated to implement demand because of the higher opportunity costs of unintended child-bearing.[6] The conclusion is that women's education is positively associated with demand for and use of contraception.

When the overall level of contraceptive use is very low and overall level of women's education is also low, more contraceptive users will be among more educated women in urban area and education do have positive effect on modern contraceptive use but in the rural area education has almost no effect.[7] In low contraception community, increased women's education causes decreased breast-feeding and abstinence durations thus have higher marital fertility for educated women than for illiterate women.[8] But this situation is likely to change during the course of socio-economic transformation, which is characterized by increasing level of women's education and relatively higher level of contraception use. Differing arguments are there that more educated women are so motivated to adopt contraception that even if there is no programme they will control fertility by use of contraception.[9] If there is family planning programme then uneducated women are also likely to use contraception and the dynamics of modern contraceptive use by educational status of women becomes more complicated.

The normally expected positive relationship between women's education and contraceptive use is under inquiry. Does the strength of such relationship change from one context to the other? What is the role of other socio-economic variables on this relationship? These questions are of sizeable importance for better understanding of nature and extent of relationship between these two variables in different social settings.

Nepal is on the way of fertility transition since 1980s. The TFR declined from 5.1 in 1986 to 3.1 in 2006[10] and further to 2.6 in 2011.[11] The current use of any modern method of contraception has been increased from 15.1 per cent in 1986 to 44.2 per cent in 2006.[10] But, this has been decreased to 43.2 per cent in 2011. From 2006 to 2011, the percentage of users of contraception of any method has slightly increased from 48 to 49.7. The decreased proportion of couples currently using modern methods have been countered by the increment in the users of withdrawal method. The educational differentials in TFR in Nepal are noticeable (in 2011, TFR is 3.7 for no education, 2.7 for primary education, 2.1 for some secondary education and 1.7 for women with higher education).[11] There is a substantial decline in TFR from 2006 to 2011 but the proportion of contraceptive users has not equally increased, rather, the proportion of current users of modern methods has slightly declined.

DHS (2006) in Nepal shows that the relationship between women's education and modern contraceptive use is not clearly negative but curvilinear. The percentage of women using any modern method of contraception with no education, primary education, some secondary education and SLC (School Leaving Certificate, an exam conducted by national board after completion of grade10) and above education are 46.4, 41.9, 38.6 and 41.7 respectively).[12] The most recent demographic and health survey of 2011 in Nepal again shows a clear decline in the percentage of currently married women using any modern method of contraception as observed from women with no education category to women attaining highest level of education.[11] In India, the percentage of women using any modern method of contraception is almost similar for all levels of education with a fluctuation rather than a clear increasing trend as one moves from uneducated category to the highly educated category of women.[13] The reason behind such relationship between women's education and the percentage using modern method of contraception has been attributed to the contrasting patterns in the use of sterilization and spacing methods due to education. At least, it can be said at this point that, the impact of education on contraceptive use is mixed in Nepal.

Based on NFHS (1992–93), Parasuraman et al., found that the prevalence of contraception among illiterates is equal or even higher compared to the most educated group in most of the Indian states. This research found substantial state level variation in the contraceptive prevalence by education of women and described it by the overall level of contraceptive prevalence.[14] As discussed earlier, the nature and extent of interrelationship between women's education and use of modern contraception appears to be a dynamic one. The same research also found a significant positive influence of education on the use of contraception after controlling for other socio-economic variables.

The curvilinear relationship between women's educational status and their adoption of contraceptive methods observed in Nepal is to be carefully studied for the better understanding of the effect of women's education on fertility regulation. At the current stage of fertility transition, whether women's education has significant effect on modern contraceptive use after controlling for other socio-economic factors? How differently the other socio-economic variables influence the modern contraceptive use among the women of different educational status? Such questions are to be cautiously answered.

This paper has a limited scope which covers studying relationship of modern contraceptive use and education in association with selected socio-economic and demographic variables, explaining the effect of selected variables on use of modern contraceptives for different levels of women's education and also to find the net effect of women's education on use of modern contraceptives controlling for the other variables.

Objectives

This paper has the following specific objectives:

- To study relationship of modern contraceptive use and education with controlling for selected socio-economic and demographic variables.
- Explaining the effect of selected variables on use of modern contraceptives for different levels of women's education.

Methods and Materials

Women's data file of Nepal Demographic Health Survey (2011), a national level sample survey has been used for analysis. Multistage sampling was adopted in this survey to get a national representative sample. Out of the total sample of 12,674 women aged 15–49, the sample of currently married women of age

15–49 which counts to 9,608 has been used in the analysis. The response variable is current use of contraceptives which is made dichotomous as: those currently using any modern method, and those not using any modern method.

Education has been coded into three categories: those respondents with no schooling (0), those with completed schooling years of up to nine years (1–9) and those who have completed at least 10 years of schooling (10+). The last category refers that respondent has at least passed school leaving certificate (SLC) in Nepalese education system. These three categories are supposed to reflect the major educational characteristics as uneducated, moderately educated and highly educated in Nepalese context.

Type of place of residence (Urban and Rural), geographical region (Mountain, Hill and Terai or Plain) and development region (Eastern, Central, Western, Mid-Western and Far Western Development Regions) are considered as spatial variables. Similarly, wealth index (measured in the well-known quintiles) has been taken as proxy to economic variable. Age (used as categorical and also continuous), living number of children (0, 1, 2 and 3+), living number of sons (0, 1 and 2+) and whether experienced any child death (No/Yes) are the demographic variables used in analysis. Exposure of women to mass media is also included in analysis. For this, the questions on specific radio or TV programmes are used. In the survey women are asked for their 'Yes' or 'No' response to ten radio and/or TV programmes which disseminate message regarding contraceptives. Based on the responses to this question, a dichotomous variable has been constructed with values: 'Heard or seen at least one programme' and 'Not heard or seen even at least one of the programmes'. I argue that this variable is better for the purpose of analysing status of use of modern contraceptives because such specific programmes disseminate message on modern contraceptives to the populace and exposure of women to such programmes really does matter. Similarly, another question related to involvement of women in four women's groups: Ama Samuha (Mother's Group), Mahila Samuha (Women's Group), Bachat Samuha (Saving Group of women) and any other women's group have been asked. Based on the responses, a dichotomous variable has been constructed with responses: 'Involved in any one of the women's groups' and 'Not involved in any one of the women's groups'. In such women's groups, women are supposed to communicate, interact and share knowledge of each other and it is expected that this has effect on adoption of modern contraception.

The percentage of respondents using any modern method of contraception by their levels of education cross-classified with other study variables has been presented to depict the scenario of modern contraceptive use by various socio-economic characteristics. Logistic regression is used to study the net effect of covariates on it. For the three different levels of education, separate logistic regressions have been fitted to make a comparative study of the net effect of other covariates on the chances of using modern contraceptive method. Also, another logistic regression model has been run by taking education and all other study variables in the model, to see the net effect of education on chances of using modern contraceptives after controlling for other variables.

Results

Figure 1 depicts that 49 per cent women with no education are using modern method and the value declines to 39 per cent for women with 1–9 years of schooling and further declines to 35 per cent for highly educated women. The pattern is just opposite in case of proportion of non-users of any modern method. The association between women's education and current use of contraception has been found highly significant, indicating gross negative association between women's education and modern contraceptive use.

Figure 1 *Percentage of Currently Married Women of Age 15–49 with Modern Contraceptive Use by Years of Schooling*

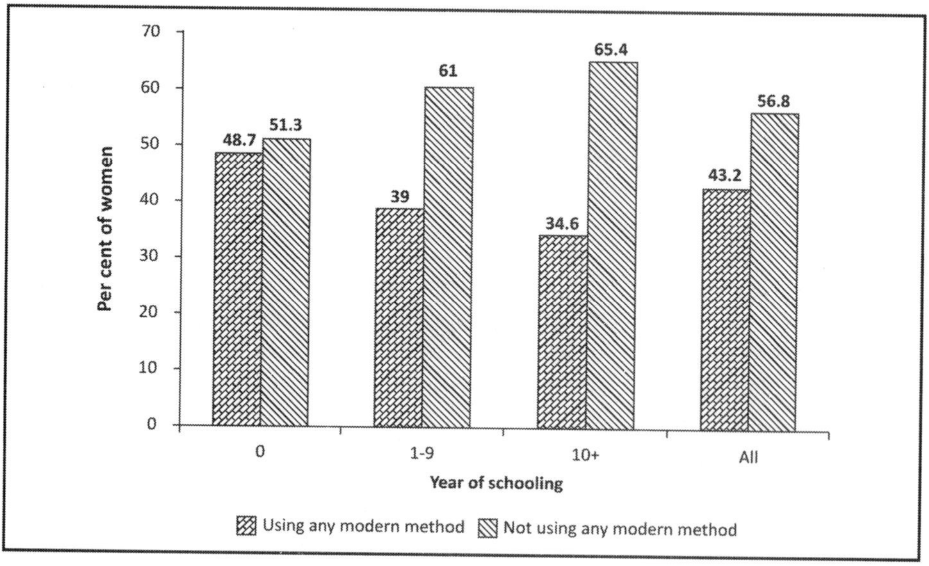

This paper tries to unfold this negative relationship between women's education and use of modern contraceptives. Only the users of modern contraceptives have been taken into account for analysis.

Table 1 shows that among uneducated and moderately educated women, there is significant positive association between belongingness of women in any women's group and modern use of contraception. But such association is not meaningful for highly educated women. Exactly similar situation has been observed for exposure of women into family planning programmes in the media. The results indicate positive role of women's social groups and specific programmes disseminating message on family planning, propagated through electronic media, especially among less educated women to have positive impact on adoption of modern contraceptives.

Experience of child death has mixed type of effect on use of modern contraceptives for women of all educational level. The association is significant for all women irrespective of their educational status as well as for women with education level 1–9 years. The number of living children and the number of living sons have significant association with response variable for all levels of education. Therefore, women of all educational background behave alike in case of the number of living children and the number of living sons and there is considerably more proportion of women using modern contraception with increasing number of living children as well as increasing number of sons. Current age has, no doubt, a significant positive relationship with contraceptive use in all educational levels of women. Highest proportions in the age group 35+ indicate higher emphasis on permanent methods. There is no educational difference among adolescent and young mothers in using modern contraceptives and their level of use is the lowest among mothers of all reproductive ages.

Table 1 *Percentage of Currently Married Women of Age 15–49 who are Currently Using any Modern Method of Contraception for Different Levels of Schooling by Selected Characteristics*

Characteristics	*Years of schooling*			*All levels (n=9,608)*
	0 (n=4,695)	*1–9 (n=3,562)*	*10+(n=1,351)*	
Belongingness to any women's group				
No	41.8	31.7	32.6	37.0
Yes	57.5	46.5	37.1	50.3
χ^2 value	113.86***	82.0***	2.94	172.82***
Exposure to any FP programme in Radio/TV				
Not exposed	45.8	36.5	37.3	42.7
Exposed	55.5	40.6	33.9	43.6
χ^2 value	37.76***	6.18*	1.65	0.78
Ever experienced child death				
No	48.6	38.3	34.1	42.0
Yes	49.0	45.1	45.8	48.1
χ^2 value	0.05	6.35*	3.37	21.36***
Number of living children				
0	5.1	8.5	12.4	8.9
1–2	39.5	37.9	39.4	38.8
3+	56.8	57.0	59.2	56.9
χ^2 value	307.3***	335.1***	114.6***	863.66***
Number of living son				
0	17.1	17.6	20.8	18.3
1	43.7	41.2	43.0	42.6
2+	61.1	62.7	59.5	61.4
χ^2 value	447.99***	439.0***	115.0***	1107.0***
Development region				
Eastern	43.9	32.6	27.5	36.2
Central	52.3	49.0	43.0	49.9
Western	46.0	35.6	29.9	38.7
Mid-Western	45.9	38.4	39.5	42.8
Far Western	52.5	40.1	29.7	47.0
χ^2 value	25.26***	63.88***	28.07***	127.23***

Cont'd...

...Cont'd

Geographical region				
Mountain	47.2	35.8	34.9	43.0
Hill	44.8	37.1	37.6	40.6
Terai	51.5	40.9	32.1	45.0
χ^2 value	18.9***	6.0*	4.33	17.88***
Type of place of residence				
Urban	56.8	50.3	42.0	49.8
Rural	48.0	37.2	31.9	42.1
χ^2 value	10.94**	31.57***	12.21***	26.22***
Wealth Index				
Poorest	38.4	27.2	33.3	35.7
Poorer	49.5	26.7	19.4	41.1
Middle	51.0	36.2	22.1	43.3
Richer	56.4	41.3	30.6	45.3
Richest	57.9	53.0	40.1	48.9
χ^2 value	86.9***	137.33***	29.0***	27.69***
Age				
15–24	20.5	21.2	20.4	20.8
25–34	48.3	45.8	37.9	45.5
35+	57.1	57.1	55.9	57.0
χ^2 value	292.1***	316.9***	97.2***	799.62***

(* indicates $p<0.05$, ** indicates $p<0.01$ and *** indicates $p<0.001$)

Table 2 *Result of Logistic Regression Showing the Odds Ratios of Using Modern Method of Contraception by Currently Married Women of Age 15–49 for Various Levels of Schooling by Selected Covariates*

Covariates	*Odds ratios*			*Including education in the model (n=9,608) (Model-II)*
	For level of schooling (Model-I)			
	0 (n=4,695)	*1–9 (n=3,562)*	*10+ (n=1,351)*	
Belongingness to any women's group				
No (Ref.)				
Yes	1.51***	1.3**	0.88	1.34***
Exposure to any FP programme in Radio/TV				
Not exposed (Ref.)				
Exposed	1.36***	1.68	0.97	1.21***
Ever experienced child death				
No (Ref.)				
Yes	0.83**	1.01	1.18	0.87*
Number of living children				
0 (Ref.)				
1–2	4.8***	2.7***	2.6***	2.8***

Cont'd...

...Cont'd

3+	6.5***	3.8***	4.1***	4.1***
Number of living son				
0 (Ref.)				
1	2.32***	1.8***	1.58**	1.9***
2+	4.42***	3.8***	2.64***	3.8***
Development region				
Eastern (Ref.)				
Central	1.67***	2.0***	1.66**	1.83***
Western	1.08	1.12	1.06	1.07
Mid-Western	1.46**	1.77***	1.88*	1.58***
Far Western	1.64***	1.81***	1.07	1.67***
Geographical region				
Mountain (Ref.)				
Hill	0.84	0.86	0.65	0.88
Terai	1.15	0.84	0.53	0.98
Type of place of residence				
Urban (Ref.)				
Rural	0.75*	0.86	0.99	0.81**
Wealth Index				
Poorest (Ref.)				
Poorer	1.52***	0.96	0.56	1.41***
Middle	1.6***	1.45*	0.6	1.65***
Richer	1.87***	1.68**	1.06	1.9***
Richest	1.02**	2.32***	1.32	2.37***
Education				
0 (Ref.)	–	–	–	
1–9	–	–	–	0.96
10+	–	–	–	0.86
Current age (continuous)	1.02**	1.02*	1.03**	1.02***
Constant	0.02***	0.03***	0.09**	0.03***
–2 Log Likelihood	5,706.6	4,030.6	1,527.0	11,343.0

(* indicates $p<0.05$, ** indicates $p<0.01$ and *** indicates $p<0.001$)

The important result is that, the proportion of women using modern contraceptives without having any living children increases from five per cent for uneducated women to 8.5 per cent to moderately educated women and it further increases to 12.4 per cent for highly educated women. A new pattern of use is emerging in which more educated women are better planning their fertility by starting their use of contraceptives from the beginning of their effective reproductive period. Same scenario has been observed for the number of living sons. Here, the pattern of use by educational level has been reversed for women with no living children. Although such a reverse did not exactly occur for women with at least one living child (and living son), at least it has been distorted.

The variation in proportions of women using modern contraceptives by development regions has been found significant for all three levels of education and there is no change in the declining patterns of these proportions from uneducated to highly educated category. The response variable has significant association with geographical region for women in uneducated and moderately educated category and the significance is lost for highly educated group. Uneducated women of Terai region have the highest proportion of modern contraceptive users, whereas the highly educated women of the same region have the least proportion. Women of urban residence are in better position in use of modern contraceptive than their rural counterparts for all levels of education and the association is significant. The situation of anomalous relationship is retained both in rural as well as in urban area.

The response variable is significantly associated with the wealth index and this holds true for all levels of education. Economic variable has positive relationship with use of modern methods of contraception for women with no education with the highest proportion of uneducated richest women using modern contraceptives. Highly educated women of poorest wealth index are better off than women of poorer and middle category in modern contraceptive use. The anomaly in the pattern of use persists for all levels of wealth indices except for the poorest one in which proportion of users of modern contraceptives first declines and then increases again as level of education rises.

The logistic regression model for uneducated women shows that, the odds of using modern contraceptives significantly increases by 1.51 times for women who are members of any women group in comparison to non-members (Table 2). Similar result is obtained for those women who have exposed to at least one FP programme on radio/TV. But, for women with higher education, there is no significant effect of membership in such groups or exposure to FP messages. The net effect of these two variables did not drop significance in presence of education itself as a covariate. The result indicates importance of women's groups as well as that of specific radio/TV programmes targeting to women of lower educational strata to enhance their use of modern contraceptives.

The odds of using modern contraceptive among uneducated women is 5 and 6.5 times more for women with 1–2 children and three or more children respectively as compared to those with no living children. But, the amount of net effect, though it remains significant, declines in other educational categories as well as for model including education. The increase in educational level mediates the effect of number of living children on modern contraceptive use. Similar net effect has been observed for the number of living sons.

For wealth index, for uneducated women, all the odds ratios are significant. As compared to the poorest strata, the odds of using modern method of contraception are increased by 1.5, 1.6, 1.9 and 1.02 times for poorer, middle, richer and richest strata. This shows that more economically well off women are more likely to use modern contraception up to richer stratum even if they are not educated. Interestingly, the odds ratios are insignificant for the most educated categories of women, indicating that the variation in contraceptive use due to wealth does work only for up to some moderate level of education. A significant but only of a very small extent of net effect has been observed for current age in uneducated and moderately educated group and the effect became insignificant for highly educated group.

The net effect of education on the chance of using modern contraceptives can be measured through the last model. It depicts the most important result that there is no significant effect of educational level as such to affect the response variable once the other socio-economic and demographic variables are controlled. In this model, all other variables which were significant for uneducated women have retained their significance with reduced extent of effect in most of the cases but women's education has no significant influence on the probability of using modern contraceptives. Therefore, it can be said that the anomaly in the relationship between women's education and modern contraceptive use is not as mysterious as expected. It is only a gross effect and there is no significant net effect of women's education to influence modern use of contraception.

Discussion

From above analysis, it is found that the anomalous relationship between women's education and modern contraceptive use has been retained in the various categories of selected socio-economic and demographic variables. But it has been distorted in some of the categories and reversed in some others. Therefore, the findings suggest possibility of some other reasons responsible for bringing this anomalous association. Female sterilization is the mostly used modern method among Nepali women, especially by uneducated women with its 35 per cent share in total modern use of all women, whereas 46 per cent share for uneducated women.[11] Therefore, as indicated in the Nepal DHS (2011) report, it can be, to some extent, due to a high proportion of uneducated women having gone for sterilization, which is due to programme effect where government tries its best to capture those women who are less likely to get the service by themselves and they will be ultimately the women of lowest socio-economic strata and hence the least educated.

Also, the pregnancy losses are relatively higher for educated women (10+ education: 9.8%) with respect to their uneducated counterparts (No education: 4%).[11] A national facility-based abortion study has found that among the clients seeking comprehensive abortion service, 30 per cent had never been to school, 29 per cent had primary or lower secondary education and 41 per cent had secondary or higher education.[15] Therefore, higher proportion of pregnancy loss for educated women can be attributed to the increased share of induced abortion. Chances cannot be ruled out that more educated women are using abortion as a substitute for contraceptives.

Similarly, use of traditional methods among women with no education is 4.3 per cent, whereas the same for women with 10+ educations is 14.2 per cent.[11] This variation in the users of traditional methods helps to widen the gap of users of modern method and this can be a part of the answer to explain the anomalous relationship. This issue should be further studied by analysing all the methods with special focus on female sterilization, by taking more variables like age at first use and number and sex composition of living children at first use.

The results of logistic regression show that the net effects of other socio-economic variables under this study are relatively stronger for uneducated women and less educated women as compared to highly educated women. Moreover, the net effect of education on modern contraceptive use is insignificant after controlling for other socio-economic variables. This indicates that the relationship between women's education and modern contraceptive use is not really anomalous, but observed so, as combined effect of all socio-economic variables including programme effect. It is concluded that, there is not a straightforward positive relationship between women's education and modern contraceptive use in Nepal.

Conclusion

The relationship of women's education and modern contraceptive use is not straightforward. The net effects of other socio-economic variables under this study are relatively stronger for uneducated women and less educated women as compared to highly educated women, showing that socio-economic variables affect differently among women of different educational status to influence their current use of modern contraceptives. The net effect of women's education on modern contraceptive use is not significant after controlling for other socio-economic and demographic variables. Moreover, there are chances of effect of family planning and other programmes to shape relationship between education and contraceptive use in Nepal.

Notes

1. Parasuraman, S., Roy, T.K., Radha Devi, D., Paswan, B., Arokiasamy, P. and Unisa, S. 1999. Summary and Conclusions. In, *Role of Women's Education in Shaping Fertility in India: Evidences from National Family Health Survey*, Mumbai: Himalaya Publishing House, pp. 126–136.
2. Jejeebhoy, S. 1994. Women's Education, Fertility and the Proximate Determinants of Fertility. Paper Presented at the International Conference on Population and Development (ICPD), Expert Group Meeting on Population and Women, Botswana.
3. Jain, A.K. 1981. The Effect of Female Education on Fertility: A Simple Explanation. *Demography*, 18: 577–595.
4. Shabana, S. and Martin, B. 2005. Women's Autonomy, Education and Contraception Use in Pakistan: A National Study. *Reproductive Health*, 2: 8 (accessed online from http://www.reproductive-health-journal.com/content/2/1/8 on 2 November 2012).
5. Gordon, C., Sabates, R., Bond, R. and Wubshet, T. 2011. Women's Education and Modern Contraceptive Use in Ethiopia. *International Journal of Education*, 3: 1–23 (accessed online from www.macrothink.org/ije on 2 November 2012).
6. Bongaarts, J. 2010. The Causes of Educational Differences in Fertility in Sub-Saharan Africa. Poverty, Gender and Youth Working Paper No. 20, New York: The Population Council.

7. Bertrand, J.T., Mangani, N., Mansilu, M. and Landry, E.G. 1985. Factors Influencing the Use of Traditional Versus Modern Family Planning Methods in Bas Zaire. *Studies in Family Planning*, 16: 332–341.
8. Oni, G.A. 1985. Effects of Women's Education on Postpartum Practices and Fertility in Urban Nigeria. *Studies in Family Planning*, 16: 321–331.
9. Soomro, G.Y. and Mahmood, N. 2005. Female Education and Fertility: Implications for Family Planning Programme. Paper Presented at the 20th Annual General Meeting and Conference, Pakistan Society of Development Economists Programme, January 10–12.
10. MOHP. 2011. *Nepal Population Report 2011*. Kathmandu, Nepal: Ministry of Health and Population, Population Division.
11. MOHP, New ERA and ICF International Inc. 2012. *Nepal Demographic and Health Survey 2011*. Kathmandu, Nepal: Ministry of Health and Population, New ERA and ICF International Inc.
12. MOHP, New ERA and Macro International Inc. 2007. *Nepal Demographic and Health Survey 2006*. Kathmandu, Nepal: Ministry of Health and Population, New ERA and Macro International Inc.
13. IIPS and Macro International. 2007. *National Family Health Survey (NFHS–3), 2005–06: India*, Volume I, Mumbai: International Institute for Population Sciences (IIPS).
14. Parasuraman, S., Roy, T.K., Radha Devi, D., Paswan, B., Arokiasamy, P. and Unisa, S. 1999a. Education and Fertility Regulation. In, *Role of Women's Education in Shaping Fertility in India: Evidences from National Family Health Survey*, Mumbai: Himalaya Publishing House, pp. 90–109.
15. MOHP and CREHPA. 2006. *Nepal Comprehensive Abortion Care (CAC): National Facility-Based Abortion Study 2006*. Kathmandu, Nepal: Ministry of Health and Population (MOHP), Centre for Research on Environment Health and Population Activities (CREHPA).

Section IV

Population Dynamics and Environment

17

Nexus Between Population Growth, Economic Growth and Poverty Reduction and Its Implications on Sustainable Development in India

M. Soundha Rajan and C. Satheesh Kumar

Poverty reduction and human development have been the major constituents of each Five-Year Plans. Though most of the developed countries achieved higher human development index through rapid economic growth coupled with its stabled growth of population, India has been struggling to achieve higher economic growth rate and stabilizing its population since independence. India, which started introducing major economic reforms in the early 1990s, has experienced GDP growth rates of around 8 per cent and 9 per cent[1] in recent years, far above the growth rates of Western industrialized nations like the USA or European Union member states[2] but it is still facing the challenges in controlling the growth of population. While higher economic growth considerably reduced the percentage of population living in Below Poverty Line (BPL) over the last two decades, India is still home to the largest percentage of people living in BPL. Currently, the poverty eradication is one of the essential components of the sustainable development. This paper aims to analyse the nexus between the population growth, economic growth and poverty reduction and its implication on sustainable development in the Indian states. The following hypothesis has been tested in this study. That is, 'in order to arrest increase in poverty, the economy must grow at rates in excess of population growth rates'.[3]

Review of Literature

This section details the existing literature in the field of population growth, economic development, poverty and sustainable development. On 11 May 2000

India became the world's second demographic billionaire. If current trends continue, India may overtake China in 2045 to become the most populous country in the world.[4] Two-thirds of India's population growth in the 20th century took place after 1971.[5] Given the rather poor state of the Indian economy and the very low level of living standards for most of its population, this fact puts a great strain on the government's efforts to promote social development.[5] Population growth (positive or negative) is caused exclusively by the operation of fertility, mortality and migration.[6]

Problems of the Population Growth

The rate of population growth is not only a demographic phenomenon; it also has a broad impact on the society and people's lives. For instance, researchers have found relationships between population growth and economic growth.[7, 8, 9] In a relatively short period of time, an increase in fertility tends to have a negative effect on the economy, while in the long run the opposite relationship is true.[7] Population growth can also lead to a rising demand for food. Problems of instability in food production are particularly difficult for some developing countries with high population growth rate and low technological changes in agriculture.[10] Furthermore, a high rate of population growth is likely to increase population density in certain geographic areas, particularly urban settings. As a result overcrowding, unemployment, and poverty are likely to lead to social problems in some localities.[11]

Population Growth and Poverty Reduction

Population growth has a substantial impact on any country's economic performance. For example, the declining fertility rates in the industrialized nations may lead to labour shortages and put strain on their pension systems. On the other hand, the rapidly expanding population in the developing nations has been viewed as a potential impediment to their socio-economic development, which prompted some countries (e.g. China, Singapore) to introduce policies aimed at decreasing the fertility rates.[12]

There is still no consensus whether population growth is beneficial or detrimental to the economic performance of a developing nation. The relationship between the upward demographic trend and economic growth has been described as 'a complex one, and the historical evidence is ambiguous, particularly concerning what is cause and what is effect'.[13] During the past few decades, rapid population growth has been accompanied by an unparalleled decline in mortality rates and by an increase in income per capita in India and China.[14] Whether population growth is good or bad for a country's sustained per capita income growth, depends on that country's human capital and technology levels.[15]

With the level of development not being uniform across the country, the reduction in poverty is expectedly unevenly distributed. In the rural areas, in terms of the percentage point decline in the Head Count Ratio (HCR), a significant decline was observed in the states of Orissa (Odisha), Jharkhand,

Uttranchal, Madhya Pradesh, Gujarat, Maharashtra and Tamil Nadu. In the low-income states of Bihar, Jharkhand, Odisha and Rajasthan, a significant decline is observed in the urban HCR (Although rural poverty has declined in Odisha and Jharkhand, the fall in urban poverty estimates is more). It is quite plausible that the immediate benefits of high growth in these low-income states were mostly felt in the urban areas.[16]

The steps in the argument used to support the propagation of population control policies can be reduced to mainly three. First, rapid growth of population means the spread of poverty and is a main obstacle to economic growth in poor countries, reducing or cancelling potential improvements in living standards, and aggravating such conditions as poor health, malnutrition, illiteracy and unemployment. Second, the political implications of such trends threaten government stability in developing countries and encourage the confrontation between developed and developing countries. Finally, the rapid growth of population pushes future generations to scarcity and an unsustainable environment carrying capacity.[17]

Economic Growth and Poverty Reduction

Government spending can have direct and indirect effects on poverty. The direct effects are the benefits the poor receive from expenditures on employment programmes. The indirect effects arise when government investments in rural infrastructure, agricultural research, and the health and education of rural people stimulate agricultural and non-agricultural growth, leading to greater employment and income-earning opportunities for the poor and to cheaper food.[18] Thus, to increase the government spending on welfare programmes, it needs to mobilize enough resources, which ultimately comes from the performance of the economy of any given state. By increasing the Gross State Domestic Product (GSDP) rate, the states can mobilize more resources and fund the poverty reduction programmes. Growth is the only sure way of providing a permanent solution to the poverty problem and increasing the overall welfare of rural people.[18]

Economic Growth and Human Development

The literature on the relationship between Economic Growth and Human Development is quite rich, indicating that the causality might work in both directions. In other words, while the process of high growth might facilitate the augmentation of Human Development in a country, the latter also contributes positively towards ensuring the former.[19]

The cross-country relationship between Per Capita GDP {in purchasing power parity (PPP) USD} and the HDI (Human Development Index) score (obtained from UNDP, 2009) shows that from the cross-country perspective (for 144 countries), as the per capita income increases, the HDI score increased up to a level beyond which it reaches a plateau. The result indicates that in a multi-country framework, the per capita income is necessarily an ingredient for achieving a higher level of HDI.[19]

The National Human Development Report (NHDR), 2001, brought out by the Planning Commission of India, is worth mentioning in this regard. While the report ranked Kerala, Punjab and Tamil Nadu as the toppers, Bihar, Madhya Pradesh and Uttar Pradesh were placed at the other extreme on the HD scale.[20]

Population Growth, Economic Growth and Sustainable Development

Due to the consequences of economic growth on the environment and society, the United Nations (UN) in 1987 created the World Commission on Environment and Development (WCED), also known as the Brundtland Commission. The objective of that commission was to study the sustainability of economic development, spreading the definition of sustainable development as 'development that meets the needs of the present generations without compromising the ability of the future generations to meet their own needs'.[21] More recently, the United Nations, 2005 World Summit stated the three mutually and interdependent reinforcing pillars of sustainable development: economic development, social development and environmental protection.[22]

The United Nations (UN) and other organizations such as Bretton Woods have taken an active role in defining 'sustainable development'. By attaching a specific interpretation, they have made population control the overriding approach to development. An illustration of such policy-making is the recent 'Five-year review and appraisal of implementation' of the International Conference on Population and Development (ICPD) Programme of Action (ICPD+5). As will be seen, such population policies have become the primary tool used to 'promote' economic development in developing countries and to protect the environment. However, these policies have failed to achieve either goals.[17]

The idea of achieving the maximum level of economic growth compatible with environmental care, so that future generations could have equal opportunities to achieve economic growth and well-being, has been linked also with sustainability and GDP.[23] Economic growth and social sustainability must be combined with environmental sustainability in order to guarantee a better future for next generations.[24]

Objective

The main objective is to study the nexus between economic growth, population growth and poverty reduction and impacts of these components on the sustainable development in India.

Methodology

The secondary data of the post-liberalization of the Indian economy between the years of 1994–95 and 2003–04 on population growth, Gross State Domestic Product (GSDP) and population living under the Below Poverty Line (BPL) of different states have been compiled to test the hypothesis. The states that have the population of more than one crore in Census 2011 were chosen and then they were ranked, based on the percentage of BPL population for the year 2009–10. From this, the top five and lowest five of the BPL states have been selected for the analysis. The states that have highest BPL population are Uttar Pradesh, Bihar, Chattisgarh, Jharkhand, and Assam. Tamil Nadu, Kerala, New Delhi, Punjab and

Jammu and Kashmir are coming under the lowest BPL population states. These two categories have been selected to find out the linkage between population growth and economic growth. Microsoft Excel software was used for the analysis.

Results and Discussion

Figures 1 and 2 presents the population growth of the states having high and low BPL population. Both figures show the increase in the growth of the population. The mean growth rate of the population in the states that have highest BPL population is higher (1.019%) than the states that have lowest BPL population (1.004%). Bihar and Uttar Pradesh posted the highest population growth of 1.02 per cent compared to the other states such as Chattisgarh, Jharkhand and Assam that posted the 1.01 per cent. Although Chattisgarh, Jharkhand and Assam stabilized their population growth, the GSDP growth rate in these states were highly unstable and mean GSDP rate is comparatively lower than Bihar and Uttar Pradesh.

Figure 1 *Population Growth of the States Having High BPL Population*

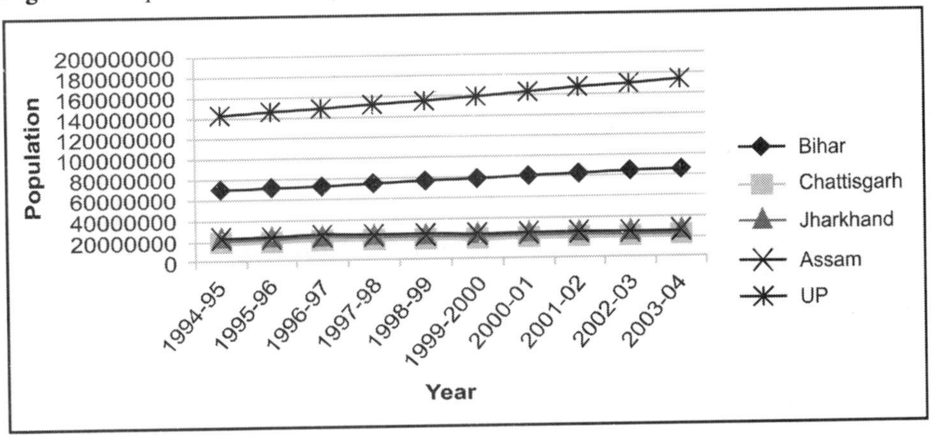

Source: compiled from www.indiastat.com

Figure 2 *Population Growth of the States Having Low BPL Population*

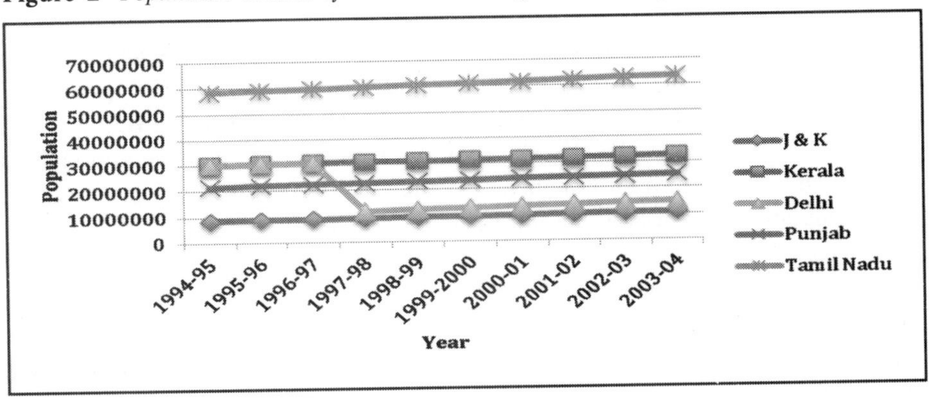

Source: compiled from www.indiastat.com

Figure 3 *GSDP Growth Rate of the States Having High BPL Population*

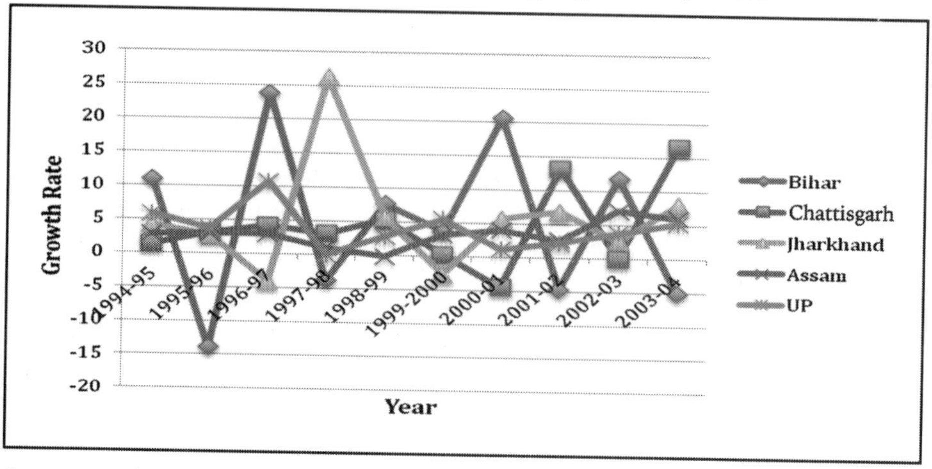

Source: compiled from www.indiastat.com

Figure 4 *GSDP Growth Rate of the States Having Low BPL Population*

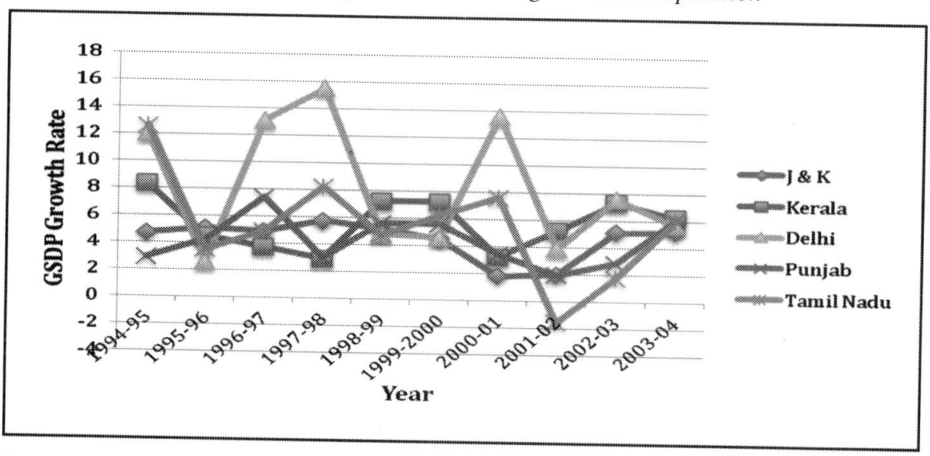

Source: compiled from www.indiastat.com

In the lowest BPL population category, Delhi recorded the lowest mean population growth rate of 0.958 per cent and posted highest GSDP growth of 8.33 per cent. Except Tamil Nadu that recorded negative GSDP growth (–1.56%) in the year 2001–02, all other states posted the positive and stabled growth rate in the decade. For instance, the GSDP growth rate in the highest BPL population category is highly unstable and recorded negative growth in many years. This stabled economic growth is major reason for sustained reduction of poverty in the lowest BPL population category. Conversely, high unstable economic growth is the reason for lack of poverty reduction in the highest BPL population category states despite stabilization of the population in some states.

Mean population growth rate of states having highest BPL population = 1.02%
Mean population growth rate of states having lowest BPL population = 1.00%
Mean GSDP growth rate of states having highest BPL population = 4.43%
Mean GSDP growth rate of states having lowest BPL population = 5.60%

In both the categories, the economic growth is higher than the population growth. But the economic growth is substantially higher and stable in the low BPL population category. The following data gives evidence to this. The mean GSDP growth rate of lowest and highest BPL population category is 5.6 per cent and 4.43 per cent respectively. The mean population growth rate is 1.019 per cent and 1.004 per cent in highest and lowest BPL population categories respectively. From the above result, it is inferred that those states, which have consistently higher rate of economic growth coupled with lower growth rate of population considerably reduced the poverty level. The human development index of those states is also prominently higher than the other states. Thus, for sustaining the development and poverty reduction, it is important to ensure that population growth is lower than the economic growth of the states.

Conclusion

Since the growth of population concerns with socio-economic development issues, strict measures should be taken to improve the quality of existing population.[25] It is also necessary to stabilize and reduce the rate of population growth and having stable economic growth. Because, this study shows that unstable economic growth is one of the major reasons for lack of poverty reduction in high BPL population category states. So, there is need to increase the government spending on the welfare programmes. It is possible only if the state government improves its economic growth by adopting suitable policies.

Notes

1. Homlong, N. and Springler, E. 2009. *Markteintritt in Indien*. Vienna: LexisNexis.
2. Springler, E. 2010. Economic Development and Foreign Direct Investment: How to Create Sustainable Development: An Analysis of the Potential for Sustainable Development on the Indian Subcontinent. *Panoeconomicus*, 3: 333–347.
3. Development EaSCfAatP. 2004. *Integrating Economic and Environmental Policies: The Case of Pacific Island Countries*. New York: United Nations Publications.
4. Government of India. 2000. *National Population Policy*. New Delhi: Ministry of Health and Family Welfare.
5. Aspalter, C. 2002. Population Policy in India. *International Journal of Sociology and Social Policy*, 22 (11): 48–72.
6. Hinde, A. 1998. *Demographic Methods*. New York: Oxford University Press.
7. Barlow, R. 1994. Population Growth and Economic Growth: Some More Correlations. *Population and Development Review*, 20: 153–165.
8. Blanchet, D. 1992. *Reversal of the Effects of Population Growth on Economic Growth Since the End of the 1970s: Reality or Artefact?* United Nations: Department of Economic and Social Affairs, Population Division.

9. Coale, A.J. 1986. Population Trends and Economic Development. In J. Menken (ed.), *World Population and the US Policy: The Choices Ahead*, New York: W.W. Norton.
10. Mellor, J.W. 1982. The World Development: Food, Employment, and Growth Interactions. *American Journal of Agricultural Economics*, 64: 304–311.
11. Sibly, R.M. and Hone, J. 2002. Population Growth Rate and its Determinants: An Overview. *Philosophical Transactions: Biological Sciences*, 357: 1153–1170.
12. Furuoka, F. and Munir, Q. 2010. Is Population Growth Beneficial or Detrimental to Economic Development? A New Evidence from Pakistan. *Journal of Population and Social Studies*, 18 (2): 25–38.
13. Thirlwall, P.A. 1994. *Growth and Development*. London: Macmillan Press.
14. Bloom, D.E. 2011. Population Dynamics in India and Implications for Economic Growth. PGDA Working Paper No. 65.
15. Liddle, B. 2001. The Population-Development Nexus: Insights from a Multi-Country Simulation Model. 2nd Workshop on Population and the Environment: Modelling and Simulating This Complex Interaction, Rostock, Germany: Planck Institute for Demographic Research.
16. Shukla, R., Bakshi, I. and Baruah, P. 2011. Trends in Poverty and Inequality: An Analysis of the High Growth Period in India. *Indian Journal of Human Development*, 5 (2).
17. Aguirre, M.S. 2002. Sustainable Development: Why the Focus on Population? *International Journal of Social Economics*, 29 (12): 923–945.
18. Fan, S., Hazell, P. and Thorat, S. 2000. Government Spending, Growth and Poverty in Rural India. *American Journal of Agricultural Economics*, 82 (4): 1038–1051.
19. Mukherjee, S. and Chakraborty, D. 2011. Is There Any Interdependence between Economic Growth and Human Development? Evidence from Indian States. *Indian Journal of Human Development*, 5 (2): 467–494.
20. Government of India. 2001. *National Human Development Report*. New Delhi: Planning Commission.
21. World Commission on Environment and Development. 1987. *From One Earth to One World: An Overview*. Oxford: Oxford University Press.
22. United Nations. 2005. *World Summit Outcome*. New York: United Nations.
23. United Nations. 2010. *Summit on the Millennium Development Goals*. New York: United Nations.
24. Aguado, R. and Martinez, J. 2012. GDP and Beyond: Towards New Measures of Sustainability Based on Catholic Social Thought. *Asia-Pacific Journal of Business Administration*, 4 (2): 124–138.
25. Singha, K. 2011. Does Population Growth Matter in Bhutan's Economic Development? *International Journal of Economics*, 5 (2): 155–165.

18

Population Dynamics and Environmental Degradation in India

H.C. Srivastava and Palani Murugesan

Environmental degradation is becoming an increasing ominous threat to the well-being of India's population and excessive population growth is the primary cause of the environmental degradation. Population growth increases the need to produce consumer products and this need, in turn, intensifies the trend to overexploit and misuse environmental resources. Efforts to control population growth with contraceptive technology, the expansion of family planning services and the control of environmental deterioration via management will meet with little success. A prerequisite for controlling these dual problems is the improvement of living for the masses.[1]

There are many environmental issues in India. Air pollution, water pollution, garbage and pollution of the natural environment are all challenges for the country. The situation was worse between 1947 through 1995, according to data collection and environment assessment studies of World Bank experts; between 1995 through 2010, India has made one of the fastest progresses in the world in addressing its environmental issues and improving its environmental qualities. Still, India has a long way to go to reach environmental quality similar to those enjoyed in developed economies. Pollution remains a major challenge and opportunity for India.[2] Some believe that economic development is causing the environmental issues. Others believe economic development is key to improving India's environmental management and prevailing pollution in India. It is also suggested that India's growing population is the primary cause of India's environmental degradation. Systematic studies challenge this theory. Empirical evidence from countries such as Japan, England and Singapore, each with population density similar to or higher than India, yet enjoying environmental quality vastly superior than India, suggests population density may not be the only factor affecting India's issues.[3]

Major environmental issues are forest and agricultural degradation of land, resources depletion (water, mineral, forest, sand, rocks), environmental degradation, public health, loss of biodiversity, loss of resilience in ecosystems, livelihood security for the poor.[4] Besides, water supply and sanitation issues are related to many environmental issues in the country. Also, the environmental issues are one of the primary causes of diseases, health issues and long-term livelihood impact for the country. In addition, some of the major issues associated with environmental degradation that India faces today are air pollution, poor management of waste, growing water scarcity, falling groundwater table, water pollution, preservation and quality of forests, biodiversity loss and land/soil degradation.[5]

There is a long history of study and debate about the interactions between population growth and the environment. According to the British thinker Malthus, for example, a growing population exerts pressure on agricultural land, causing environmental degradation, and forcing the cultivation of land of poorer and poorer quality. This environmental degradation ultimately reduces agricultural yields and food availability, causes famine, disease and death, thereby reducing the rate of population growth.[6]

Objective of the Paper

The paper aims to review levels and trends in population dynamics and its linkages with the selected issues of environmental degradation in the country. In addition, attempt has been made to throw light on changing scenario of land-use pattern and degradation namely; agricultural land, settlement pattern, population below poverty line, availability of infrastructure facilities and their association with environmental degradation in the country.

Source of Data

The necessary data and information for the paper has been compiled on the above-mentioned aspects namely; levels and trends of population growth, density, proportion of increasing urban population, infant mortality rates, expectation of life at birth over a period of time, changing land-use pattern, changing forest cover in the country, availability of drinking water as well as infrastructure facility in households, from different census reports as well as from the Sample registration system reports produced by the Registrar General of India, Compendium of Environment Statistics, India, India State Forest Survey Report and Statistical Abstract, India. In addition relevant information available through internet, pertaining to the desired area of investigation, has also been used.

Population Density in the States of India

Density of population is defined as the number of persons per square kilometre. It is an important index of population which shows concentration of population in a particular area. As per the provisional population totals of Census–2011 the population density of India has gone up to 382 persons per square kilometre from 325 persons per square kilometre in 2001.[7]

The population density of India from 1901 to 2011 is shown in Table 1. As evident from the Table in the beginning of the 20th century, i.e. 1901 the density of population in India was as low as 77 per cent per square kilometre. However, over the decades the density steadily increased and soon after the independence of the country it reached 117 persons per sq km in 1951; subsequently it rose to 325 persons per sq km according to the Census of 2001, and it has reached 382 persons per square kilometre in the latest Census of 2011. This constitutes 17.5 per cent increase over 2001.

Table 1 *Density of Population, India: 1901–2011*

Census Year	*Density (per sq km)*	*Absolute Increase*	*% age Increase*
1	2	3	4
1901	77		
1911	82	5	6.5
1921	81	–1	–1.2
1931	90	9	11.1
1941	103	13	14.4
1951	117	14	13.6
1961	142	25	21.4
1971	177*	35	24.6
1981	216**	39	22
1991	267**	51	23.6
2001	325**	58	21.7
2011	382**	57	17.5

Source: Census of India 2011, Provisional Population Totals.

Note: * While working out the density of India, Jammu & Kashmir has been excluded as comparable figures of area and population are not available for that state.
** The density has been worked out on comparable data.

Further, Table 2 provides ranking among the states by density of population for the decade 2001–2011. The lowest density was observed in both the Censuses 2001 and 2011 for Arunachal Pradesh, 13 and 17 people per square kilometre respectively.

While considering density of population amongst the states during the decades 2001 and 2011 it was observed that West Bengal with density of 903 persons and 1,029 persons per square kilometre for the year 2001 and 2011 respectively occupied the first rank followed by Bihar(881 persons per square kilometre for 2001 and 1,102 persons for 2011). It is interesting to note that both the states Bihar and West Bengal have interchanged their places during the two consecutive Census of 2001 and 2011. Kerala and Uttar Pradesh have retained their ranks of third and fourth respectively, in both the censuses. Interestingly, Himachal Pradesh dropped by one rank, Nagaland dropped by four ranks, Some of the states having low population density are Arunachal Pradesh, Mizoram, Sikkim, Jammu & Kashmir, and Manipur (Table 2).

Table 2 *Ranking of States of India by Density: 2001 and 2011*

Rank in 2011	*States*	*Density (per sq km)*		*Rank in 2001*
		2011	*2001*	
1	*2*	*3*	*4*	*5*
	INDIA	382	325	
1	Bihar	1,102	881	2
2	West Bengal	1,029	903	1
3	Kerala	859	819	3
4	Uttar Pradesh	828	690	4
5	Haryana	573	478	7
6	Tamil Nadu	555	480	6
7	Punjab	550	484	5
8	Jharkhand	414	338	10
9	Assam	397	340	9
10	Goa	394	364	8
11	Maharashtra	365	315	11
12	Tripura	350	305	12
13	Karnataka	319	276	14
14	Andhra Pradesh	308	272	13
15	Gujarat	308	258	15
16	Orissa (Odisha)	269	236	16
17	Madhya Pradesh	236	196	17
18	Rajasthan	201	165	18
19	Uttarakhand	189	159	19
20	Chhattisgarh	189	154	20
21	Meghalaya	132	103	23
22	Jammu & Kashmir	124	100	25
23	Himachal Pradesh	123	109	22
24	Manipur	122	103	24
25	Nagaland	119	120	21
26	Sikkim	86	76	26
27	Mizoram	52	42	27
28	Arunachal Pradesh	17	13	28

Source: Census of India 2001 and 2011.

Table 3 *Poverty Lines and Poverty Head Count Ratio for 2004–05 Using Tendulkar Methodology*

S.N.	*State*	*Poverty line(₹)*		*Poverty head count Ratio(%)*		*Total*
		Rural	*Urban*	*Rural*	*Urban*	
1	Andhra Pradesh	433.43	563.16	32.3	23.4	29.9
2	Arunachal Pradesh	547.14	618.45	33.6	23.5	31.1
3	Assam	478	600.03	36.4	21.8	34.4
4	Bihar	433.43	526.18	55.7	43.7	54.4
5	Chhattisgarh	398.92	513.7	55.1	28.4	49.4
6	Delhi	541.39	642.47	15.6	12.9	13.1
7	Goa	608.76	671.15	28.1	22.2	25
8	Gujarat	501.58	659.18	39.1	20.1	31.8
9	Haryana	529.42	626.41	24.8	22.4	24.1
10	Himachal Pradesh	520.4	605.74	25	4.6	22.9
11	Jammu & Kashmir	522.3	602.89	14.1	10.4	13.2
12	Jharkhand	404.79	531.35	51.6	23.8	45.3
13	Karnataka	417.84	588.06	37.5	25.9	33.4
14	Kerala	537.31	584.7	20.2	18.4	19.7
15	Madhya Pradesh	408.41	532.26	53.6	35.1	48.6
16	Maharashtra	484.89	631.85	47.9	25.6	38.1
17	Manipur	578.11	641.13	39.3	34.5	38
18	Meghalaya	503.32	745.73	14	24.7	16.1
19	Mizoram	639.27	699.75	23	7.9	15.3
20	Nagaland	687.3	782.93	10	4.3	9
21	Orissa (Odisha)	407.78	497.31	60.8	37.6	57.2
22	Pondicherry (Puducherry)	385.45	506.17	22.9	9.9	14.1
23	Punjab	543.51	642.51	22.1	18.7	20.9
24	Rajasthan	478	568.15	35.8	29.7	34.4
25	Sikkim	531.5	741.68	31.8	2.9	31.1
26	Tamil Nadu	441.69	559.77	37.5	19.7	28.9
27	Tripura	450.49	555.79	44.5	22.5	40.6
28	Uttar Pradesh	435.14	532.12	42.7	34.1	40.9
29	Uttarakhand	486.24	602.39	35.1	26.2	32.7
30	West Bengal	445.38	572.51	38.2	24.4	34.3
	All India	446.68	578.8	41.8	25.7	37.2

Source: Press note on Poverty Estimates Govt of India Planning Commission January 2011. Planning Commission – Press_pov_27Jan11.pdf
http://planningcommission.nic.in/reports/genrep/Press_pov_27Jan11.pdf

Land Degradation

'Land is degraded when it suffers a loss of intrinsic qualities, decline in its capabilities or loss in its productive capacity. Land degradation may be due to natural causes or human causes or it may be a combination of both. Soil erosion is the major cause of land degradation.[8] Table 4 presents land-use pattern in India for the period from 1950–51 to 2006–07, i.e. for a period of more than

Table 4 *Land Use Patterns in India from 1950–51 to 2006–07*

Unit (Million Hectare)[2]

Classification	*1950–51*	*1960–61*	*1970–71*	*1980–81*	*1990–91*	*2000–01*	*2006–07(P)*
I. Geographical area	328.7	328.7	328.7	328.7	328.73	328.73	328.73
II. Reporting area for land utilization statistics(1 to 5)	284.32	298.46	303.76	304.15	304.86	305.17	305.51
1. Forests	40.48	54.05	63.91	67.47	67.81	69.53	69.81
2. Not available for cultivation(a+b)	47.52	50.75	44.64	39.62	40.48	41.62	42.63
(a) Non-agricultural uses	9.36	14.84	16.48	19.66	21.09	23.86	25.19
(b) Barren and unculturable land	38.16	35.91	28.16	19.96	19.39	17.76	17.44
3. Other uncultivated land (excluding fallow land) (a+b+c)	49.45	37.64	35.06	32.31	30.22	27.7	27.05
(a) Permanent pasture and other grazing land	6.68	13.97	13.26	11.97	11.4	10.66	10.36
(b) Land under miscellaneous tree crops and groves not included in net area sown	19.83	4.46	4.3	3.6	3.82	3.43	3.45
(c) Culturable wasteland	22.94	19.21	17.5	16.74	15	13.61	13.24
4. Fallow land (a+b)	28.12	22.82	19.88	24.75	23.36	25.08	25.72
(a) Fallow land other than current fallows	17.44	11.18	8.76	9.92	9.66	10.1	10.48
(b) Current fallows	10.68	11.64	11.12	14.83	13.7	14.77	15.24
5. Net area sown	118.75	13.2	140.27	140	143	141.4	140.3
6. Gross cropped area	131.39	152.77	165.79	172.63	185.74	185.37	193.72
7. Area sown more than once	13.14	19.57	25.52	32.63	42.74	43.97	53.72
8. Cropping intensity	110.1	114.7	118.2	123.3	129.9	131.1	138.1
III. Net irrigated area	20.85	24.66	31.1	38.72	48.02	55.08	60.86
IV. Gross irrigated area	22.56	27.98	38.2	49.28	63.2	75.97	85.78

Source: Agricultural Statistics at a Glance, 2008. Directorate of Economic and Statistics, Ministry of Agriculture, cf compendium of Environment Statistics, India 2008/2009 (Tenth Issue), Central Statistics office, Govt. of India, Ministry of Statistics and programme implementation.

five decades, the data suggests that out of geographical area of the country 328.73 million hectare, only 305.51 million hectare as per 2006–07 year, is reporting area for land utilization statistics while the rest being non-administrative for various reasons.

Further, the land being utilized for non-agricultural uses has shown systematic increase form 1950–51(9.36) to 2006–07(25.19) million hectare. Likewise baron and uncultivable land shown declined from 38.16 million hectare for 1950–51 to 17.34 million hectare during 2006–07. The area sown has shown the increasing trend from 1950–51(118.75 million hectare) to 1970–71(140.27 million hectare) however, it did not show appreciable increase in 2006–07 as during this period the corresponding figure for the same area was 140.30 million hectare. Therefore, this trend requires adequate measures for further land reclamation.

Land Degradation Scenario of India

The land serves as storage for water and nutrients required for plants and other living micro- and macro- organisms. The demand for food, energy and other human requirements depends upon the preservation and improvement of productivity of land. India has about 18 per cent of world's population, 15 per cent of live-stock population to be supported from only 2 per cent of geographical area and 1.5 per cent forest and pasture lands. The increasing human and animal population has reduced the availability of land over the decades. The per capita availability of land has declined from 0.89 hectare in 1951 to 0.37 hectare in 1991 and is projected to slide down to 0.20 hectare in 2035. This decline in per capita land availability in the country is mostly on account of rising population.

The information on the extent of soil degradation in the country has been assessed by various agencies. The estimates of these agencies vary widely i.e. 63.9 m.ha. to 187.0 m.ha. due to different approaches in defining the degraded soil and adopting various criteria for delineation. The main agencies that have estimated soil degradation are: National Commission on Agriculture (NCA 1976), Society for Promotion of Wastelands Development (SPWD, 1984), National Remote Sensing Agency (NRSA, 1985), Ministry of Agriculture 1985 and National Bureau of Soil Survey and Land Use Planning (NBSSLUP, 1984 and 2005).

The problems of land degradation are prevalent in many forms throughout the country. In most cases, a combination of such problem exists. According to National Bureau of Soil Survey and Land Use Planning (NBSS and LUB) of Nagpur and Indian Council of Agricultural Research (ICAR) has published that 146.82 million hectare area is reported to be suffering from various kinds of land degradation. It includes water erosion 93.68 million hectare, wind erosion 9.48 million hectare, waterlogging/flooding 14.30 million hectare, salinity/alkalinity 5.94 million hectare, and soil acidity 16.04 million hectare and complex problems 4.3 million hectare.[9]

The state-wise details of extent of various kind of land degradation are presented in Table 5. It is evident from the table that with regard to the degraded

Table 5 *State-Wise Extent of Various Kinds of Land Degradation in India*

(As per NBSS&LUP-ICAR–2005 on the Scale of 1:250000)

(Area in thousand hectares)

Name of the States	*Water Erosion*	*Wind Erosion*	*Water-logging*	*Salinity Alkalinity*	*Soil Acidity*	*Complex Problem*	*Degraded Area*	*Geographical Area*	*Degraded Area (%)*
Andhra Pradesh	11,518	0	1,896	517	905	156	14,992	27,505	54.5
Arunachal Pradesh	2,372	0	176	0	1,955	0	4,503	8,374	53.8
Assam	688	0	37	0	612	876	2,213	7,844	28.2
Bihar+Jharkhand	3,024	0	2,001	229	1,029	0	62,83	17,387	36.1
Goa	60	0		76	0	2	24	162	370
Gujarat	5,207	443	523	294	0	1,666	8,133	19,602	41.5
Haryana	315	536	146	256	0	214	1,467	4,421	33.2
Himachal Pradesh	2,718	0	1,303	0	157	0	4,178	5,567	75
Jammu & Kashmir	5,460	1,360	200	0	0	0	7,020	22,224	31.6
Karnataka	5,810	0	941	110	58	712	7,631	19,179	39.8
Kerala	76	0	2,098	0	138	296	2,608	3,886	67.1
Madhya Pradesh + Chattisgarh	17,883	0	359	46	6,796	1,126	26,210	44,345	59.1
Maharashtra	11,179	0	0	1,056	517	303	13,055	30,771	42.4
Manipur	133	0	111	0	481	227	952	2,233	42.6
Mizoram	137	0	0	0	1,050	694	1,881	2,108	89.2
Meghalaya	137	0	7	0	1,030	34	108	2,243	53.9
Nagaland	390	0	0	0	127	478	995	1,658	60

Cont'd...

...Cont'd

Orrisa	5,028	0	681	75	263	75	612	15,571	39.3
Punjab	372	282	338	288	0	0	1,280	5,036	25.4
Rajasthan	3,137	6,650	53	1,418	0	110	11,368	34,224	33.2
Sikkim	158	0	0	0	76	0	234	710	33
Tamil Nadu	4,926	0	96	96	78	138	5,334	13,006	41
Tripura	121	0	191	0	203	113	628	1,049	59.9
Uttar Pradesh + Uttarakhand	11,392	212	2,350	1,370	0	0	15,324	29,441	52
West Bengal	1,197	0	710	170	556	119	2,752	8,875	31

Source: There are several estimates for the extent of degraded lands reported by various agencies in the country. These estimates vary largely due to activation in approaches and methodologies of estimation. In absence of comprehensive and periodic scientific surveys, the figures reported by National Bureau of Soil Survey and Land Use Planning, Nagpur based on studies and several estimates (2005) for various land degradation have been considered as logically concluded and are being used for various purpose.

cf - http://www.agrcoop.nic.in/nrm/statrm.pdt-MicrosoftInternetExplorer.

areas among the states and union territories is concerned there are drastic variations. State of Madhya Pradesh has shown the highest degraded area 26,210 thousand hectares followed by for combined Uttar Pradesh and Uttarakhand (15,324 thousand hectares), whereas in case of Delhi the corresponding figure is only 82 followed by Goa with 162 thousand hectares respectively. Also, while comparing percentage of degraded areas one may find that State of Meghalaya has shown highest percentage (89.2), on the contrary in case of Punjab it has shown the lowest corresponding figure of only 25.4 per cent. In brief, it may be stated that there exists wide variation among different states and union territories within the country as far as various kinds of land degradations are concerned. With regard to the extent of various kinds of land degradation in country as a whole was concerned, the table reveals that the existing levels of degradation were found as water erosion (93.48 m.ha), wind erosion (9.48 m.ha), water logging/flooding (14.3 m.ha), salinity/alkalinity (5.94 m.ha), soil acidity (16.04 m.ha) and complex problems (7.38 m.ha).

Comparative Situation of Forest Cover in India

The comparative situation of forest cover in India for the period 1999 to 2007 for the states and union territories has been depicted in Table 6. The table insinuates that a significant decrease in the forest cover is reported from the states of Andhra Pradesh, Arunachal Pradesh, Assam, Chandigarh, Nagaland and Tripura, whereas the states of Jharḳhand, Manipur, Meghalaya, Mizoram and Odisha have shown increase in forest cover. It may be emphasized that maximum increase in this regard has been noticed in case of Mizoram (640 sq km), followed by Manipur (328 sq km) and Jharkhand(172 sq km) and so on.

Human Settlements

The root cause of environmental degradation in India may be attributed to rapid growth of population. India has approximately 18 per cent of the world's population, whereas only 2 per cent of the geographical area. Human development is also adversely affected by the environmental degradation. Two of the environmental indicators viz., access to the safe drinking water and sanitation are closely linked with two of the very important human development indicators namely, infant mortality rate and life expectancy. Polluted air and poor hygienic conditions in settlements contribute to reduction in life expectancy and increase in infant mortality. Life expectancy in India is still on very low ebb, and infant mortality rate is much more than desired. The poor, therefore, take fertility decisions to compensate for all those factors and avoid risks. The expectation of life at birth of females which was lower than that of males till 1980 has shown an upward trend during the decade 1981–90 and thereafter the combined expectation of life at birth in the country during 1901–11 was only 22.9 years, showing continuous increase over the decades and reached 63.4 years during 2002–06 . Larger population leads to more poverty, worsens the environment and create various cycles.[10]

Table 6 *Comparative Situation of Forest Cover in India (sq km)*

States/Uts	*Assessment*					*Change in*			
	2007	*2005**	*2003*	*2001*	*1999*	*2001*	*2003*	*2005*	*2007#*
2	*3*	*4*	*5*	*6*	*7*	*8*	*9*	*10*	*11*
Andhra Pradesh	45,102	45,231	44,412	43,195	44,229	–1,034	1,217	819	–129
Arunachal Pradesh	67,353	67,472	67,692	69,760	68,847	913	2,068	–220	–119
Assam	27,692	27,758	27,735	25,290	23,688	1,602	2,445	23	–66
Bihar	6,804	6,807	5,573	5,375	4,830	545	198	1,234	–3
Chattisgarh	55,870	55,929	55,992	57,730	56,693	1,037	1,738	–63	–59
Delhi	177	177	174	125	88	37	49	3	0
Goa	2,151	2,156	2,164	1,565	1,251	314	599	–8	–5
Gujarat	14,620	14,604	14,814	12,913	12,965	–52	1,901	–210	16
Haryana	1,594	1,604	1,576	1,135	964	171	441	28	–10
Himachal Pradesh	14,668	14,666	14,359	12,907	13,082	–175	1,452	307	2
Jammu & Kashmir	22,686	22,689	21,273	19,886	20,441	–555	1,387	1,416	–3
Jharkhand	22,894	22,722	22,569	22,531	21,644	887	38	153	172
Karnataka	36,190	36,200	35,246	33,296	32,467	829	1,950	954	–10
Kerala	17,324	17,284	15,595	13,417	10,323	3,094	2,178	1,689	40
Madhya Pradesh	77,700	77,739	76,145	75,282	75,137	145	863	1,594	–39
Maharashtra	50,650	50,661	47,514	45,040	46,672	16,32	2,474	3,147	–11
Manipur	17,280	16,952	17,259	17,889	17,384	505	–630	–307	328
Meghalaya	17,321	17,205	16,925	16,535	15,633	902	390	280	116

Cont'd...

...Cont'd

Mizoram	19,240	18,600	18,583	16,397	18,338	1,941	2,186	17	640
Nagaland	13,464	13,665	14,015	13,980	14,164	–184	35	–350	–201
Orissa (Odisha)	48,855	48,755	48,353	49,044	47,033	2,011	–691	402	100
Punjab	1,664	1,660	1,545	1,628	1,412	216	–83	115	4
Rajasthan	16,036	16,012	15,821	14,542	13,871	671	1,279	191	24
Sikkim	3,357	3,357	3,262	3,164	3,118	46	98	95	0
Tamil Nadu	23,338	23,314	23,003	20,992	17,078	3,914	2,011	311	24
Tripura	8,073	8,173	8,123	8,869	5,745	3,124	–746	50	–100
West Bengal	12,994	12,970	12,389	10,392	8,362	2,030	1,997	581	24

Source: India State of Forest Report, 2009

* Revised

The change in the above table refers to change in the area with respect to revised assessment for 2005.

Slum Population

A total of 42.6 million people living in 8.2 million households have been enumerated in slums of 640 cities/towns spread across 26 states and union territories in 2001 Census. The slum population constitutes 4 per cent of the total population of the country, whereas the slum dwellers in the country constitutes nearly a seventh of the total urban population of the states and union territories. About 17.7 million population lives in the cities with population above one million, which is 41.6 per cent of the total slum population in the country. In absolute numbers, Greater Mumbai has highest slum population of around 6.5 million followed by Delhi, 1.9 million and Kolkata, 1.5 million. The slum areas of Surat, Hyderabad, Chennai and Nagpur have more than half a million population each.

Solid Waste and Hazardous Material

Due to rapid growth of urbanization in the country there is a substantial increase in the generation of solid waste in both absolute and per capita terms. Surveys have been conducted to assess solid waste generation, collection, treatment and disposal of 291 class I cities and 345 class II cities. It has been indicated that very little amount of waste generated is treated. The problems may be seen with regard to its management, collection, handling, transportation and disposal.

When this solid waste is not collected and disposed off efficiently and effectively, it attracts rodents and flies which spread diseases. It also pollutes and degrades land and water resources. If these wastes are untreated it would ferment slowly and produce biogas which could be distributed in the atmosphere. The biogas contains 65–70 per cent Methane gas which is a green-house gas, has a global warming potential 34 times more than that of carbon dioxide. Therefore, development of suitable technologies for utilization of waste is essential to minimize adverse health and environment consequences.[11]

Summary and Conclusion

In view of the interpretation of data and discussion presented above, it may be stated that present high rate of growth of population of the country continues to be a matter of concern, as it has many foul effects associated with degradation of the environment namely; change in land use pattern, considerable increase in non-agricultural land, rise in fallow land, steep decrease in area under tree crop and groves. Besides, area under non-agricultural use have grown fast at the cost of agricultural land.

Despite prevailing National Forest Policy in the country it appears that forests have been neglected in planning and adequate measures are required for their protection. Agencies working to manage them are poorly funded; consequently forests are subjected to overexploitation, encroachments, illegal felling and so on, leading to their degradation. To check forest degradation and to fulfil the need of the people dependant on forest, rehabilitation of degraded forests and afforestation of waste land, forest management through involvement of local communities are the strategies that need to be taken up.

Human development is also adversely affected by environmental degradation and in this regard, access of safe drinking water and sanitation are closely linked with the two important human development indicators namely; infant mortality rate and expectation of life at birth. Further, polluted air and poor hygienic condition in settlements seems to be directly associated with the same, therefore, efforts need to be made to improve the prevailing conditions of the human settlements by providing basic needs.

Another area of concern for degradation of environment could be attributed to rapid growth of urbanization which poses variety of problems, including environmental degradation in the country. In order to check the prevailing high rate of growth of urbanization it would be pertinent to provide necessary infrastructure in the cities and towns to cater for the needs of the people.

Apart from developing infrastructure in cities and towns, it is also important that alternative employment is generated in villages itself to control urbanization. This measure may help in avoiding formation of slum settlements in the cities. Consequently, it would ensure a more even development, as well as better quality of life in both rural and urban areas.

Besides, lack of adequate measures for management of solid waste in relation to its collection, handling, transportation and disposal results in formation of biogas which pollutes the environment and causes various health hazards. Therefore, there is a need for development of suitable technologies for utilization of waste to minimize adverse health and environmental consequences.

In addition to the above measures, some action points may be suggested to protect or improve the environment: (1) Observe World Population Day on 5th June and sincerely pledge to take some remedial measures beneficial for improvement of the environment. (2) Plant trees, they will help to absorb excess carbon dioxide. (3) Do not burn any waste, especially plastic, for the smoke may contain polluting gases. (4) Dispose the waste after separating them into biodegradable and non-biodegradable waste material. (5) Never put any leftover chemicals, used oils down the drain, toilet or dump them on the ground or in water or burn them in the garden. If you do so, it will cause pollution. (6) Avoid fast starts and sudden braking of automobiles. (7) Send your waste oil, old batteries and used tyres to a garage for recycling or safe disposal; all these can cause serious pollution, and (8) Use public transport whenever you can, or form a car pool for everyday travel.

To sum up, in order to check environmental degradation various speedy measures are required to be taken up in the country and some amongst them could be checking the prevailing high rate of growth of the population, educating people about harmful consequences of environmental degradation through different communication strategies, In this regard, youth may be encouraged to extend their help and support in educating the people about serious consequences of environmental degradation and its effects on living condition and well-being of the people.

Efforts need to be made to generate more resources and innovative models for improving economic status of the people and for controlling various types of environmental degradations in the country. Public-private partnership may be enhanced for the improvement in deteriorating situation of environment in the country. The most important measure we need is political will at national and state levels, congenial political and economic environment to use appropriate measures to mitigate the issues related to environment degradation in larger interest of the individual in particular and society in general.

Notes

1. Mitra, A. 1984. Rising Population and Environmental Degradation. *Yojana*, October 1–15, 28 (18): 4–8.
2. Environment Assessment, Country Data India. http://data. worldbank.org/country/india
3. The World Bank. 2011. http://worldbank.org/country/india
4. Urdal, Henrik. 2005. People vs. Malthus: Population Pressure, Environmental Degradation and Armed Conflict Revisited. *Journal of Peace Research*, July, 42 (4): 417–434.
5. Chandrappa, R. and Ravi, D.R. 2009. *Environmental Issues, Law and Technology: An Indian Perspective*. Delhi: Research India Publication.
6. European External Action Services. 2007. *India: Country Strategy Paper, 2007-13*. European Union. http://eeas.europa.eu/india/csp/07_13_en.pdf
7. Registrar General and Census Commissioner of India. 2011. Census of India 2011, Provisional Population Totals, New Delhi.
8. Central Statistical Office. 2008/2009. Government of India, Ministry of Statistics and Programme Implementation, New Delhi: Compendium of Environment Statistics India (Tenth Issue), p. 137 and pp. 221–222.
9. http://www.agricoop.nic.in/nrm/statnrm.pdf-microsoftinter net explorer
10. Government of India. 2006. Ministry of Environment and Forests: National Environment Policy.
11. Central Statistical Organization. 2004. Ministry of Statistics and Programme Implementation, Government of India, New Delhi, Statistical Abstract, India.

19

Fuel Consumption and Kitchen Environment in Female Headed Households

An Analysis from Census 2011

Avijit Mistri and Nasrin Banu

Around 1.5 million excess deaths per annum occurred globally due to exposer of smoke by the combustion of solid fuel (ISEE, 2005). Exposure levels are usually much higher among women especially of childbearing age and children up to five years. Even at the period of pregnancy, women usually are attached to the domestic and cooking work, hence the developing foetus is indirectly exposed that causes stillbirth and low birth weight (LBW). Mavalankar et al. (1991) first highlighted the significant association between biofuel use and stillbirth in the Indian context.

Later on, Mishra et al. (2005)[1] strongly argued that those Indian women (15–49 years) who cooked only with biomass fuels were twice as likely to have experienced two or more stillbirths as those who cooked with clean fuels. Study from developing countries, especially in rural Guatemala (Boy et al., 2002), Zimbabwe (Mishra et al., 2004), Southern Pakistan (Siddiqui et al., 2008) and India (TERI and AIIMS joint research, 2011)[2] revealed an association between LBW and the use of biomass fuels in open fire for cooking. TERI and AIIMS joint research team (2011) reported that nearly 82 per cent of pregnant women are exposed to biomass related indoor air pollution in India and approximately 12 to 28 per cent of low birth weight babies being exposed to the same. Cooking with solid fuel more than doubles the risk of acute lower respiratory infection (ALRI) mortality among children under five (Rehfuess et.al., 1979). Along with this, there have been significant correlation with kitchen location, fuel quality and room ventilation (Rehfuess et al., 1979). In India, approximately .05 to .08 million post-neonatal deaths (24 to 39%) in a year caused by acute respiratory infection (ARI) are attributed by indoor air pollution (TERI and AIIMS, 2011).

Around half of the world's population (3.0 billion) still depend on solid fuels for everyday energy needs, of which 2.4 billion on biomass (wood, animal dung, crop wastes) and 0.6 billion on coal (ISEE, 2005). In India 70 per cent households use unclean fuel and near about one-third of households have no separate kitchen inside the room as per the Census 2011. Firewood, crop residue and cow dung cake are the major source of energy need. These fuels are typically used inside the houses or in partly enclosed cooking areas, burnt in poorly vented, inefficient stoves and leading to very high levels of exposure to smoke which contains products of incomplete combustion. In this context, the present study is an attempt to investigate the trend and pattern of the fuel consumption and kitchen environment of Indian households. The whole study is based on Census of India, 2001 and 2011 data sources with bit of help taken from District Level Health Survey, 2007–08 (DLHS–3) data sets. This study basically examines some prime elements of the kitchen environment of households such as use of fuels, availability of different kinds of kitchen and building material of kitchen stock and so on and so forth. It also tries to explain the inter-censual changes (2001 to 2011) and regional pattern of the same. Besides, this study focuses on the condition of female headed households as compared to male headed households in terms of the kitchen environment. It is an important issue in gender studies, especially on the grounds of women empowerment in the context of contemporary India. In traditional Indian societies, aged person in a household is considered as a head of the household. They highly influence the household decision making. Census 2011, for the first time reported that a substantial proportion of households in India are headed by females (11%) and expects faster growth in the near future indicating women empowerment in the so-called patriarchal Indian society. Two facts strongly argue in support of that. Firstly, the robust growth of the elderly population[3] (aged 60 and above) is becoming a major concern in India during last two decades (1991 to 2001). The size of the elderly population has been increasing at a faster rate[4] where the female share is not only higher than male but growth also surpasses the male population. Secondly, female life expectancy at birth (70.0 year) is higher than male (67.1 years) and it has also been increasing in trend (in 2002–06, SRS, 2008). As a result, India will get more females as drivers of households in the near future. In this situation, what would be the social structure, what kind of social institutions would exist and what changes would come into a household are the matters of future gender study. For this kind of gender study there is need for obtaining proper data sets on regular basis. Census, 2011 first time separately provides gender information, especially of women headed households. The present study tries to provide some insight into that.

Since 1960, Census of India began to collect the household information, especially the quality and quantity of housing stocks in the country (Kundu, 2011). With the growing demand, its scope had been broadened and basic amenities as well as assets possessed by the households were gradually brought under the ambit of house listing and housing census. In the Census 1991, the question related to type of fuel used for cooking by the households was first time canvassed to assess the impact of fuel consumption pattern on the environment and forest resources.[5] In next Census 2001, another question related to availability of separate kitchen within the house was added to intensively investigate the indoor environment of households. Recent Census 2011, provides a wide range of household information collected by standardized schedule where schedule of Census 2001 was considered as reference one (Kundu, 2011). Use of fuel, availability of kitchen, material of kitchen stock and other kitchen related information is included within basic amenities of house listing and housing census.

Research Techniques

Cross tabulation, cartographic methods, arithmetic growth rate and some descriptive statistics are used to analyse the data sets. Apart from these, the kitchen environment index is constructed with the help of range equalization (normalization) technique. Negative aspects of the kitchen are chosen to make the index, hence higher the score indicates the more worsened condition of the kitchen and vice versa for the good condition of that.

Discussion

Fuel Used for Cooking

Since 1991, Census of India has provided nine types of fuel use such as firewood, crop residue, cow dung cake, coal/lignite/charcoal, kerosene, Liquefied Petroleum Gas (LPG)/Piped Natural Gas (PNG), electricity, biogas and any other on a uniform basis. Around 70 per cent households in India used unclean fuel in 2011, though it has substantially declined from previous Census 2001 (Table 1). This fall is highly predominant in urban areas compared to rural. Near about 87 per cent rural households use unclean fuel, whereas only 34 per cent urban households use it. The rural urban gap is 53 per cent. Unclean fuel use is more or less same between male and female headed households but rural to urban difference is also high.

In India, firewood is the major source of kindling. Near about 49 per cent households use it meanwhile crop residue, cow dung cake, kerosene and coal/lignite/charcoal were used by households 8.9, 7.9, 2.9 and 1.4 per cent respectively in 2011. These fuel usages have declined in 2011 from the previous census (Table 2). In female headed households (FHHHs), use of firewood (52.2%) is higher than male headed households (MHHHs) (48.6%). Basically patriarchal society in India, females in a household are engaged in collecting firewood from their neighbourhood which is considered as a part of their domestic work. This practice is highly pronounced where the female is the head of the household. Besides, income of the households is also a crucial factor for use of fuel. Head of the household always tries to save their income in her own fashion that may be in the form of using cheap and ubiquitous fuel such as firewood for cooking, which are easily available in rural India. Hence, the tendency of firewood use is comparatively higher among FHHHs. One important thing is noticed especially in urban areas, that FHHHs use substantially higher proportion (41%) of unclean fuel compared to MHHHs (33%), where firewood use also plays a significant role to make the distinction between them.

On the other hand, only 29 per cent households used clean fuel in 2011 and it is highly predominant in urban India (66%). Here rural-urban difference is also high. LPG/PNG (29%) is second highest fuel consumption after firewood

Table 1 *Fuel Used (Percentage) for Cooking by the Household*

	2011			*2001*			*MHHHs 2011*			*FHHHs 2011*		
	Total	*Rural*	*Urban*	*Total*	*Rural*	*Urban*	*Total*	*Rural*	*Urban*	*Total*	*Rural*	*Urban*
Unclean fuel*	70.1	87.2	33.6	80.9	92.7	50.6	70.1	87.3	32.7	70.6	86.6	40.9
Clean fuel**	29.0	11.9	65.5	18.1	6.3	48.6	29.1	11.8	66.6	28.6	12.4	58.4
Any other	0.5	0.6	0.2	0.6	0.8	0.2	0.5	0.6	0.2	0.5	0.6	0.2
No cooking	0.3	0.2	0.5	0.3	0.2	0.6	0.3	0.2	0.5	0.3	0.2	0.5
	100.0	100.0	100.0	100.0	100.0	100.0	100.0	100.0	100.0	100.0	100.0	100.0

Source: Census of India, 2001 and 2011; * Unclean fuel includes firewood, crop residue, cow dung cake, coal/lignite/charcoal and kerosene. ** Clean fuel includes LPG/PNG, electricity and biogas.

Table 2 *Different Kinds of Clean and Unclean Fuel Used for Cooking by the Households*

		2011			*2001*			*MHHHs 2011*			*FHHHs 2011*		
		Total	*Rural*	*Urban*	*Total*	*Rural*	*Urban*	*Total*	*Rural*	*Urban*	*Total*	*Rural*	*Urban*
Unclean fuel	Firewood	49.0	62.5	20.1	52.5	64.1	22.7	48.6	62.1	19.3	52.2	66.3	26.3
	Crop residue	8.9	12.3	1.4	10.0	13.1	2.1	9.1	12.6	1.4	7.2	10.3	1.4
	Cow dung cake	7.9	10.9	1.7	9.8	12.8	2.0	8.2	11.2	1.7	6.0	8.5	1.5
	Coal, Lignite, Charcoal	1.4	0.8	2.9	2.0	1.1	4.6	1.4	0.8	2.9	1.5	0.7	3.1
	Kerosene	2.9	0.7	7.5	6.5	1.6	19.2	2.8	0.7	7.4	3.5	0.9	8.5
Clean fuel	LPG/PNG	28.5	11.4	65.0	17.5	5.7	48.0	28.6	11.3	66.0	28.1	12.0	57.9
	Electricity	0.1	0.1	0.1	0.2	0.1	0.3	0.1	0.1	0.2	0.1	0.1	0.1
	Biogas	0.4	0.4	0.4	0.4	0.5	0.4	0.4	0.4	0.4	0.3	0.3	0.4
	Any other	0.5	0.6	0.2	0.6	0.8	0.2	0.5	0.6	0.2	0.5	0.6	0.2
No cooking		0.3	0.2	0.5	0.3	0.2	0.6	0.3	0.2	0.5	0.4	0.3	0.5

Source: Census of India, 2001 and 2011.

(49%) in 2011. LPG/PNG consumption not only has increased among the other fuel consumption but also made rapid stride, that is a 11 per cent point change and growth is 11 per cent per annum between 2001 and 2011. Other clean fuel consumption is very minimal and changes are negligible. It is found that there is more or less the same proportion of households that use LPG/PNG in MHHHs as well as in FHHHs.

It has already been mentioned that, on an average, 70 per cent households use unclean fuel in the country. Whole of Central States, Eastern States and North-Eastern States barring Mizoram, Manipur and Sikkim and including one Western State namely, Rajasthan altogether make a strip extend from West to East where more than 70 per cent households use unclean fuel (Figure 1). Firewood, crop residue and cow dung cake are highly used here. These usages are widely varied, region to region and highly depend on residential communities in these regions. In North-Eastern States, 66.07 per cent of its geographical areas are covered by forest in comparison to the national average of 21.05 per cent (Forest Survey of India, 2011). Besides, most of the households belong to Scheduled Tribes community whose economy and socio-cultural practice are woven around the forest from the historical past (ibid.). In the Gangatic plain like Uttar Pradesh, Bihar and West Bengal, the use of crop residue and cow dung cake are comparatively higher. On the other hand in Chhattisgarh, Odisha, Jharkhand,

Figure 1 *India: Use of Unclean Fuel by the HHs Census, 2011*

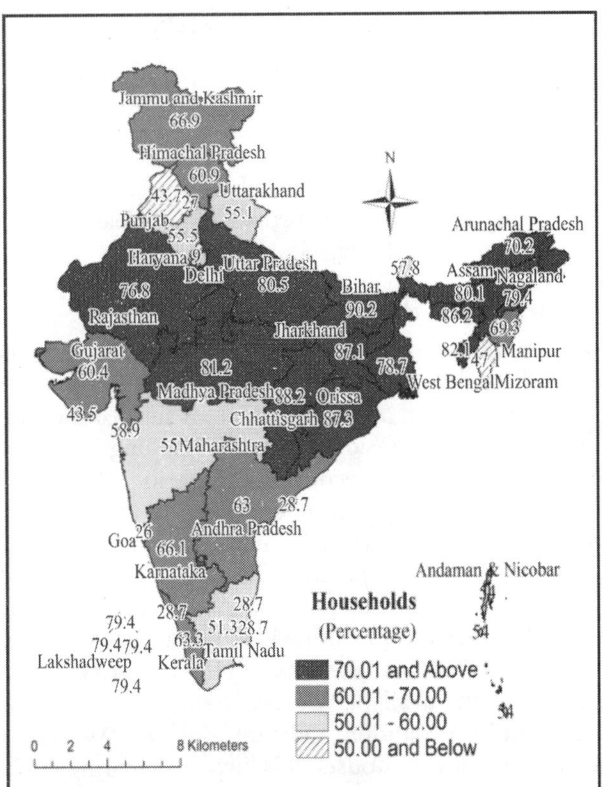

Figure 2 *India: Use of Clean Fuel by the HHs Census, 2011*

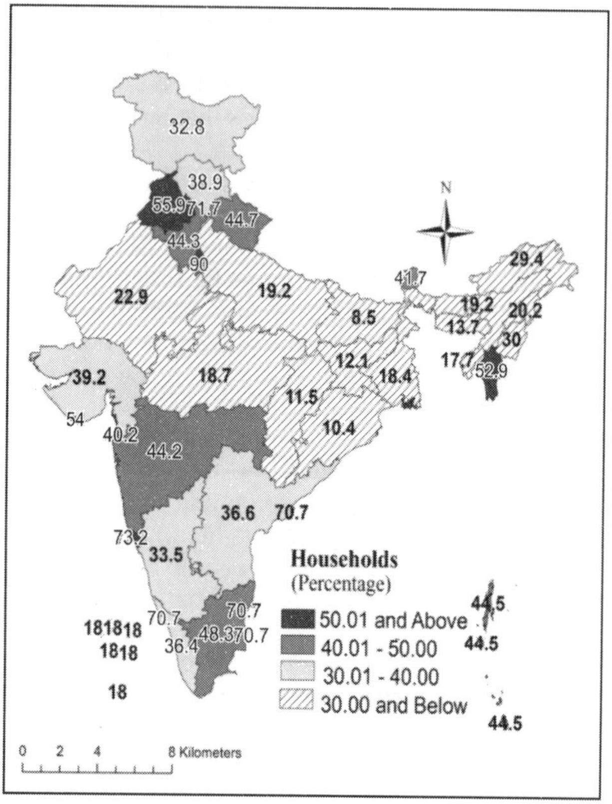

Madhya Pradesh and Rajasthan, the use of firewood is comparatively higher where a substantial proportion of geographical areas are under forest cover[6] and Scheduled Tribe[7] people also reside. The proportion of clean fuel use is comparatively higher in South and North Indian States (Figure 2).

Availability of Kitchen Facility

Near about 61 per cent households had separate kitchen inside the house in 2011 which has declined (three per cent point) from previous Census 2001 (Table 3). This fall is mainly found in rural areas. Urban areas have shown slightly positive achievement of separate kitchens inside the house. Cooking in open space has also declined both in urban and rural areas during this period. But, near about 32 per cent households do not have separate kitchen inside the house as yet. It has increased by eight per cent point to 2011 from 2001 which is mainly concentrated in rural areas; growth 12 per cent point at the rate of 7.6 per cent per annum. FHHHs (63%) use a slightly higher proportion of separate kitchen inside the house compared to MHHHs (61%) meanwhile, not available of separate kitchen among MHHHs (32%) is slightly higher than FHHHs (29%).

Regional pattern of the availability of kitchen reveals that in the whole of Central and Eastern India (excluding Odisha) and one Western State namely Rajasthan, more than 30 per cent households have no separate kitchen inside the

Table 3 *Availability of Separate Kitchen (Percentage) Within the House*

	2011			*2001*			*MHHHs 2011*			*FHHHs 2011*		
	Total	*Rural*	*Urban*	*Total*	*Rural*	*Urban*	*Total*	*Rural*	*Urban*	*Total*	*Rural*	*Urban*
Available	61.3	52.8	79.4	64.0	59.4	76.0	61.0	52.5	79.6	63.3	55.1	78.3
Not available	31.5	37.9	18.0	23.9	26.1	18.0	31.9	38.3	17.9	28.7	34.1	18.7
Cooking in open	6.8	9.1	2.0	11.8	14.2	5.5	6.7	9.0	2.0	7.6	10.4	2.5
No cooking	0.3	0.2	0.5	0.3	0.2	0.6	0.3	0.2	0.5	0.4	0.3	0.5
Total	100.0	100.0	100.0	100.0	100.0	100.0	100.0	100.0	100.0	100.0	100.0	100.0

Source: Census of India, 2001 and 2011.

Figure 3 *HHs Having No Separate Kitchen Inside the House Census, 2011*

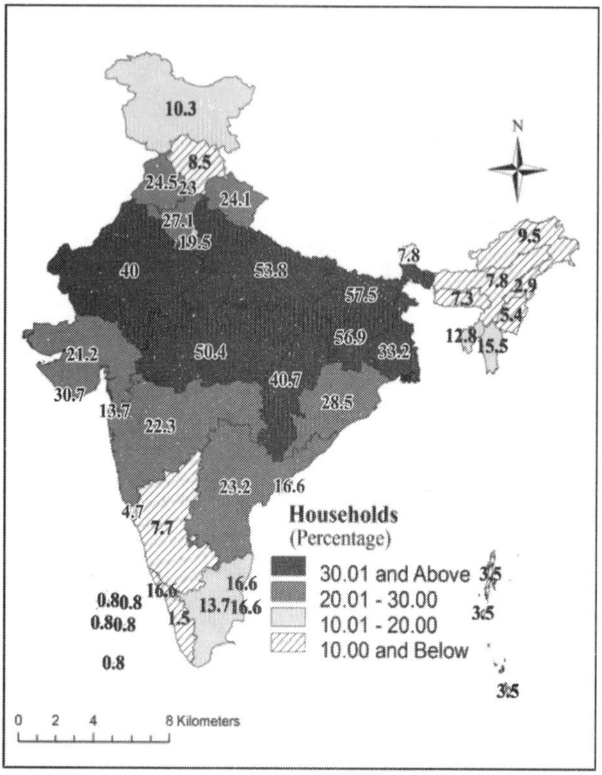

house for cooking (Figure 3). Meanwhile more than 80 per cent households in the whole of North-Eastern States, two Southern States namely Karnataka and Kerala and two Northern States namely Jammu and Kashmir and Himachal Pradesh have separate kitchen inside the house for cooking (Figure 4). Besides, in the states along the Eastern Coastal regions, namely Odisha, Andhra Pradesh and Tamil Nadu and two states in plain areas, Bihar and Rajasthan, more than eight per cent households cook in open (Figure 5). Among them Andhra Pradesh (22%) strides far ahead from the rest of them.

Actually, use of different kinds of kitchen is highly influenced by climatic, demographic, geographical factors as well as economic factors of that region. In North-Eastern States due to high rainfall over the year (average 100–200 cm), attack of poisonous insects from extensive vegetation cover and higher rate of urbanization[8] in 2011, use of separate kitchen by the households are comparatively higher. On the other hand, in Central and Eastern States, most of the people are marginal farmers (Agricultural Census, 2005–06).[9] Somehow they manage within their limited amount of land. Somewhere population density[10] is so high that cooking in open is not possible. Very high incidence of poverty is also found in these regions. On an average 41.03 per cent people in the Central States (Uttar Pradesh, Madhya Pradesh and Chhattisgarh) and 39.03 per cent people in the Eastern States (West Bengal, Bihar, Jharkhand, and Odisha) belong to Below Poverty Line (BPL), whereas all-India average is 29.8 per cent (Planning

Figure 4 *India: HHs Having Separate Kitchen Inside the House Census, 2011*

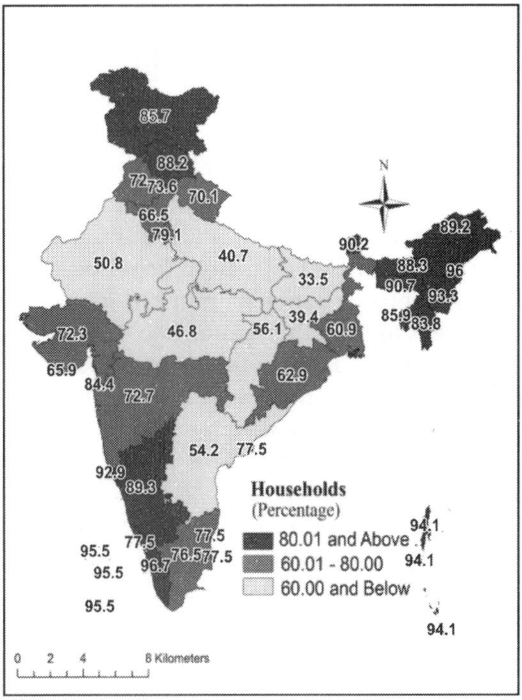

Figure 5 *India: Cooking in Open Census, 2011*

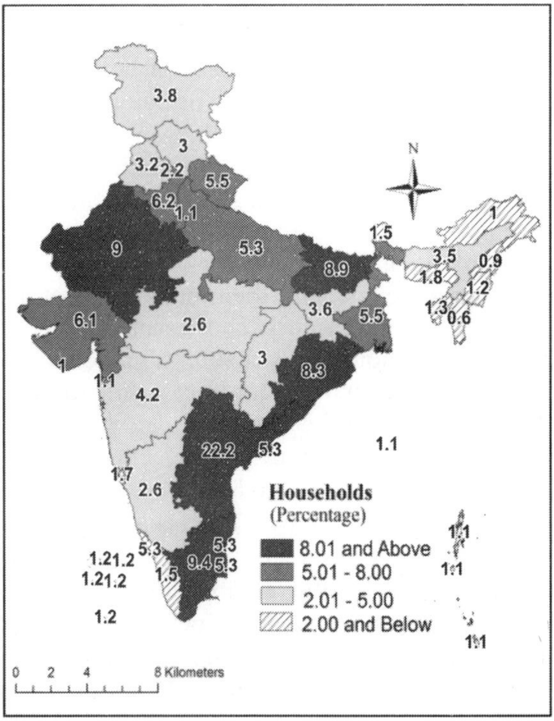

Commission, 2012). Besides, climate also plays a significant role, some places with bright sunshine all through the year, others where rainfall and sunshine both are severe. As a result, they obligate to cook inside the house but use of separate kitchen within the house is very low. In case of Eastern coastal states, pleasant weather and availability of firewood induce the households to cook in the open.

Availability of Kitchen by Type of Fuel Used for Cooking

Near about 57 per cent and 42 per cent households used unclean and clean fuel in separate kitchens respectively in 2011 (Table 4). These are more or less equally shared by MHHHS and FHHHs. Both firewood (43%) and LPG/PNG (42%) in near about same proportionately are used for cooking in the separate kitchens inside the house. On the other hand, one harmful practice is observed that near about 91 per cent Indian households use unclean fuel for cooking in non-separate kitchens inside the house. Here also, more than half of the households (57%) use firewood for cooking followed by crop residue (14%), cow dung cake (14%) and LPG/PNG (9 %). This practice is more or less same in MHHHs and FHHHs. Along with it, use of unclean fuel is higher in open cooking (94%) and use of firewood (69%), crop residue (14%) and cow dung cake (eight %) are also predominant one.

Building Material of Kitchen Stock

The building material of kitchen stock is an important factor for kitchen environment. Cooking by unclean fuel in kutcha[11] (temporary) kitchen or semi-pucca (semi-permanent) is not as harmful as cooking in pucca[12] (permanent) kitchen because the materials of kutcha kitchen or semi-pucca kitchen's walls and roof can easily suck the heat and smoke out. On the other hand, if Pucca kitchen has no proper exhaust, Carbon dioxide (CO_2), Carbon monoxide (CO) and other harmful particles of smoke make the environment inside the kitchen toxic. It causes lots of health hazards.

Census of India as well as District Level Health Survey does not provide data related to building material of kitchen stocks as such. But it is assumed that those households which have pucca or semi-pucca or kutcha housing stock, their kitchen would be of the same type. In case of households cooking inside the house but do not have separate kitchens, their building material of housing stock and that of kitchen stock would obviously be the same because one part of their house is used for cooking. Though this assumption would not be always true because those households which have pucca houses sometimes construct kutcha kitchen by extending some part of their house.

However, now in India, near about 62 per cent households live in pucca houses followed by semi-pucca (25%) and kutcha (12%) in the Census 2011. These are more or less equally shared by MHHHs and FHHHs.[13] According to DLHS–3, more than half of households having pucca houses (56.0%) used clean fuel in 2007–08 (Table 5). But a substantial proportion of households having pucca houses (43.5%) used unclean fuel for cooking in this period. In rural areas, the tendency of unclean fuel use in pucca houses is higher than clean fuel use and it is vice versa for urban areas. Moreover, most of the Indian

Table 4 *Availability of Kitchen by Type of Fuel Used for Cooking, 2011*

	Availability of separate kitchen inside the house			*Not-availability of separate kitchen inside the house*			*Cooking in open*		
	Total	*MHHHs*	*FHHHs*	*Total*	*MHHHs*	*FHHHs*	*Total*	*MHHHs*	*FHHHs*
Unclean fuel	57.4	57.1	59.5	90.6	90.6	89.7	93.5	93.5	94.0
Clean fuel	42.3	42.5	40.2	8.8	8.7	9.5	5.5	5.6	5.1
Any other	0.3	0.3	0.3	0.7	0.7	0.8	0.7	1.0	0.9
No cooking	0.0	0.0	0.0	0.0	0.0	0.0	0.0	0.0	0.0
Total	100.0	100.0	100.0	100.0	100.0	100.0	99.7	100.0	100.0

Source: Census of India, 2011.

households use unclean fuel both in semi-pucca (83%) and kutcha (96%) houses. This practice is highly pronounced in rural areas compared to urban. Regional pattern of unclean fuel use in pucca houses portrays that Northern, Central, Western and Eastern Indian states use higher proportion of the same as compared to Southern and North-Eastern States (Figure 6).

Table 5 *Use of Fuel by Different Kitchen Stocks, 2007–08*

	Pucca (permanent)			*Semi-pucca (semi-permanent)*			*Kutcha (temporary)*		
	Total	*Rural*	*Urban*	*Total*	*Rural*	*Urban*	*Total*	*Rural*	*Urban*
Clean fuel	56.2	24.9	77.4	16.7	7.8	40.3	3.6	1.7	17.8
Unclean fuel	43.5	74.9	22.3	82.8	91.8	59.1	96.1	98.0	81.8
Other	0.3	0.2	0.3	0.4	0.3	0.7	0.3	0.3	0.5
Total	100.0	100.0	100.0	100.0	100.0	100.0	100.0	100.0	100.0

Source: Districts Level Health Survey (DLHS–3). *Note – all figures are unweighted cases.*

Figure 6 *India: Unclean Fuel Use in Pucca Houses, DLHS–3*

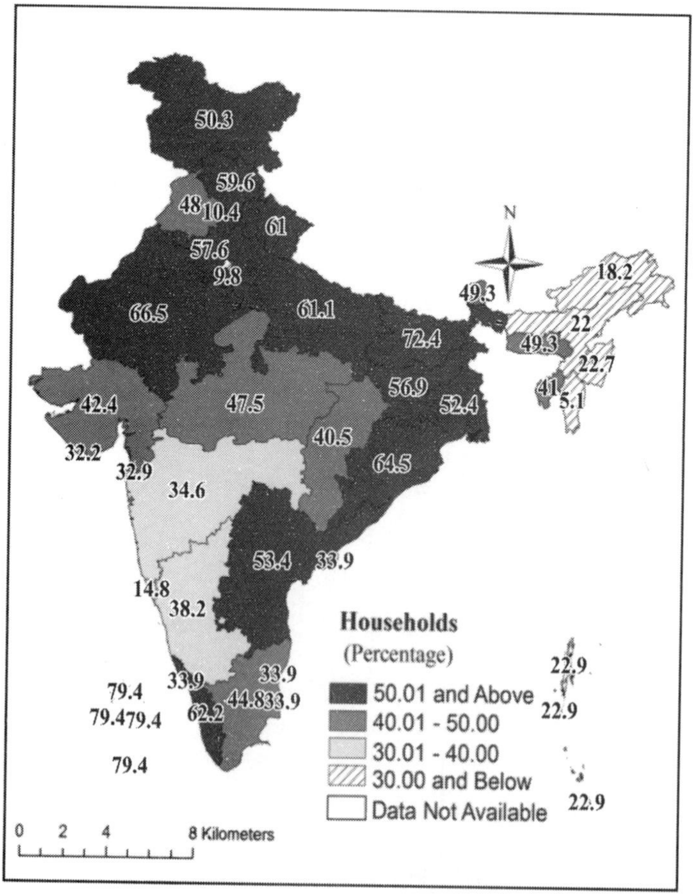

A kitchen environment index for the Indian households (Figure 7) has been prepared with the help of range equalization technique (normalization) through using the following variables: households have no separate kitchen inside the house, use of unclean fuel and unclean fuel use in pucca house. Number of variables is three hence, the score of the States/UTs walks from zero to three. All unidirectional variables of the Index denote the negative aspect of the kitchen environment. So, higher the score indicates the more worsened condition of the kitchen. First two variables are taken from the population Census 2011 and the last one from DLHS–3.[14] But, DLHS–3, did not collect the data for the Nagaland State, therefore, Nagaland is excluded from the Index.

The index reveals that whole of Central and Eastern States and one Western State namely Rajasthan possess higher score of the index that indicates the very worst condition of the kitchen environment (Figure 7). Whole of North-Eastern States barring Meghalaya and Tripura show very good condition of that. Whole Southern, Northern and Western India (excluding Rajasthan) demonstrate the moderate condition of the kitchen environment where Southern and Western Indian condition is comparatively better than Northern India.

Figure 7 *India: Kitchen Environment Index*

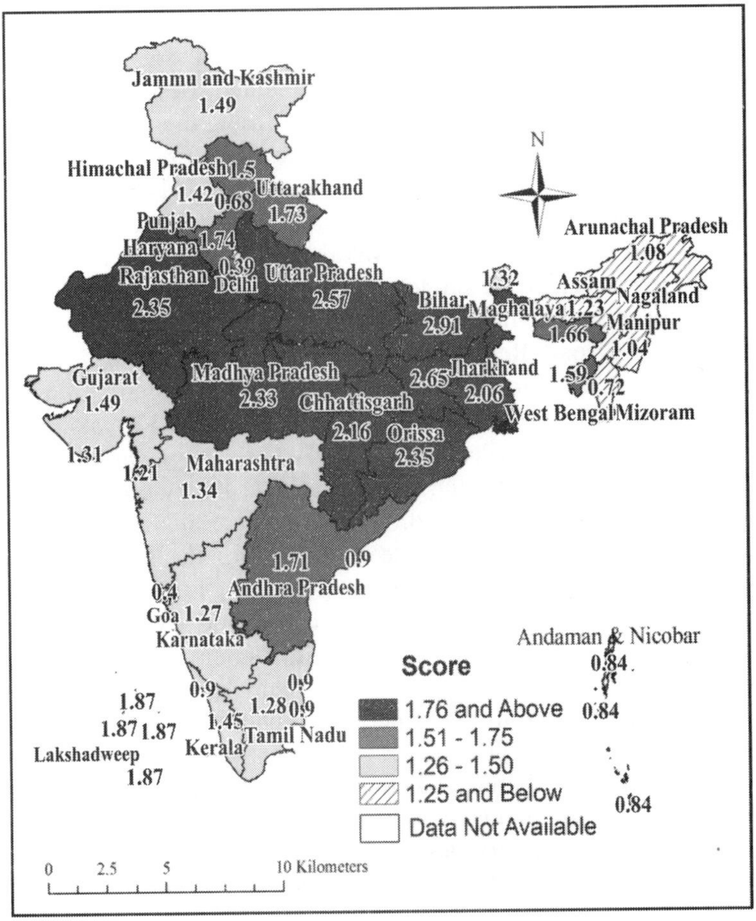

Policy Issues and Conclusion

Finally, it can be concluded that most of the Indian households have separate kitchen but most of them use unclean fuel – especially firewood, crop residue and cow dung cake are most common fuel for combustion for everyday household energy needs. Besides, more than one-third of households with pucca houses use unclean fuel for cooking as yet. The rural-urban gap is highly pronounced for availability of kitchen as well as for the use of fuel and nature of kitchen stocks. There is a wide spatial variation of the kitchen environment in India. Western, Central and Eastern Indian kitchen environmental conditions are worse as compared to the rest of India.

These outcomes point out that there have been huge threats of the high prevalence rate of low birth rate (LBW), acute respiratory infection (ARI) and tuberculosis (TB) in India where rural areas suffer more as compared to urban. While ARI and LBW are recognized as priority health problems in children as well as pregnant women, the kitchen environment has not widely received the attention which with its magnitude that it deserves. Only few national and international agencies such as WHO and UNICEF have been focusing on this issue through limited number of intervening programmes. Policy interventions such as the supply of clean fuels for cooking, improved stoves, separate kitchen used inside and outside the house, proper ventilation and use of high quality of building materials should be funded and implemented. Besides campaigning for consciousness is also an integral part of that. In India, there are a half dozen of Ministries such as Ministry of New and Renewable Energy, Petroleum and Natural Gas, Human Resource Development, Rural Development, Urban Development and Ministry of Health and Family Welfare which are responsible for the citizens' health, services and development but none of these have taken the issue seriously as yet. Not a single initiative is incorporated into the so-called famous and success schemes like National Rural Health Mission (2005), Jawaharlal Nehru Urban Renewal Mission (2005), Janani Suraksha Yojana (2005) and Mahatma Gandhi National Rural Employment Guarantee Act (2005) and the recently launched Janani Shishu Suraksha Karyakaram (2011). During the Eleventh Five-Year Plan (2007–12), the Central Government launched some mega projects such as the National Policy on Biofuels (2009), Rajiv Gandhi Gramin LPG Vitrak (2009) and Jawaharlal Nehru National Solar Mission (2010), but they are not able to enter into the kitchen of common people. Rajiv Gandhi Gramin LPG Vitrak (RGGLV) is directly linked to fuel consumption in the kitchen but it was limited within eight states and State Governments were not able to properly implement it except the Delhi Government. In 2012, Delhi Government launched 'kerosene-free Delhi scheme' as part of RGGLV under which .36 million households will get LPG cylinder and a gas stove free of cost.

There are very few differences between MHHHs and FHHHs in terms of fuel consumption and kitchen environment. Actually in Indian society, an aged person is considered as honourable head of the household, irrespective of his/her income, leadership and power of decision making within the household.

This kind of headship is defined as distressed headship. Oldest person in a family holds some belongings till his/her death. Family members always try to show their respect for the expectation of these belongings. Sometimes after the death of father, mother becomes head of the household. In this case, basic kitchen condition does not change for the shifting of headship. When study regarding female headship is considered as an indicator of women empowerment, women active participation in family decision making, her leadership and income contribution should be brought under ambit of the study, not imposing them as an honourable head. For these, proper data sets are essential. Census 2011 was not able to capture it. There is wide lacuna in the definition of headship. When data regarding the head of the household is collected, it is not justified how much he or she plays the role over the household, it is just an opinion of the informant. Besides, age-wise headship data are also essential. When aged people are traditionally honoured as the head of the household in Indian society then, an elderly woman automatically would be the head of the household in the absence of her male partner. If an older woman is head of the household, then it may be a sign of respect or change of status after the death of the husband. However, when younger woman leads the household, then this type of ambiguity does not exist. Hence, further study related to above-mentioned aspects is essential to explore the additional facts.

Notes

1. Mishra et al.'s (2005) study was based on Indian National Family Health Survey (NFHS–2) 1998–99: sample size was 92,486 households that covered more than 99 per cent of Indian population.
2. A joint research on healthy cooking fuel options for India was carried out by The Energy and Resources Institute (TERI) and All India Institute of Medical Sciences (AIIMS) during 2009–10 with funding support from UNICEF.
3. The size of the elderly population is 7.4 per cent of total population in India where female share i.e. 7.8 per cent is higher than the male share of 7.1 per cent in Census 2001.
4. Elderly population has increased 3.5 per cent per year during inter-censual period, 1991 to 2001. Elderly female population has increased at a faster rate i.e. 4.2 per cent per year than the male 2.9 per cent per year during that period.
5. Census of India. 2011. *History of Census in India.* Retrieved on 18 April 2013 from http://www.censusindia.gov.in/ad_campaign/drop_in_articles/05history_of_census_in_india.pdf
6. Areas under forest of total geographical areas of Chhattisgarh, Odisha, Jharkhand, Madhya Pradesh and Rajasthan are 41.2, 31.4, 28.8, 25.2 and 4.7 per cent respectively (Forest Survey of India, 2011: 7).
7. The proportion of Scheduled Tribe population in Chhattisgarh, Odisha, Jharkhand, Madhya Pradesh and Rajasthan is 30.6, 22.8, 26.2, 21.1 and 13.5 per cent respectively in Census 2011.
8. The rate of urbanization in North-Eastern States is 37.5 per cent per decade between 2001 and 2011 Census.

9. Agricultural Census. 2005–06. Agricultural Census Data Base. Retrieved on 18 April 2013 from http://agcensus.dacnet.nic.in/stateholdingsize class.aspx.
10. Population density of Bihar, West Bengal and Uttar Pradesh is comparatively higher i.e. 1102, 1029 and 828 persons per sq km respectively, whereas Indian average is 382 persons per sq km in Census 2011. In Jharkhand, Odisha, Madhya Pradesh and Chhattisgarh population density is 414, 269, 236 and 189 persons per sq km respectively in 2011.
11. The kachha or temporary house's wall may be made of grass, thatch, leaves, reeds, bamboo, mud, plastic/polythene, unburnt bricks or wood. Roof may be made from grass, leaves, bamboo, thatch, mud, unburnt bricks or wood (Census 2001).
12. The pucca or permanent house's material of wall can be burnt bricks, GI/metal/asbestos sheets, stone with lime or cement or cement concrete. Roof may be made of tiles, slate, shingle, corrugated/galvanized iron or zinc/other metal or asbestos sheets, bricks, lime and stone, stone, RBC/RCC or concrete (Census 2001).
13. In MHHHs, 62 per cent, 25 per cent and 12 per cent households lived in pucca, semi-pucca and katcha houses respectively, in Census 2011. Likewise, in FHHHs, 60 per cent, 26 per cent and 12 per cent households lived in these housing stocks respectively in 2011.
14. To compare with Census data, the weight cases of DLHS–3 are used rather than absolute.

References

Boy, E., Bruce, N. And Delgado, H. 2002. Birth Weight and Exposure to Kitchen Wood Smoke During Pregnancy in Rural Guatemala. *Environmental Health Perspectives*, 110 (1): 109–114.

International Society for Environmental Epidemiology (ISEE). 2005. *Indoor Air Pollution from Solid Fuel and Risk of Low Birth Weight and Still Birth*. Johannesburg, South Africa and Switzerland: World Health Organisation,S September.

Kundu, Amitabh. 2011. *Report of the Technical Group on Urban Housing Shortage (TG-12) (2012–17)*. New Delhi: Ministry of Housing and Urban Poverty Alleviation, National Building Organization, Government of India.

Mavalankar, D.V., Trivedi, C.R. and Gray, R.H. 1991. Levels and Risk Factors for Perinatal Mortality in Ahmedabad, India. *Bulletin of World Health Organization*, 69 (4): 435–442.

Ministry of Environment and Forests, Government of India. 2011. *Forest Survey of India, State of Forest Report 2011: Executive Summary*. Dehradun: Ministry of Environment and Forests, Government of India.

Ministry of Health and Family Welfare, Government of India. 2005. *Janani Suraksha Yojna*. Retrieved on 13 July 2013 from http://jknrhm.com/pdf/jsr.pdf

Ministry of Health and Family Welfare, Government of India. 2005. *National Rural Health Mission*. Retrieved on 13 July 2013 from http://jknrhm.com/guideline/frame_work.pdf

Ministry of Health and Family Welfare, Government of India. 2011. *Janani Shishu Suraksha Karyakaram*. Retrieved on 13 July 2013 from http://statehealthsocietybihar.org/rch/goi-guideline-jssk.pdf

Ministry of Home Affairs, Government of India. 2008. *Sample Registration System Compendium 1971–2007*. New Delhi: Registrar General of India.

Ministry of New and Renewable Energy, Government of India. 2009. *National Policy on Biofuels*. Retrieved on 13 July 2013 from http://mnre.gov.in/filemanager/userfiles/biofuel_policy.pdf

Ministry of New and Renewable Energy, Government of India. 2010. *Jawaharlal Nehru National Solar Mission*. Retrieved on 13 July 2013 from http://www.mnre.gov.in/solar-mission//jnnsm/inroduction-2/

Ministry of Petroleum and Natural Gas, Government of India. 2009. *Rajiv Gandhi Gramin LPG Vitrak*. Retrieved on 13 July 2013 from http://www.hindustanpetroleum.com/upload/en/updf/rgglv_brochure.pdf

Ministry of Rural Development, Government of India. 2005. *Mahatma Gandhi National Rural Employment Guarantee Act*. Retrieved on 13 July 2013 from http://nrega.nic.nic.in/netnrega/writereaddata/circulars/operational_guidence-4thedition_eng_2013.pdf

Ministry of Urban Development, Government of India. 2005. *Jawaharlal Nehru Urban Renewal Mission*. Retrieved on 13 July 2013 from http://jnnurm.nic.in/wpcontent/uploads/2011/01/uigoverview.pdf

Mishra, V., Dai, X., Smith, K.R. and Mika, L. 2004. Maternal Exposure to Biomass Smoke and Reduced Birth Weight in Zimbabwe. *Ann Epidemiol*, 14 (10): 740–747.

Mishra, V., Retherford, R.D. and Smith, K.R. 2005. Cooking Smoke and Tobacco Smoke as Risk Factors for Stillbirth. *International Journal of Environmental Health Research*, 15 (6): 397–410.

Planning Commission, Government of India. 2012. *Press Note on Poverty Estimates, 2009–10*. New Delhi: Press Information Bureau, Government of India.

Pokhrel, A.K., Bates, M.N., Verma, S.C. and Joshi, H.S. 2010. Tuberculosis and Indoor Biomass and Kerosene Use in Nepal: A Case Control Study. *Environmental Health Perspective*, 118 (4): 558–564.

Rehfuess, E.A., Tzala, L., Best, N., Briggs, DJ. and Joffe, M. 1979. Solid Fuel Use and Cooking Practices as a Major Risk Factor for ALRI Mortality among African Children. *Journal of Epidemiology and Community Health*, 63 (11): 887–892.

Siddiqui, A.R., Gold, E.B., Brown, K.H., Lee, K. and Bhutta, Z. 2008. Preliminary Analysis of Indoor Air Pollution and Low Birth Weight (LBW) in Southern Pakistan. In, International Society for Environmental Epidemiology (ISEE), *Indoor Air Pollution from Solid Fuels and Risk of Low Birth Weight and Stillbirth*, Johannesburg, South Africa and Switzerland: World Health Organization, 5 September, 11–14.

The Energy and Resources Institute (TERI) and All India Institute of Medical Sciences (AIIMS). 2011. *Indoor Air Pollution: A Case for Change*. Retrieved on 12 May 2013 from http://www.unicef.org/india/policy_brief_1-Indoor- air_pollution.pdf

Windham, G., Eaton, A. and Hopkins, B. 1999. Evidence for an Association between Environmental Tobacco Smoke Exposure and Birth Weight: A Meta Analysis and New Data. *Paediatric and Perinatal Epidemiology*, 13 (1): 35–57.

World Health Organization. 2008. *Global Tuberculosis Control: Surveillance, Planning, Financing*. Geneva: World Health Organization.

20

Examining Changes in Food Consumption and Its Implications Towards Calorie Undernourishment in India

Balakrushna Padhi

Indian economy has witnessed a significant change over the last few decades. One such change in this case, is that of paradoxical change in the nature of food consumption and declining in calorie norms in India. As proper food consumption and proper level of nutrient intakes is essential for the proper development of human metabolic activities, the decline in it raises the problem of food and nutritional security in the country. This also leads to rising level of calorie deprivation in India. This basically poses two questions – why such shift and what are its consequences. So, to find out the main reasons of this phenomenon the present study has looked through it in a broad prospective manner. In this present study we look into the observed trend through choice and inadequacy prospect. It is because food and nutritional security has been imperative both for an individual and for the economy. Also, healthy nutritional population status is vital for economic growth and also has both demand and supply effect. On the demand side, health and nutrition have an effect on fertility and mortality of the population and in supply side it affects individual productivity, thereby having an effect on human capital formation (Sinha, 2005). So by looking at its importance, it is essential to learn the status of these issues with changes in the nature of production and consumption pattern of the households.

In a developing country like India, where the achievement of food security is a challenge, the consequent decline in nutritional intake of the households raises the problem of nutritional security as well. The structural shift in the consumption pattern of the households has serious implications in terms of ensuring food security and combating poverty because, as shown by

Meenakshi and Viswanathan (2003), only income poverty has declined, while the calorie deprivation has increased. The main concern here is that, the average calorie consumption in India is already low by international standards and it declined despite much acclaimed economic growth of the country (Nasurudeen et al., 2006). As most of the direct food consumption items, like cereals which consist of the lion's share of the total nutrition and a cheap source of energy to Indians, the decline in it will have severe deleterious effects on the nutritional status of the people.

Yet, there is a growing body of literature which claims that the decline in the calorie consumption in the Indian diet is not a sign of declining welfare; rather it is a sign of improving economic status of the population (Deaton and Dreze, 2009; Dreze, 2003). Arguments that range from moving up the curve on Engel's law and sedentariness owing to shifting employment structure claim that the decline in calorie consumption is a positive feature of the growing economy. In this context the present study examines the extent of calorie deprivation in rural and urban households, its magnitudes and distribution. In our discussion of food and nutritional security, we are largely concerned with the issues relating to hunger, poverty and undernutrition.

Calorie Consumption Puzzle in India

One of the enduring puzzles related to economic development in India over the past two decades depicted in most of the studies is the calorie consumption puzzle, a key feature of which is the changes in nature of the Indian diet pattern. The recent consumer expenditure survey (NSSO-CES 2009–10) shows a shift in expenditure pattern away from food to non-food items in both the rural and urban areas. It also suggests that non-food consumption expenditure increased, but along with it there was widening inadequacy in essential nutrient intakes like calorie and protein for lower income/expenditure classes. Several studies have equally observed a declining trend in the level of consumption of food, along with structural shift of economy (Gopalan, 1992; Deaton and Dreze, 2009). However, these studies have varied rationalizations of the observed pattern. It also poses the problem of food and nutritional security in the country, because food security necessitates not only the provision of sufficient food to meet the market demand but also to create conditions for acquiring sufficient food for healthy life (Kumar and Dey, 2007; Suryanarayana, 2003). The decline in essential food consumption raises the problem of calorie inadequacy in India. The growing body of literature regarding this puzzle can be divided into two broad prospects. That is examining the calorie undernourishment in both welfare and non-welfare centric. Whereas some economists argue the changes in the calorie intake is due to increase in the standard of living and improvement in human health, this proposition is vehemently criticized by other economists. While study of, Deaton and Dreze (2009), depicts that the decline in food consumption as well as calorie norms shows improvement in human welfare, this argument has a counter by others such as Patnaik (2003). According to her the changing average consumption is a necessary condition but not a sufficient condition for assessing human welfare. It could also be due to insufficient increment of income among the lower expenditure groups, which basically make them incapable of increasing the spending on food consumption. Lastly, the inefficiency of PDS may also lead to the occurrence of the above phenomena. But in terms of choice which has been put forward by some economists depicts the scenario in a different prospective. Their main argument in this regard is that choice is the main factor which shapes their consumption profile. Summarizing the literature on declining calorie intake and the structural shift, the arguments can be classified as of two roots, namely arguments on inadequacy and arguments on choice. While some studies examine these phenomena as improvement of human welfare, others have criticized this argument. If we synthesize the arguments based on the above analysis we can get a picture of rising income and nutritional insufficiency in terms of inadequacy and choice prospective.

Three sets of aspects which may lead to changes in consumption profile are sedentariness, demonstration effect and occurrence of Engels law phenomena as defined by Deaton and Dreze (2009). The various rationalizations given in the literature is summarized below in the chart (Figure 1).

Figure 1 *Structural Shift and Calorie Intake*

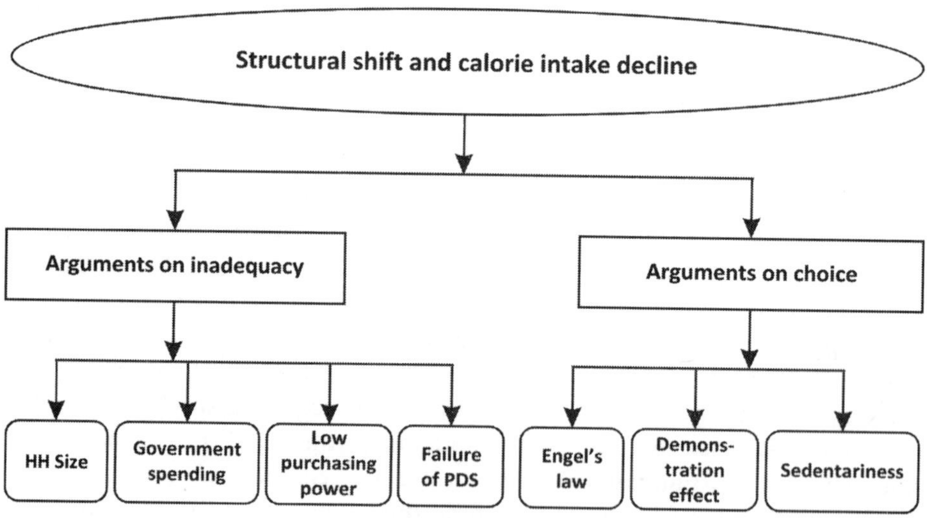

From the above literature review it can be noted that a wide spectrum of change has occurred in the consumption habits of the households over the last three decades. Although it assumes that structural transformation of the economy leads to improving the health status of the people, this argument does not hold over, if we look at the nutritional standard of the population? It may be possible in the higher expenditure class but it may not be possible in the bottom level category, which is already at the subsistence level. The distinction related to diet diversification in different expenditure groups may throw some light on the question of whether it is choice or inadequacy that leads to this diet diversification. However, this question has only been peripherally addressed in the past literature. Because for the bottom households, this may not be the true connotation of improving welfare.

Keeping these issues in mind, this study enquires into the following specific research questions. First, we look at the determinants behind this structural shift in consumption pattern and prevalence of undernutrition. Second, we try to find out the factors behind this trend through choice vs inadequacy perspective. The underlying objective is to understand the level of food and nutritional security in terms of rising calorie undernourishment, when the country is experiencing high economic growth.

Data Source and Methodology

This study is based on secondary data. To analyse the structural shift in the food and non-food consumption expenditure of the households, this study uses the NSSO major thick quinquennial rounds of consumption expenditure survey (Unit level data on dietary patterns and consumer expenditure, NSSO-CES). The present analysis is based on the NSSO-CES of, 50th, 61st and 66th rounds. We abstain from the use of NSS-CES of 55th round for comparative analysis, because of changes in methodology adopted to perform the survey in that particular round, which made the round less comparable with the other rounds. Due to the unavailability of income data, the per capita expenditure of sample households was used as a proxy for per capita income. For converting nominal prices to real prices in rural and urban area, the CPI index for agricultural labour for rural area and industrial worker for urban area has been used respectively to deflate the series, which has been obtained from the labour bureau, ministry of labour and employment, Government of India. Calorie intakes are calculated by applying conversion factor as mentioned in Nutritional Intake of India Report, which are reported as having been consumed by the sample households during the last 30 days. To learn about the long-term changes in nutritional intake we consider nutritional data based on previous rounds from the Nutritional Intake of India Report. The calorie deprivation/undernutrition analysis is based on the information from the NSSO's 50th, 61st and 66th rounds consumption expenditure survey. We have used comparative analysis to conceive the food and nutritional security in India. In order to consider household calorie undernourishment, we take the cut-off point of 2,400 kcal for rural area and 2,100 kcal for the urban area.

Consumption and Nutrition Profile of Indian Households

Indian economy has undergone a great transition with the structural transformation of the economy. With this, the per capita income in India has grown manifolds during the last two decades. During this period the total consumption expenditure of average Indian household also has increased substantially. Due to nutritional significance of essential food grains like cereals, the decline in it

Figure 2 *Percentage Break-up of MPCE Over Broad Groups of Consumption*

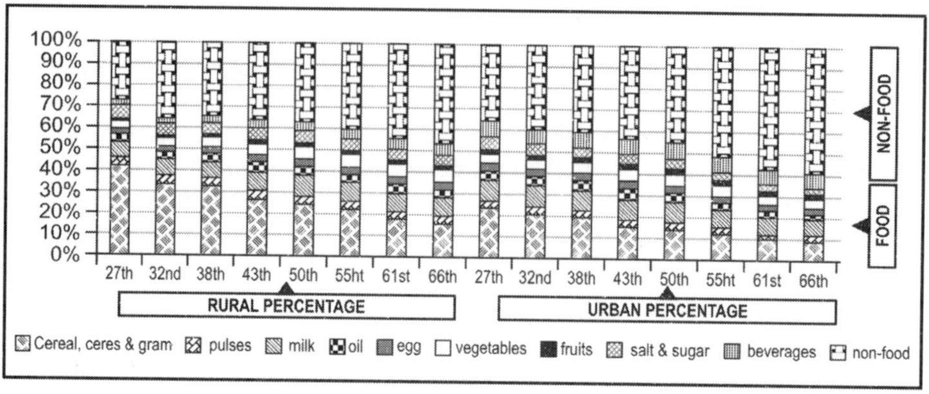

Source: Various NSSO reports on consumer expenditure.

raises the problem of nutritional security in the country. With this change the food expenditure share has declined while that of non-food increased.

It is very clear from Figure 2 that since last four decades there is a steady decline in expenditure share on food intake in urban areas as compared to rural areas. Although the share of non-food expenditure has been increasing since 1972–73, this trend is more evident in the post-liberalization area. The non-food item shows a higher percentage increase in the post-1990s. In the 66th round the expenditure on total urban food expenditure share reached below 40 per cent mark, which is a matter of concern in nutrition front. The decline in expenditure on food intake is mainly due to the decline in expenditure on cereal consumption. With the diversification of food intakes, the households are moving towards non-cereals food items. Within non-food groups also, some of the consumption expenditure on durables, education and other items is increasing over the period of time.

The decline in expenditure on cereal intakes is clearly visible both in rural and urban area. Not only food consumption but also food expenditure of cereals is declining. The cereal consumption which had a major share in the total expenditure in 1993–94 (24.5) has declined to only 13.9 per cent in 2009–10 in rural areas. With the decline in expenditure share the consumption level of cereal intakes also declining both in rural and urban India. The consumption of egg, vegetables, fruits and spices has increased during the period in the rural area, whereas in urban area the picture is different. While the expenditure on food has shown a continuous decline as a proportion of total expenditure, expenditure on durables and other items increased during this period (NSSO, 2009–10). Similar to our results Radhakrishna et al. (2004) shows that, over NSSO percentile groups while total consumption expenditures have increased for all classes for three decades since the 1970s, consumption expenditure on food shows a negative growth over 1990s. During the same period there have been large changes in the expenditure pattern of food consumption as well. Expenditure on direct food consumption is declining while indirect food consumption (egg, meat, oil, etc.) is showing increasing trend overtime. Besides providing necessary energy, adequate calorie level is thus equally important in permitting the protein to perform its prime function for body maintenance.[1] In terms of food consumption, direct food intakes are the cheapest source of energy. People, mostly in India, prefer the direct food intakes like cereals and pulses for obtaining adequate energy, as shown in 1993–94 that these food intakes almost provides 90 per cent of nutrient consumption. Hence, changes in the essential food norms may affect the nutritional status of the households, which is an important area of attention. This is followed by the Bennett's law, which basically shows that with increasing income, households will move from the cheaper source of calorie to a dearer source of calories. The food budget also got squeezed due to rise in the share of non-food expenditure in the consumption profile.

Factors Behind Decline in Calorie Intakes

For examining the main factors behind decline in calorie and protein intakes we took an exercise of examining the changing share of nutrient based food products. It is found that the essential food items share to total calorie and protein intakes is declining since last two decades, both in rural as well as urban area. This is largely due to decline in the share of food intakes, which contains a large share of calorie and protein. In rural India, calorie intake declined between 1993–94 and 2009–10. Most of it is attributed to the decline in calories from cereals and pulses. In rural area the percentage of calories from cereals is declining from 71 per cent to 64 per cent and that for pulses from 7 per cent to 4 per cent (Figure 3).[2] This is true for urban area also, where the percentage has declined from 58 per cent to 54 per cent. With the decline in essential food intakes the percentage share of calorie as well as protein intakes in cereals and pulses are showing declining trend both in rural and urban area. There is a small

Figure 3 *Percentage of Calorie and Protein Intakes by Food Commodities*

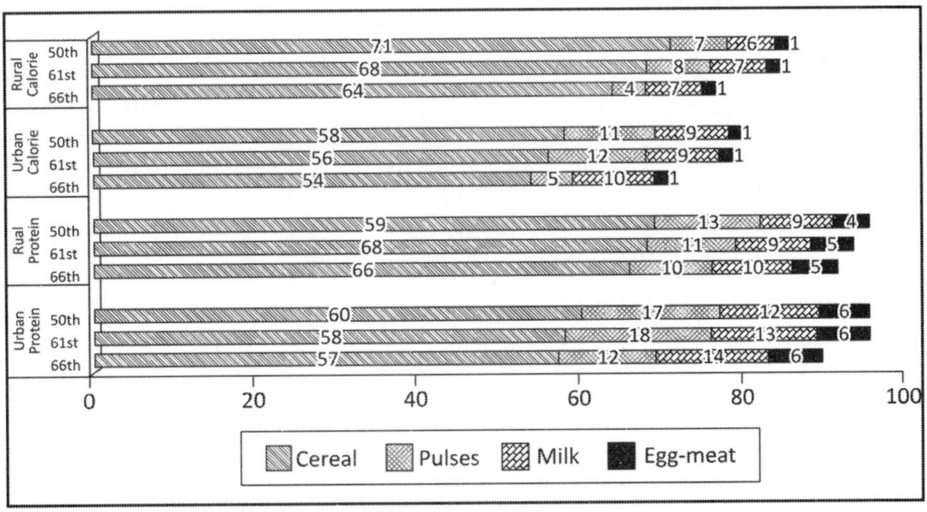

Source: Various NSSO reports on Nutritional Intakes in India.

increase in the indirect consumption nutrient intakes. Both in rural and urban area, the percentage share of calorie and protein in case of milk and egg/meat consumption is also very small. The percentage derived from milk intakes increased from 6 to 7 per cent in rural calorie and 9 to 10 percentage in urban calorie during 1993–94 to 2009–10. The same trend is also observed in case of distribution of egg/meat intakes.

Calories obtained from cereals declined from 1530 in 1993–94 to 1296 in 2009–10 (NSSO, 2009–10). The contribution of other indirect consumption is almost unchanged in these periods. The contribution of calorie intake from oil has increased. Similar results are also found for urban areas as well. There is a drastic decline in cereal and pulses contribution to total calorie intakes in urban areas. As there is a close relationship between cereal consumption and nutrition, the decline in one affects the others, which is clearly shown from the above analysis.

Changes in Aggregate Food Consumption, Calorie Norms and Implications on Poverty in India

From the following analysis we observe that there is a drastic decline in essential food consumptions since 1993–94. The income growth is not visualizing in terms of rising nutrition. As most of the cereal and pulses based items has a major proportion in the total nutrition, the decline in it leads to decline in nutrient norms in terms of calorie and protein intakes. It can be seen from the Figure 4, that although the real MPCE has increased substantially over last two decades, the essential nutrients like, calorie and protein is declining in the rural area. There is a growing body of literature on this persisting puzzle. Patnaik (2005, 2009, 2010),

Figure 4 *Average Calorie Intake and Real MPCE-Rural*

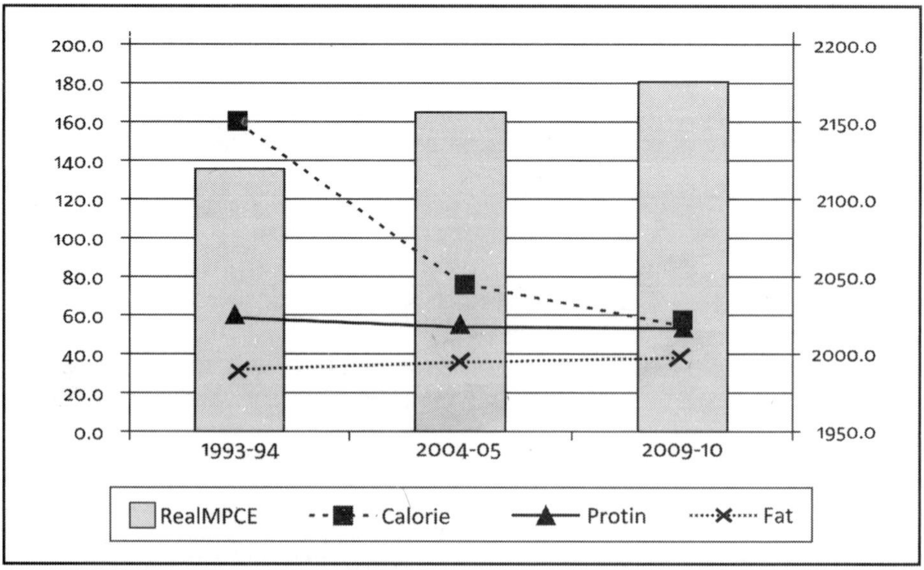

Source: Computed from NSSO unit level data.[3]

states that this puzzle does not exist in the real sense. For her the decline in average calorie intake is a direct outcome of impoverishment, i.e. the decline in real income and expenditure of majority of the population. Others like Deaton and Dreze (2009), and Li and Eli (2010) on the other hand take recourse to the Engel's law to argue the existence of this puzzle of declining nutrient with increase in income and decline in nutrition, while Basu and Basole (2012), argue that this phenomena is the outcome of food budget squeeze and declining home-grown consumption. So the question remains, what causes the reduction of essential food intakes which leads to fall in basic nutrient requirements?

It is very clear from Figure 4 over the last four decades the average per capita per day calorie intake is declining from 2,266 kcal in 1972–73 to 1,946 kcal. As per the recent NSSO round (2009–10), only fat consumption is increasing, both protein and calorie consumption is showing a declining trend. The proportion of average per capita per day calorie intake is showing an increase only in 1999–00 in the urban area, but in the rest of the years it is showing a declining trend both in rural and urban area. Going by the specified norm of 2,400 kcal and 2,100 kcal calorie norm in rural and urban areas over the last two decades the percentage share of households, those having above the specified norm has declined from 28.5 per cent in the 50th round to only 18.8 per cent in 2009–10 in the rural area and 39 per cent to 35 per cent in urban areas. This leads to wide variation in money-metric and calorie-metric poverty estimation in rural and urban India.

Changing Nature of Nutrient Intakes in Rural and Urban India

In the last two decades, a drastic decline is shown in nutrient intakes and also essential food intakes. The decline is not only confined to calories but also to other nutrients as well. If we look at the long-term trends in the nutrient intakes, we can find that over the last four decades the average per capita per day calorie intake is declining from 2,266 kcal in 1972–73 to 1,946 kcal. As per the recent NSSO round (2009–10), only fat consumption is increasing (Table 1).

Table 1 *Changing Average Per Capita Nutrient Intake Per Day over NSS Rounds*

	Rural			*Urban*		
	Calorie	*Protein*	*Fat*	*Calorie*	*Protein*	*Fat*
1972–73	2,266	62	24	2,107	56	36
1983–84	2,221	62	27	2,089	57	37
1993–94	2,153	60.2	31.4	2,071	57.2	42
1999–00	2,149	59.1	36.1	2,156	58.5	49.6
2004–05	2,047	57	35.5	2,020	57	47.5
2009–10	2,020	55	38.3	1,946	53.5	47.7

Source: Computed from NSSO unit level data.

The proportion of average per capita per day calorie intake is showing an increase only in 1999–00 in the urban area. But in the rest of the years it is declining both in rural and urban area. The long-term trend in calorie, protein and fat intakes indicates that except for fat, both protein and calorie intakes are declining substantially both in rural and urban area. After examining the long-term trends in nutrient intakes, in the next section, we will discuss state-wise variation in different nutrient intakes.

Interstate Variation in Nutritional Content

In order to study the trends in nutrient intake in rural and urban India, we have taken three time periods in our analysis. The time period 1993–94 to 2004–05 is taken as the first period, 2004–05 to 2009–10 is considered as second period and the whole period 1993–94 to 2009–10 is the third period. From Table 2, we can observe that there has been a drastic decline in calorie and protein intakes, only fat intake has shown an increasing trend. The overall increase in fat intake is larger between the period 1993–94 and 2009–10 for rural and urban area (it is 22% for rural and 14% for urban). Now we will discuss the variation of states in these three periods, among the nutrient intakes in rural and urban areas.

From Table 2, we can find that although there is some percentage increases in calorie intake in rural in the second period in Karnataka, Maharashtra and Tamil Nadu, during the third period there is a little improvement only in Tamil Nadu in rural areas and Maharashtra, Tamil Nadu in urban areas. Only Tamil Nadu, Maharashtra and Karnataka are showing improvement in protein intakes in rural India.[4] But with this increment also, it is far from the required norms. In terms of percentage changes in average calorie intakes and protein intakes although some states are showing improvement as compared to the first period, only few states exhibit growth in the third period in rural area. But in terms of fat intakes almost all the states exhibit a positive change in all three periods in rural area. If we will look at the average percentage changes in urban area we can find that although most of the states such as Andhra Pradesh, Gujarat, Karnataka, Madhya Pradesh, Maharashtra, Odisha, Rajasthan, Tamil Nadu show an improvement but by third period only Maharashtra and Tamil Nadu show a positive change in calorie intakes. But similar to rural area both of the states are far away from the required norms (2,100 kcal urban area). This change leads to rise in the level of calorie undernourished population, both in rural and urban households.

Measuring Nutrition According to Different Calorie Cut-off Points

From the above analysis we can find that there is a drastic decline in terms of nutrient intakes in India. By keeping the 2,400 kcal for rural and 2,100 kcal for urban (as per the planning commission norm of 1979), the undernourished population has increased substantially. As the prescribed norm has been questioned by several economists, in this present context, we tried to put different norms for quantifying the level of undernourishment in India.[5] But, if we divide the households into different calorific norms, i.e. from 0 to 1,800 kcal, 1,800 to 2,400 kcal and 2,400 to 3,000 kcal and more in rural area and 0 to 1,700 kcal, 1,700 to 2,100 kcal, 2,100 to 2,600 kcal and 2,600 kcal and above, we can get some interesting features.

Table 2 *Rate of Changes in Essential Nutrient Intakes in Rural and Urban India*

	Changes in calorie intakes						*Changes in protein intakes*						*Changes in fat intakes*					
	Rural			*Urban*			*Rural*			*Urban*			*Rural*			*Urban*		
	50th–61st	*61st–66th*	*50th–66th*	*50th–61st*	*61st–66th*	*50th–66th*	*50th–61st*	*61st–66th*	*50th–66th*	*50th–61st*	*61st–66th*	*50th–66th*	*50th–61st*	*61st–66th*	*50th–66th*	*50th–61st*	*61st–66th*	*50th–66th*
AP	0.4	–1.3	–0.9	–2.8	2.6	–0.2	–2	1.8	–0.2	2.6	–0.2	2.4	23.2	13.1	39.3	24	0	23.8
AS	1.7	–6.5	–5	4.2	–4.5	–0.5	6.5	–7.6	–1.6	4.5	–5.9	–2	27.1	–5.2	20.5	20	–9	8.8
BR	0.1	–8.1	–8	–3.1	–5.8	–8.7	–4	–7.3	–11	1.3	–9.2	–8	23.5	–0.4	23	24	-13	7.6
GR	–1.8	–0.4	–2.2	–3.6	3.1	–0.6	–4.1	1.3	–2.9	4.4	–7	–3	7.4	11.8	20	9.7	3.8	13.8
HR	–5	–4.6	–9.3	–10.6	–2.1	–13	–11	–3.7	–15	–4.9	–4.8	–9	3.4	6	9.5	10	0	10.1
KR	–4	2.2	–1.9	–11	3.1	–8.2	–11	0.4	–11	–1.7	–0.8	–2	18.5	18	39.9	15	8.3	24.7
KE	1.5	–2.8	–1.3	2.5	–2.5	–0.1	9.1	–4.9	3.7	8.2	–4.8	3.1	24.8	4.9	30.9	21	1.6	23.2
MP	–6.1	–5.1	–11	–10.9	0.5	–10	–6.7	–0.7	–7.3	–2.7	–7	–10	24	4.8	30	7.7	6.9	15.1
MH	–7.1	2.9	–4.4	–0.3	6.1	5.8	1.6	0.9	2.6	–6.1	1.2	–5	23.9	16.4	44.2	4.6	8.4	13.4
OR	–5.4	–2	–7.3	–8	5.1	–3.3	–8.3	2.9	–5.7	–3.5	–4.9	–8	20.3	30.3	56.8	0.7	11	11.4
PN	2.9	–4.1	–1.3	–7.4	–0.8	–8.1	–11	–1.9	–12	2.6	–4.7	–2	–1.8	5.5	3.5	14	1.5	15.3
RJ	–3.1	–4.8	–7.8	–11.7	0.5	–11	–12	–2.6	–15	–3.8	–5.5	–9	–3.6	8.1	4.2	9.3	–1.2	7.9
TN	0.7	1.4	2.1	–2.2	4.5	2.2	–4.1	5.3	1.1	1	2	3.1	19.8	24.3	49	21	7.1	29.8
UP	0.5	–9.5	–9	–4.6	–6.2	–11	–6.4	–9	–15	3	–14	–11	5.6	–2.4	3.1	12	–8.2	2.7
WB	–5.6	–8	–13.1	–6.4	–6.9	–13	–5.1	–7.9	–13	–2.7	–11	–13	23.8	7.2	32.7	14	-1.8	12.3
IND	–2.5	–3.7	–6	–4.9	–1.3	–6.2	–5.3	–3.5	–8.6	–0.3	–6.1	–7	13.1	7.9	22	13	0.8	14

Figure 5 *Calorie Distribution in Rural and Urban India*

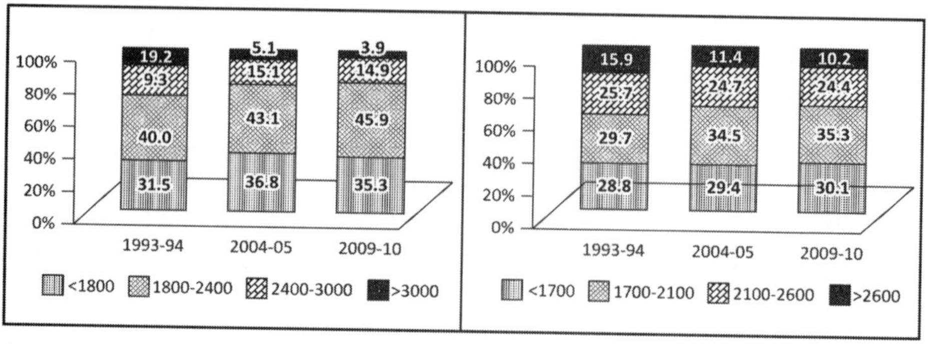

Source: Computed from NSSO unit level data.

We can find that in the rural area most of the households nutrient compliance fall within the range of 1,800 to 2,400 whereas in the urban area most of the households are coming under 0–1,800 range (Figure 5). This may be due to more diet diversification in urban area as compared to the rural area (Ray, 2007). Indian states are shown a wide range of variation in terms of average per capita calorie intake norm. Although at the all-India level, the mean per capita calorie intake has reduced from 2,156 in1993–94 to 2,020 in 2009–10 in rural areas and similar decline is also found in urban areas, but if we divide the states according to different calorie norms as we discussed above, we will get some interesting picture. The percentage of well-nourished households have declined from 28.5 per cent in the 50th round to 18.8 per cent in the 66th round in rural areas, whereas this decline in urban area is from 41.6 per cent to 34.5 per cent. This clearly indicates the decline in calorie intakes is higher in rural area as compared to urban. By this shift in calorie norms, none of the states are able to qualify the required amount of calorie norms both in rural and urban India. With this we found a vast difference between money-metric and calorie-metric poverty norms.

Figure 6 *Differences in Calorie-Metric and Money-Metric Poverty Norms in India*

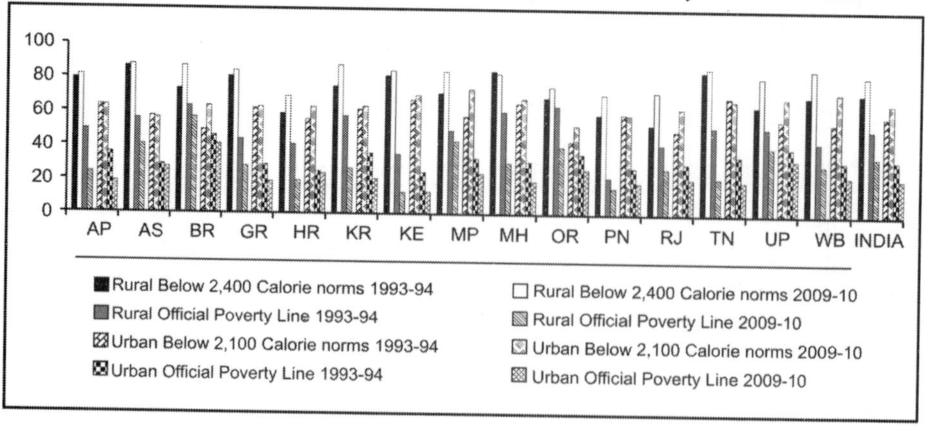

Source: Computed from CSO and NSSO unit level data.

Table 3 *Percentage Distribution of Well-nourished and Undernourished Households According to Different Quintile Groups*

	Rural				*Urban*				*Rural*				*Urban*				*Rural*				*Urban*			
	50th								*61st*								*66th*							
	Q1	*Q3*	*Q5*	*Total*	*Q1*	*Q3*	*Q5*	*Total*	*Q1*	*Q3*	*Q5*	*Total*	*Q1*	*Q3*	*Q5*	*Total*	*Q1*	*Q3*	*Q5*	*Total*	*Q1*	*Q3*	*Q5*	*Total*
Undernourished (<2400–Rural, 2100–Urban)	19.5	15.4	6.9	71.5	18	12	4.5	58.4	20	17.3	9.5	79.8	19	13	5.9	63.9	20	17	10	81.2	18	14	6.5	65.4

From the above figure it is clear that both money-metric and calorie-metric poverty are showing an opposite trend. Although the money-metric poverty is showing a declining trend over the last two decades, the calorie*metric deprivation showing an increasing trend over this period. The estimates of undernourishment are much higher than the expenditure-based poverty estimates using the official poverty line (Ray and Lancaster, 2005; Osmani, 1992). Table 3 depicts that over one and half decades, there has been rising calorie-metric deprivation, i.e. an increasing failure to meet the calorie requirement at the household level. This shows rising calorie undernourishment in rural and urban India. The calorie undernourishment also presents in top expenditure classes also (Table 3). So this rise in the share of calorie deprivation classes with decline in essential food expenditure share has an important issue to look into. This also calls for a serious policy initiatives on this ground.

Conclusion

In the present study we have analysed the spatial aspect of consumption profile (both food and non-food) and nutritional standard since 1990s. Here we examine a puzzling or paradoxical trend in terms of declining food consumption and nutrition in apparent economic growth. Our study shows that there was a drastic decline in essential food intakes both in rural and urban areas, but the former is larger than the latter. The larger reduction in commodity goods has reduced the disparity in terms of food consumption across states. As there is a close link existing between food consumption and nutrition, the decline in cereal consumption, which constitute lion's share of the total nutrients, increased the nutritional deprivation in India. It is also found that the increase in indirect food consumption does not adequately compensate the decline in cereal consumption. The large reduction in direct food consumption reduced the cereal consumption disparity between rural and urban area. With this decline in nutrients the percentage of calorie deprived population has risen substantially. In most of the Central Indian states, the overall decline in total cereal consumption is due to the absolute reduction in the coarse cereal consumption. The percentage of non-food consumption expenditure is increasing in most of the states, in our analysis. The southern states are showing more calories deficiency as compared to other states. The calorie undernourishment also showed a raising trend while taking different calorie cut-off points also. Rising undernutrition is also attributable to inadequate increase in indirect food consumption in recent periods. We also found a large divergence in terms of money-metric and calorie-metric norms, although the money-metric poverty is declining but the calorie-metric norm increasing in the recent periods in most of states. In concluding we can say that in the phase of significant economic change and structural transformation of the economy, one needs to go beyond the standard expenditure based money-metric measures to assess the changes in the living standard of households.

Notes

1. Adatte, A.C. 2010. Food Grains Consumption in India: An Analysis of Trends and Patterns. M.Phil Thesis (Unpublished) submitted at Centre for Development Studies, Trivandrum (now Thiruvanthapuram).
2. It is also possible that if low level of cereals calorie consumption is compensated by calorie rich non-cereal items, but in actual practice the shares are not compensating, through which we are finding declining level of total nutrition.
3. Note that real MPCE is in rupee terms and Protein and fat in gms.
4. For details please see Table 2.
5. Even recent studies talk about lower calorie requirements.

References

Adatte, A.C. 2010. Food Grains Consumption in India: An Analysis of Trends and Patterns. M.Phil Thesis (Unpublished) submitted at Centre for Development Studies, Trivandrum.

Basu, Deepankar and Basole, A. 2012. *The Calorie Consumption Puzzle in India: An Empirical Investigation*. Amherst: Political Economy Research Institute, University of Massachusetts, http://www.aae.wisc. edu/mwiedc/papers/2013/ basole_amit.pdf

Deaton, Angus and Dreze, Z. 2009. Food and Nutrition in India: Facts and Interpretations. *Economic and Political Weekly*, 44 (7): 42–65.

Dreze, J. 2003. Food Security and Right to Food. In S. Mahendra Dev, K.P. Kannan and Ramachandran Nira (eds), *Towards a Food Secure India: Issues and Policies*, New Delhi: Institute for Human Development.

Gopalan, C. 1992. Food Production and Consumption Trends. In *Nutrition in Development Transition in South East Asia*, New Delhi: WHO and SEARO, pp. 7–18.

Kumar, Praduman and Dey, M.M. 2007. Long-Term Changes in Indian Food Basket and Nutrition. *Economic and Political Weekly*, 42 (35): 3567–3572.

Li, N. and Eli, S. 2010. In Search of India's Missing Calories: Energy Requirements and Calorie Consumption. http//emlab.berkeley.edu/ webfac/emiguel/e271_f10/li.pdf

Meenakshi, J.V. and Viswanathan, B. 2003. Calorie Deprivation in Rural India: 1983–1999/2000. *Economic and Political Weekly*, 25 January: 369–375.

Nasurudeen, P., Kuruvila, A., Sendhil, R. and Chandrasekhar, V. 2006. The Dynamics and Inequality of Nutrient Consumption in India. *Indian Journal of Agricultural Economics*, 61 (3): 362–373.

Osmani, S.R. 1992. *Nutrition and Poverty*. New Delhi: Oxford University Press.

Patnaik, U. 2003. Food Stocks and Hunger: Causes of Agrarian Distress. *Social Scientist*, 31 (7–8): 15–41.

——. 2005. Theorizing Food Security and Poverty in the Era of Economic Reforms. *Social Scientist*, 33 (7–8): 50–81.

——. 2010. A Critical Look at Some Propositions on Consumption and Poverty. *Economic and Political Weekly*, XLV (6): 74–80.

Radhakrishna, R., Rao, K.H., Ravi, C. and Reddy, B.S., 2004. Chronic Poverty and Malnutrition in 1990s. *Economic and Political Weekly*, pp. 3121–3130.

Ray, R. 2007. Changes in Food Consumption and the Implications for Food Security and Undernourishment: India in the 1990s. *Development and Change*, 38 (2): 321–343.

Ray, R. and Lancaster, G. 2005. On Setting the Poverty Line Based on Estimated Nutrient Prices: Condition of Socially Disadvantaged Groups During the Reform Period. *Economic and Political Weekly*, 40 (1): 46–56.

Sinha, K., 2006. Household Characteristics and Calorie Intake in Rural India: A Quantile Regression Approach. https://digitalcollections.anu.edu.au/bitstream/1885/43190/2/WP2005_02.pdf

Suryanarayana, M.H. 2003. Is Targeting the Poor a Penalty on the Food Insecure? Poverty and Food Insecurity in India. *Journal of Human Development*, 8 (1): 89–107.

Contributors

Nasrin Banu, Ph.D. Scholar, Department of Geography, Aligarh Muslim University (AMU), Aligarh, Uttar Pradesh. nasringeo@gmail.com.

Montu Bose, Research Associate, Public Health Foundation of India, Delhi. monbose@gmail.com

Aalok Ranjan Chaurasia, 'Shyam' Institute, Bhopal. aranjan@hotmail.com

Arutselvi Devarajan, Research Scholar, Centre of Social Medicine and Community Health, School of Social Sciences, Jawaharlal Nehru University, New Delhi. darutselvi@gmail.com

Komal Prasad Dulal, Assistant Professor, Centre for Population and Development (CPAD), Purbanchal University, Nepal. Currently, Research Scholar, Centre for Study of Regional Development (CSRD), Jawaharlal Nehru University, New Delhi. komal.dulal@gmail.com

Garima Dutta, Ph.D Scholar, International Institute for Population Sciences, Mumbai. garimadutta03@gmail.com

Gunjan Gaurav, Masters in Health Administration (MHA), Tata Institute of Social Sciences (TISS), Mumbai.

K.B. Gotpagar, Former Faculty, International Institute for Population Sciences (IIPS), Mumbai.

Sandhya Gupta, a postgraduate in Public Health from TISS, Mumbai, is India CCM Coordinator for the Global Fund in Ministry of Health and Family Welfare. sandhya27pisces@gmail.com.

Jyotsna Jha, Director, Centre for Budget and Policy Studies (CBPS), Bangalore. jyotsna@cbps.in

Suhas Kadam, Masters of Public Health in Social Epidemiology (MPH), Tata Institute of Social Sciences (TISS), Mumbai. skadam86@gmail.com

Ramesh Babu Kafle, Assistant Professor, Centre for Population and Development (PAD), Purbanchal University, Nepal. Currently Research Scholar, Centre for the Study of Regional Development (CSRD), School of Social Sciences, Jawaharlal Nehru University, New Delhi. rbkafle@gmail.com

Divya Krishnaswamy, Research Advisor, Centre for Budget and Policy Studies (CBPS), Bangalore.

C. Satheesh Kumar, Assistant Professor, Department of Social Work, Pondicherry University, Puducherry. satheeshsw@gmail.com

Avijit Mistri, Ph.D. Scholar, Centre for the Study of Regional Development (CSRD), Jawaharlal Nehru University (JNU), New Delhi. avijit.mistri@gmail.com

M.S.R. Murthy, Emeritus Professor, Department of Population Studies, Sri Venkateswara University, Tirupati, Andhra Pradesh.mocherla_s@hotmail.com

Palani Murugesan, Senior Researcher, Department of Fertility Studies, IIPS, Mumbai. pmuruiips@gmail.com

D.A. Nagdeve, Professor and Head, Department of Fertility Studies, International Institute for Population Sciences, Mumbai. dnagdeve@iips.net

Balakrushna Padhi, Doctoral Scholar in Economics, Centre for the Study of Regional Development, Jawaharlal Nehru University, New Delhi. padhicds@gmail.com

Sarang Pedgaonkar, Assistant Professor, International Institute for Population Sciences, Mumbai. sarang@iips.net

Manas Ranjan Pradhan, Assistant Professor, International Institute for Population Sciences (IIPS), Mumbai. manas@iips.net

M. Soundha Rajan, Ph.D Research Scholar, Department of Social Work, Pondicherry University, Puducherry. soundharajanm@gmail.com

Abhishek Saraswat, Ph.D Scholar, International Institute for Population Sciences, Mumbai. abhi.srswt@gmail.com

Varun Sharma, Research Advisor, Centre for Budget and Policy Studies (CBPS), Bangalore. varun.srf@gmail.com, varun@cbps.in

Chander Shekhar, Professor, International Institute for Population Sciences (IIPS), Mumbai. buddhab@iips.net

H.C. Srivastava, Former Professor, International Institute for Population Sciences (IIPS), Mumbai. harishcsrivastava@gmail.com

Dipika Subba, School of Social Sciences, Centre for the Study of Regional Development, Jawaharlal Nehru University, New Delhi. subba.dipika@gmail.com

Sayeed Unisa, Professor, International Institute for Population Sciences, Mumbai. unisa@iips.net

Index